'This impressive book is indispensable for anyone who wants to understand the COVID-19 crisis from a human rights perspective. Through a comprehensive exploration of the impact of the coronavirus on diverse issues, the authors demonstrate why human rights are indeed an essential compass to guide our reactions and our policy to this unprecedented crisis.'

Kathryn Sikkink, *Harvard University, USA*

'The COVID-19 pandemic constitutes one of the major contemporary human rights challenges to governments and the international community. The current volume provides compelling insights to how we will be better prepared for similar challenges in the future. Governments had to take far-reaching measures which drastically restricted the rights to personal liberty, to work, to freedom of movement, privacy, property, the right to education, and freedom of assembly. In addition, governments had to protect the most vulnerable groups and ensure that the pandemic did not increase existing social and economic inequalities. After one year of trial and error, we need to admit that neither governments nor the international human rights community were prepared. This book offers ideas and inspiration for how to reach a scientifically sound and balanced human rights-based approach.'

Manfred Nowak, *Vienna University and Secretary General of the Global Campus of Human Rights, Austria*

'The COVID-19 pandemic has provoked unprecedented restrictions to human rights even in democratic regimes and highlighted the obstacles to international cooperation. But it also underscored the crucial importance of protecting the right to health and other social rights to preserve human life and dignity as well as functioning economies and states. This timely book illuminates how pandemics can be fought from a human rights-based approach and what can be done to seize this opportunity to adopt transformative policies to overcome structural inequalities.'

Manuel José Cepeda Espinosa, *Former President of the Constitutional Court of Colombia*

'Amid a flood of scholarly work on the human rights dimensions of the pandemic, this book stands out. Although written as events continue to unfold, the volume is remarkable for the penetrating analyses by leading scholars, which both cover an array of human rights issues, and raise critical, enduring questions regarding gaps not just in compliance but also in normative frameworks. While illuminating the sweeping devastation and upending of progress that the pandemic has wrought, the volume also offers hope that human rights frameworks can and must play a central role in transforming our social and international orders in light of the stark truths this crisis has laid bare.'

Alicia Ely Yamin, *Petrie-Flom Center, Harvard Law School, USA*

COVID-19 AND HUMAN RIGHTS

This timely collection brings together original explorations of the COVID-19 pandemic and its wide-ranging, global effects on human rights.

The contributors argue that a human rights perspective is necessary to understand the pervasive consequences of the crisis, while focusing attention on those being left behind and providing a necessary framework for the effort to 'build back better'. Expert contributors to this volume address interconnections between the COVID-19 crisis and the human rights to equality and non-discrimination, including historical responses to pandemics, populism and authoritarianism, and the rights to health, information, water and the environment. Highlighting the dangerous potential for derogations from human rights, authors further scrutinize the human rights compliance of new legislation and policies in relation to issues such as privacy, the rights of persons with disabilities, freedom of expression, and access to medicines. Acknowledging the pandemic as a defining moment for human rights, the volume proposes a post-crisis human rights agenda to engage civil society and government at all levels in concrete measures to roll back increasing inequality.

With rich examples, new thinking, and provocative analyses of human rights, COVID-19, pandemics, crises, and inequality, this book will be of key interest to scholars, students, and practitioners in all areas of human rights, global governance, and public health, as well as others who are ready to embark on an exploration of these complex challenges.

Morten Kjaerum is Director of Raoul Wallenberg Institute of Human Rights and Humanitarian Law, Lund, Sweden and Adjunct Professor at the University of Aalborg, Denmark.

Martha F. Davis is University Distinguished Professor at Northeastern University School of Law, USA.

Amanda Lyons is Executive Director of the Human Rights Center at the University of Minnesota Law School, USA.

ROUTLEDGE STUDIES IN HUMAN RIGHTS

The Routledge Studies in Human Rights series publishes high quality and cross-disciplinary scholarship on topics of key importance in human rights today. In a world where human rights are both celebrated and contested, this series is committed to create stronger links between disciplines and explore new methodological and theoretical approaches in human rights research. Aimed towards both scholars and human rights professionals, the series strives to provide both critical analysis and policy-oriented research in an accessible form. The series welcomes work on specific human rights issues as well as on cross-cutting themes and institutional perspectives.

Series Editors: *Mark Gibney, UNC Asheville, USA*, *Thomas Gammeltoft-Hansen, University of Copenhagen, Denmark*, and *Bonny Ibhawoh, McMaster University, Canada.*

Why Human Rights Still Matter in Contemporary World Affairs
Edited by Mahmood Monshipouri

Actualizing Human Rights
Global Inequality, Future People, and Motivation
Jos Philips

Protecting Human Rights Defenders at Risk
Edited by Alice M. Nah

COVID-19 and Human Rights
Edited by Morten Kjaerum, Martha F. Davis, and Amanda Lyons

COVID-19 AND HUMAN RIGHTS

Edited by Morten Kjaerum, Martha F. Davis, and Amanda Lyons

Routledge
Taylor & Francis Group
LONDON AND NEW YORK

First published 2021
by Routledge
2 Park Square, Milton Park, Abingdon, Oxon OX14 4RN

and by Routledge
605 Third Avenue, New York, NY 10158

Routledge is an imprint of the Taylor & Francis Group, an informa business

British Library Cataloguing-in-Publication Data
A catalogue record for this book is available from the British Library

Library of Congress Cataloging-in-Publication Data
Names: Kjaerum, Morten, editor.
Title: COVID-19 and human rights / edited by Morten Kjaerum,
Martha F. Davis, and Amanda Lyons.
Description: Milton Park, Abingdon, Oxon; New York, NY: Routledge, 2021. |
Series: Routledge studies in human rights |
Includes bibliographical references and index.
Identifiers: LCCN 2021003628 (print) | LCCN 2021003629 (ebook) |
ISBN 9780367688059 (hardback) | ISBN 9780367688035 (paperback) |
ISBN 9781003139140 (ebook)
Subjects: LCSH: COVID-19 (Disease)–Political aspects.
Classification: LCC RA644.C67 C68317 2021 (print) |
LCC RA644.C67 (ebook) | DDC 362.1962/414–dc23
LC record available at https://lccn.loc.gov/2021003628
LC ebook record available at https://lccn.loc.gov/2021003629

ISBN: 978-0-367-68805-9 (hbk)
ISBN: 978-0-367-68803-5 (pbk)
ISBN: 978-1-003-13914-0 (ebk)

Typeset in Bembo
by Newgen Publishing UK

This book is dedicated to the courageous people on all continents working on the frontlines to stem the impacts of the COVID-19 pandemic, some of whom paid the ultimate price.

CONTENTS

CONTRIBUTORS

Zarizana Abdul Aziz is a human rights lawyer and co-founder of the Due Diligence Project. She has been involved in legal reform initiatives on gender equality and anti-violence as well as training of judges, lawyers, civil society advocates, religious scholars, and government officials in several countries. She was twice shortlisted for the UN Working Group on Discrimination against Women in Law and Practice. She was a Human Rights Fellow and visiting scholar at Columbia University and is currently adjunct professor at George Washington University.

Brook K. Baker teaches at Northeastern University School of Law, is an honorary research fellow at the University of KwaZuluNatal, and is a senior policy analyst for Health GAP, which campaigns for universal access to HIV treatment. Recently he is working on equitable access to COVID-19 health products and is a civil society representative to the Therapeutics Pillar of the Access to COVID-19 Tools Accelerator. He writes and consults extensively on intellectual property rights, trade, access to medicines, and related issues.

Sanchita Banerjee Saxena, PhD in political science from UCLA, is the Executive Director of the Institute for South Asia Studies and the Director of the Chowdhury Center for Bangladesh Studies at UC Berkeley. She is the editor of *Labor, Global Supply Chains, and the Garment Industry in South Asia: Bangladesh after Rana Plaza* (2019) and author of *Made in Bangladesh, Cambodia, and Sri Lanka: The Labor Behind the Global Garments and Textiles Industries* (2014).

Elina Castillo Jiménez is a feminist human rights lawyer. After completing her JD (*summa cum laude*) in the Dominican Republic, she pursued an LLM in Public International Law and Human Rights (Distinction) at the University of Nottingham as a Chevening Scholar. She has worked at the intersection of human rights, gender, migration, and public policy with government, grassroots collectives, and international organizations. Her research interests include critical legal theory, state compliance with international law, and the Inter-American human rights system.

Martha F. Davis is University Distinguished Professor of Law at Northeastern University in Boston, Massachusetts, where she is a faculty co-director of the Program on Human Rights and the Global Economy. Davis's publications include *Human Rights Advocacy in the United States* (co-author) and *Global Urban Justice: The Rise of Human Rights Cities* (co-editor). She is co-editor of the Human Rights at Home Law Profs Blog and an affiliated scholar of the Raoul Wallenberg Institute of Human Rights and Humanitarian Law.

Olivier de Schutter is a professor at UC Louvain and SciencesPo and the United Nations Special Rapporteur on extreme poverty and human rights. He was formerly the UN Special Rapporteur on the right to food (2008–2014) and a member of the Committee on Economic, Social and Cultural Rights (2015–2020).

Claudia Ituarte-Lima, PhD, University College London and MPhil University of Cambridge. For twenty years, she has specialized on human rights, biodiversity, and climate law. As an international public lawyer and scholar, her focus is on environmental justice and the transformation of international law into new governance forms that support healthy ecosystems and people's wellbeing. Claudia is Senior Researcher at the Raoul Wallenberg Institute of Human Rights and Humanitarian Law (RWI) and is also affiliated to Stockholm University and the University of British Columbia.

Steven L. B. Jensen, PhD in History, is Senior Researcher at The Danish Institute for Human Rights. His publications include the prize-winning book *The Making of International Human Rights. The 1960s, Decolonization and the Reconstruction of Global Values* (CUP 2016). His forthcoming book *Social Rights and the Politics of Obligation in History* (co-edited with Charles Walton) will be published by Cambridge University Press in 2021.

Harpreet Kaur holds a PhD in Anthropology from the University of Delhi, India. She is the Business and Human Rights Specialist at the UNDP's Asia Pacific Regional Centre. Harpreet led Ashoka University's Genpact Centre for Women's Leadership where she designed cutting-edge programs that enabled women to lead with equality and dignity. She has been the South Asia Researcher at Business and Human Rights Resource Centre. Harpreet serves as a Council Member of the World Economic Forum Global Future Council on Human Rights.

Morten Kjaerum is Director of the Raoul Wallenberg Institute of Human Rights and Humanitarian Law, Lund, Sweden and Adjunct Professor at Aalborg University, Denmark. He was the first director of the European Union Agency for Fundamental

Rights, and director of the Danish Institute for Human Rights. He was member of the UN Committee on Elimination of Racial Discrimination and is a member of the Board of Trustees for the UN Voluntary Fund for Technical Cooperation in the field of Human Rights.

Ian M. Kysel is Visiting Assistant Clinical Professor of Law at Cornell University. He has previously held appointments at the University of Oxford and Georgetown University Law Center. He co-founded and directs the International Migrants Bill of Rights (IMBR) Initiative, based at Cornell. Among other things, he is a co-author of the IMBR and its accompanying legal commentaries and of *Human Mobility and Human Rights in the COVID-19 Pandemic: Principles of Protection for Migrants, Refugees and Other Displaced Persons*.

Amanda Lyons, JD, is the Executive Director at the Human Rights Center at the University of Minnesota Law School. Her research, teaching, and advocacy have focused on human rights and development, the human right to water, and gender justice. Prior to joining the university, she worked with human rights organizations in Brazil, Colombia, and the United States.

Tove H. Malloy, is Professor of European Studies at the Europa-Universität Flensburg, Germany. Her research interests include minority rights, the European human rights regime, and ethno-cultural autonomy. She has co-edited *The Framework Convention for the Protection of National Minorities, A Commentary* (2018), *Managing Diversity through Non-Territorial Autonomy* (2015) and is the author of *National Minority Rights in Europe* (2005).

Hope Metcalf, Executive Director of the Schell Center for International Human Rights and Clinical Lecturer at Yale Law School, co-teaches at the Lowenstein International Human Rights Clinic. Her teaching, research, and writing focus on the rights of people in various forms of detention, and she consults with organizations around the world on those subjects. For the past decade, her clinic has challenged ongoing violations at Connecticut's supermax prison and supports the local movement to end solitary confinement.

Helga Molbæk-Steensig is a research assistant on the 'Human Rights in the Endgame of the COVID-19 Pandemic' project at the European University Institute where she is also writing her PhD on the reform of the European Court of Human Rights. Before this, she toured Denmark with lectures on populism.

Janine Moussa is adjunct professor at The George Washington College of Law, Washington DC. She is an international lawyer with over 15 years of experience on women's human rights and access to justice. She has worked with the United Nations, the Organization of American States, and the World Bank as well as academic institutions and non-governmental organizations. She has authored several policy papers; moderated a number of high-level panels; led many multi-year multi-country research studies; and is an accomplished human rights trainer.

Juliana Nnoko-Mewanu holds a PhD in Sociology and Sustainable Agriculture from Iowa State University. She is senior researcher at Human Rights Watch and works on women's land and property rights across Africa and Asia. Her work examines the impact of government policies such as family, property, and land laws and business interests on land and property rights, highlighting disproportionate impacts on women. She previously worked at Iowa State University and the University of Buea, Cameroon.

Pedi Obani is a senior lecturer in the Department of Jurisprudence and International Law, University of Benin and a visiting research fellow in water, security, policy, and governance at University of Leeds. Her research mainly focuses on the rights to water and sanitation.

Katharina Ó Cathaoir, PhD, is assistant professor of health law at the Faculty of Law, University of Copenhagen. Her research interests span health and human rights, focusing on how legislation can protect the public's health, while respecting human rights. She is Principal Investigator of PRONTO, which examines restrictions on movement in response to Covid-19.

Gerard Quinn is the UN Special Rapporteur on the rights of persons with disabilities. He was the founding director of the Centre for Disability Law and Policy at the National University of Ireland and now holds the Wallenberg Chair at the Raoul Wallenberg Institute and a research chair at the University of Leeds. A graduate of Harvard Law School, he holds three lifetime awards for his international disability law work. He was a drafter of the UN disability convention.

Martin Scheinin is British Academy Global Professor at the Bonavero Institute of Human Rights, University of Oxford. His COVID-19 research is based at the European University Institute where he is a part-time professor. He is a member of the Scientific Committee of the EU Fundamental Rights Agency.

Ana María Suárez Franco holds a PhD from the University of Mannheim and is the permanent representative to the UN in Geneva for FIAN International. She works closely with communities affected by violations of the right to food and has coordinated FIAN's COVID-related work throughout 2020. She has a law degree from the Universidad Javeriana, postgraduate studies in public policies from the Universidad de los Andes, and an LLM from the University of Heidelberg.

Salil Tripathi is senior adviser (global issues) at the Institute for Human Rights and Business. He co-wrote the Standards of Conduct for Business with regard to LGBTI rights for the Office of the High Commissioner for Human Rights. He has been a researcher at Amnesty International and has published extensively. He is the author of three works of non-fiction and chairs PEN International's Writers in Prison Committee. He holds an MBA from the Tuck School of Business at Dartmouth College.

FOREWORD

Olivier de Schutter

By the end of 2020, the COVID-19 pandemic has already claimed more than 1.8 million lives globally, and eighty-three million people have contracted the virus. As this volume goes to press, governments are struggling to face a second wave of contaminations, which many anticipate will be deadlier than the first. Since the start of the pandemic, in their haste to control the spread of the virus, governments have improvised: during the first great lockdown between March and June 2020, schools were closed in 195 countries, depriving some 368 million children of school meals which, for many of them, was their main meal of the day; non-essential businesses were temporarily shut down, leading to the laying off of a large number of workers, often without any form of compensation; in many countries, restrictions to the freedom of movement meant that many micro businesses in the informal sector lost their source of income, and that supply chains were disrupted. The economic and social impacts are already considerable. The global economy is expected to contract by 4.4 percent in 2020. At least ninety million are more at risk of falling into extreme poverty – potentially rising to as many as 150 million in 2021, when the temporary fixes adopted to cushion the most severe impacts of the crisis will be phased out. Although the most significant contraction will be in OECD countries and in Latin America, low-income countries will be the most affected, because of their dependency on rich countries (for foreign investment, for remittances from migrant workers, and for the export of raw materials), because they face the burden of high levels of foreign debt, and because their social protection systems are unprepared for the shock.

For all these reasons, this pandemic and the enormous impacts it is having on economies and societies are putting human rights to the test. Just as after the terrorist attacks of 9/11 in 2001 and the great recession of 2008–2009, questions are raised about human rights' ability to resist the shock and to guide the recovery. I believe they can do both. Human rights, this 'Esperanto of the virtuous' in Conor

Gearty's felicitous expression, are not an impediment to effectively addressing the pandemic, nor are they a luxury we cannot afford in times of crisis: they are an essential compass to guide our reactions.

In a large number of countries, 'emergency powers' were granted to the executive to allow it to adopt measures to combat the spread of the virus and to address the impacts of the shutdown of the economy on the population. In the European Union for instance, sixteen states declared a 'state of emergency' during the first wave of the pandemic, between 31 January 2020 (when such a declaration was made by Italy) and the end of March (when Poland and France, on 20 and 23 March respectively, made similar statements). In the United States, the Trump administration declared a public health emergency on 31 January 2020 under the Public Health Service Act. It issued two national emergency declarations on 13 March under the Disaster Relief and Emergency Assistance Act (known as the Stafford Act, initially adopted in 1988 and normally designed to face natural disasters by allowing support to state and local authorities) and the National Emergency Act; and invoked emergency powers via Executive Order under the Defense Production Act on 18 March. Similar states of emergency were declared in other regions.

Such declarations served two functions during this crisis. They facilitated the swift adoption of measures to reduce the spread of the pandemic, by allowing certain restrictions to civil liberties and to political rights. Elections were postponed in seventy-three countries. Restrictions on the freedom to demonstrate were imposed. Borders were closed. In countries such as Belgium, France, and Italy, drones were used to monitor compliance with regulations concerning 'social distancing.' Many jurisdictions put in place mechanisms to track persons affected by the COVID-19 virus as well as those with whom they interacted, or to ensure that people complied with quarantine: in Poland, individuals placed in quarantine had to regularly transmit selfies to the authorities, proving that they were effectively staying at home. The 'emergency powers' allocated to the executive, however, also served another function: they allowed the speedy provision of support to collectivities facing a lack of resources to combat the pandemic and the adoption of social protection measures to protect those most affected by the closure of the economy. According to one count from July 2020, more than 1,400 social protection measures were adopted across the world, totaling approximately 590 billion US dollars in spending, to mitigate the impacts.

The attribution of emergency powers to the executive in such circumstances should not be confused with the setting aside of human rights. It is the modalities that changed, not the duty. The crisis may affect the procedures through which human rights are enforced, but not the requirement to remain within the boundaries of what human rights allow. Whether or not states formally announce that they will suspend certain guarantees to face the emergency (in the European Union for instance, three States have notified derogations under article 15 of the European Convention on Human Rights), the key obligations of necessity and non-discrimination remain applicable. The measures adopted should remain temporary and not go beyond what is required to face the circumstances of the crisis, and although they operate post hoc rather than ex ante, both parliamentary and judicial controls should ensure that the executive remains accountable to these requirements. Moreover, far from being an impediment to the effectiveness of the reaction of governments to the crisis, human rights are essential to preserve the legitimacy of public action, and thus to ensure compliance. As UN High Commissioner for Human Rights Michelle Bachelet declared on 6 March 2020, during the initial stage of the pandemic:

> [b]eing open and transparent is key to empowering and encouraging people to participate in measures designed to protect their own health and that of the wider population, especially when trust in the authorities has been eroded. It also helps to counter false or misleading information that can do so much harm by fueling fear and prejudice.

Human rights moreover should continue to define not only how much governments may do to combat the pandemic and its impacts on the population, but also how they should design the measures to ensure human rights are fully complied with. The measures adopted by States in the area of social protection illustrate this role of human rights as a guide to action. The measures adopted so far in this area seem impressive in their numbers (although the numbers themselves should be placed in the right perspective: the 590 billion US dollars figure cited above represents just about one twentieth of the total amount, approximately 12,000 billion US dollars, injected in the economy by September 2020 as part of various economic recovery plans adopted worldwide). But these social protection measures have often been in the form of short-term fixes: they have consisted of temporary unemployment schemes limiting the number of workers laid off; improvised cash transfer schemes; or the removal of conditionalities imposed for the provision of social support. In many cases, important groups have been left out, including workers in the informal sector and in precarious forms of employment (a total of 2 billion workers worldwide, among whom women are overrepresented), migrants (especially undocumented migrants), and people in poverty (who typically have weak internet access, making it difficult for them to fill in forms online, who may have insufficient information about the support measures adopted, or who may find it difficult to provide the required documentation or to prove that they comply with the required conditionalities).

A rights-based approach would allow a strengthening of social protection both by transforming temporary fixes into permanent measures guaranteeing the human right to social security and by closing the gaps in existing social protection schemes. It would redefine the support measures as based not on charity but on a relationship based on rights and duties. This makes a considerable difference. In contrast to individuals and families being provided with some form of help from authorities based on improvised solutions adopted under the pressure of the crisis, rights-holders claiming benefits before independent bodies on the basis of entitlements stipulated in domestic legislation will face less shame and stigma (major explanations for the high rates of non-take-up of rights in many jurisdictions); less discrimination; and less petty corruption. Instead of their dependency increasing, they will be empowered and have incentives to hold public bodies accountable.

Thus, human rights are not less relevant in times of crisis, nor are they an inconvenient obstacle to speedy and effective action by the executive. It is rather the opposite: they are especially important where extensive powers are granted to governments (entailing the risk that parliamentary and judicial checks will be circumvented or weakened) and when measures are taken in the name of expediency to protect the population from certain shocks. Human rights in times of crisis are both a shield against abuse, and a map for recovery.

Human rights are also relevant for a third reason: they can underpin progress in international cooperation. If the pandemic has taught us anything, it is that, in the oft-repeated slogan, 'no one is secure until everyone is secure'. The crisis has illustrated the various interdependencies between States that grew from globalization: how the virus has traveled; how economies have become dependent on global supply chains; and how the shutdown of the economies in the North affected opportunities in the Global South. All these factors have brought to light that we live in a world of semi-sovereign States, in which what each country can do depends on its ability to coordinate with others, and in which both prosperity and decline are shared across nations. In such a world, the search for solutions cannot be left to each State acting alone: it must take the form of a collective search, and lead to the provision of global public goods.

The quest for a vaccine provides the most visible example. The charity Oxfam International calculated that, by October 2020, 51 percent of the vaccine doses under preparation had been pre-empted (acquired in advance) by governments representing 13 percent of the world's population. That is vaccine nationalism: the richer you are, the more affordable it is to take measures to protect your population, even though this may be at the expense of the ability of other governments to do the same. As noted in a joint statement adopted by a number of Special Procedures of the Human Rights Council:

> If States do not coordinate globally, there is a high risk that global competition will increase the prices of medical supplies and of a potential vaccine which, in turn, will affect all countries. This will be of particular detrimental effect to the various developing countries already facing high debt and financial crises.

Alternatives are emerging, however. The World Health Organization is seeking to convince governments to join the COVAX initiative for global equitable access to COVID-19 vaccines led, in addition to the WHO, by Gavi, the Vaccine Alliance, the Coalition for Epidemic Preparedness Innovations (CEPI). Its purpose is to guarantee fair access for all countries, rich or poor, to effective immunization. On 2 October 2020, South Africa and India, who already had been leading the effort that led to the adoption in 2001 of the Ministerial Declaration on the TRIPs

Agreement and Public Health to face the AIDS crisis, petitioned the World Trade Organization to ensure the TRIPs flexibilities shall be used to combat this pandemic, where necessary by suspending the normal application of intellectual property rights and by resorting, in particular, to compulsory licenses. This again aims to avoid that the technology gap between North and South, and the widely varying purchasing powers of rich and poor populations, will result in an inequitable access to the vaccine.

Just like essential medicines should be treated as a global public good, so should the establishment of social protection floors. In Recommendation (No. 202) Concerning National Floors of Social Protection (2012), the International Labour Conference encouraged the adoption worldwide of social protection floors to 'ensure at a minimum that, over the life cycle, all in need have access to essential health care and to basic income security which together secure effective access to goods and services defined as necessary at the national level' (para. 4). The COVID-19 pandemic highlighted, however, that the pledge to adopt social protection floors universally remained unfulfilled, leaving many groups without adequate support. Adequate international support could fill that gap. In September 2020, the International Labour Organization released estimates showing that, taking into account the COVID-19 pandemic, developing countries would need to invest an additional 1.2 trillion USD each year – equivalent to 3.8 percent of their gross domestic product (GDP) – to close the financing gap, and that the gap for low-income countries is seventy-eight billion USD, equivalent to 15.9 percent of their GDP. While this may seem like a considerable amount, it is in fact almost insignificant in comparison with the sums injected in the global economy through the already adopted economic recovery plans, and it represents about half of the total official development assistance (ODA) provided by OECD countries to poor countries in 2019.

The idea of increased international support for the adoption of social protection floors therefore re-emerged during the crisis. In 2011, the Report of the Social Protection Floor Advisory Group chaired by Ms. Michelle Bachelet already had recommended, *inter alia*, that 'donors provide predictable multi-year financial support for the strengthening of nationally defined and determined social protection floors in low-income countries within their own budgetary frameworks and respecting their ownership'. The 2012 Social Protection Floors Recommendation (No. 202) itself noted that, while 'national social protection floors should be financed by national resources,' 'Members whose economic and fiscal capacities are insufficient to implement the guarantees may seek international cooperation and support that complement their own efforts' (para. 12). Later that same year, the Special Rapporteur on the right to food and the Special Rapporteur on extreme poverty and human rights made a proposal for the establishment of a Global Fund for Social Protection. The proposal was referred to by the High-Level Panel of Eminent Persons on the Post-2015 Development Agenda in the Report *A New Global Partnership: Eradicate Poverty and Transform Economies through Sustainable Development* submitted in May 2013 to the Secretary-General. Other proposals were also put forward in preparation of the Third International Conference on Financing for Development convened in Addis Ababa on 13–16 July 2015, and the Addis Ababa Action Agenda, as endorsed by the General Assembly in its resolution 69/313 of 27 July 2015, includes a pledge by the Heads of State and Government and High Representatives to provide 'strong international support' for the efforts to establish social protection floors (para. 12).

These recommendations are fully consistent with international human rights law, which recognizes a special responsibility for states to provide international assistance and cooperation in the fulfillment of economic, social, and cultural rights to other states with limited resources. It also underpins the 2030 Sustainable Development Agenda: under SDG 17, the global community has committed to supporting developing countries by means of strengthening domestic resource mobilization; increasing official development aid; and mobilizing additional resources to that effect.

Human rights, in sum, can fulfil three roles during this crisis. They can provide an essential safeguard against the risk of abuse, by the executive, of the special powers it is granted in order to allow it to combat the crisis. They can guide the post-pandemic recovery efforts, ensuring that, as expressed by UN Secretary-General Antonio Guterres, we 'build back better' following the pandemic. And they can stimulate new forms of international cooperation, based on the realization that neither the pandemic itself, nor the economic and social crises that it has caused, respect borders. Yes, the crisis has put human rights to the test. But human rights can emerge victorious, provided parliaments, human rights bodies, and civil society hold governments accountable. I welcome this timely publication as an important contribution to this objective.

PREFACE

The COVID-19 pandemic and the measures taken by States and other actors to curtail the spread of the disease have impacted most aspects of life all around the world. The disease and the responses to it have had far-reaching effects on economies, welfare systems, and individual freedoms. COVID-19 has and will continue to have an exceptional impact on the enjoyment of human rights on a global scale. The pandemic therefore presents one of the major human rights challenges of our time, highlighting many of the fundamental issues surrounding the enjoyment of human rights, including inequality and non-discrimination, the indivisibility of rights, and the necessity and proportionality of limitations and derogations from human rights.

Despite the frequent refrain that the virus does not discriminate, the pandemic dramatically heightens existing societal inequalities. The crisis impacts the rights of individuals differently based on a variety of factors and exacerbates the vulnerability of persons and groups already at risk due to, e.g., discrimination, migration status or lack thereof, homelessness, displacement, economic insecurity, and lack of access to necessities such as clean water. Just one example of the gendered impacts of the current crisis is the rise in domestic violence in many countries following the adoption of containment measures, which may effectively trap victims in close proximity to their abusers. Inequalities in access to fundamental social and economic rights such as the rights to health, education, and an adequate standard of living are made particularly serious and visible in the midst of the crisis. In many countries for example, persons belonging to minority groups are disproportionately represented among those hospitalized and deceased due to COVID-19. The economic repercussions of the crisis are likely to fall the hardest on those already living in precarious conditions and therefore risk severely undermining the enjoyment of economic and social rights. Besides the health crisis, the pandemic presents a socio-economic crisis, fueled by inequalities both within and between states.

While COVID-19 and the containment measures adopted have a clear and direct impact on rights such as the rights to life and health, freedom of movement, and freedom of assembly, the crisis also affects a myriad of other rights. These include the right to privacy, which is impacted by the wide variety of measures adopted to track the spread of the disease through mobile devices and to monitor compliance with restrictions through surveillance by drones and other tools. With the swift adoption of far-reaching derogations from and limitations to rights, there is a risk that such extraordinary measures will become normalized or used for illegitimate purposes, such as to clamp down dissent or frustrate the sharing of public information. Technology may serve as a tool for undermining human rights during the crisis, but at the same time the situation highlights the affirmative human rights dimensions of access to technology as both children and adults must increasingly rely on technological means to access education, work, public information, and basic services. These dimensions of the pandemic also bring to the fore the role and responsibilities of private actors in the respect and fulfilment of human rights related to work, medicines, food, and water.

The COVID-19 crisis presents challenges that are unprecedented in a modern and globalized society. In responding to such an urgent and exceptional situation, mistakes are bound to be made, but when human rights are so fundamentally impacted, close monitoring and evaluation of the situation is required. This book seeks to examine the first year of the COVID-19 crisis from a human rights perspective. The aim is to map out some of the wide-ranging human rights effects of the crisis in the short- and long-term and offer preliminary predictions and recommendations for what comes next. The book is based on the premise that a human rights perspective is necessary to understand and evaluate the wider consequences of the crisis, to highlight the plight of those being left behind, and to identify transformative routes forward. The chapters present these different interconnections between the COVID-19 crisis and human rights, bringing together original analyses of the pandemic and responses to it from a human rights perspective with a view to the future.

The book is divided into three parts with a concluding chapter that contemplates the post-COVID future. The first part with four chapters takes a broad look at 'Human rights during health crises' and opens with the question of what lessons from past epidemics and pandemics can offer in the context of the current and future outbreaks. Democracies and authoritarian regimes are equally hit by the pandemic, however the approaches to stemming the spread of the virus are different. Authoritarian and populist leaders pay little attention to concerns of the individual in their attempts to protect society at large whereas democracies are more inclined to apply a human rights-based approach. So, what does the human rights framework prescribe in an emergency situation as the COVID-19 crisis? This part closes with a key concern in any crisis, namely the right to information, which in the end is a matter of life and death for the individual but also for the broader community.

The second part focuses on 'Vulnerability and inequality' as the key features exposed by the pandemic. The opening chapter frames the section with a focus on digital, spatial, and racial inequalities and their profound impacts on the enjoyment of human rights. These perspectives mark the fundamental difference between the concepts of poverty and inequality, which are exemplified in five subsequent chapters on race, gender, disability, prisoners, and migrants. Systemic discrimination and vulnerability along these lines means that particular groups have been severely affected during the COVID crisis to such an extent that their situations have – finally – captured the attention of media, politicians, and policymakers.

Part 3 moves from vulnerability and inequality to discuss the cornerstones of a coherent society that have been de-stabilized or exposed as vulnerable by the COVID-19 crisis. The opening chapter addresses the key question of whether the UN Sustainable Development Goals can continue on the track laid out prior to the pandemic or if a paradigm shift is needed and possible. The pandemic underscores the importance of the public sector's role in guaranteeing basic rights, challenging the idea that states can simply sit back and prune the landscape for the private sector to maximize profit. The chapters that follow address the challenges related to the right to food, water and sanitation, land, and medicine as well as the right to decent work and global supply chains. Part 3 closes with a focus on the environment we live in as a key element of any future policy.

While all chapters are oriented toward recommendations for the next phase, the closing chapter is dedicated to offering a forward-looking perspective, foreseeing a future human rights agenda where all civil, economic, social, political, and cultural rights are finally seen as equally important. This is a precondition for addressing in a profound manner the future equality agenda, i.e., tackling inequality based on economy and status.

We are very much in the midst of the pandemic as we send this collection to print; cases are still soaring in most countries, distribution of the vaccines is just beginning, and the economic toll and lasting social consequences are still to be seen. Our aim with this early volume is to offer an array of assessments grounded in human rights principles and standards. The contributors draw expertise from academia and activism, as well as a range of regional perspectives. In this way, we wish to contribute to the debate and construction of transformative responses that empower claims by rights-holders, that advance substantive equality, and that strengthen democracy and the rule of law.

We would like to thank Elina Hammarström from the Raoul Wallenberg Institute of Human Rights and Humanitarian Law, who skillfully assisted us through the compressed editorial process with great dedication and commitment.

We also want to thank Colm Kelly Ryan of Lund University, Genevieve M. Kinder of Suffolk University Law School, James Levine of Northeastern Law School, and Verónica Cadavid Gónzalez, Cooper Christiancy, and Kristin Trapp from the University of Minnesota Law School for their expert research assistance, as well as Jennifer True (Northeastern Law School) for technical assistance during the editing process. In addition, we are grateful to the many scholars and colleagues who served as peer reviewers and sounding boards, sharpening individual chapters and contributing to the volume's overall shape. Developed through two online workshops and intensive virtual individual consultation, this book reflects the deep commitment of all participants to work together for a more just world. We look forward to continuing this work together in person as well as virtually in the coming years.

Morten Kjaerum, Martha F. Davis, Amanda Lyons

PART 1

Human rights during health crises

1

'HUMAN RIGHTS AGAINST HUMAN ARBITRARINESS'

Pandemics in a human rights historical perspective

Steven L. B. Jensen

Time and history are woven into the fabric of our responses to COVID-19. We see this when the current pandemic is described as a 'hundred-year event' and when the economic impacts are described as 'unprecedented' or spark comparisons to the 1930s Depression Era. Diseases and epidemics have always defined the history of humanity – although in recent decades many in more privileged parts of the world may have forgotten the extent of this.

Health is also a human rights battlefield. This reality has been made abundantly clear throughout the COVID-19 pandemic. We have witnessed the cost incurred from decades of negligent treatment of economic and social rights. The disproportionate impacts on mortality and morbidity have been severe with clear human rights implications. The experience of lockdowns has varied significantly from country to country as well as within countries depending on social class, economic conditions, ethnicity and legal status. These factors – and the battlefield itself – all have historical roots or trajectories that can help illuminate the current situation.

This chapter therefore looks at the relationship between epidemics and the right to health from a longer historical perspective highlighting three historical phases which encompassed new or existing outbreaks of typhus, cholera, the influenza of 1918,[1] and HIV/AIDS. The chapter starts with the emergence of social medicine and human rights thinking about public health in the 1840s focusing on the highly influential German doctor and politician Rudolf Virchow (1821–1902), whose writings and actions almost single-handedly changed how we should approach this aspect of the historical evolution of human rights. The chapter concludes by tracing the inclusion of the right to health in international legal conventions in the twentieth century and global health developments in the twenty-first century, showing how Virchow's legacy has remained an influence. In the 1840s, the political choice in an age with typhus and cholera epidemics was defined by Virchow as being 'human rights against human arbitrariness' (Virchow 1848b, p. 9). That framing speaks with surprisingly clarity to the current age of COVID-19 and HIV/AIDS.

In his 2020 book *American Contagions: Epidemics and the Law from Smallpox to COVID-19*, Yale Law Professor John Fabian Witt argues:

> If the past is a guide, how our law responds to contagion now and in the future will help decide the course of our democracy. Historically, the law of epidemics has prompted Americans to make choices about basic values. People who know their history make better choices.
>
> *(Witt 2020, pp. 2–3)*

A historical approach, however, does not necessarily capture an evolution in the form of progress. It is more complex than that. In the 1946 Constitution of the World Health Organization, the right to health was defined as a 'fundamental right' (WHO 1946). This represented historical wisdom and experience in the aftermath of the Second World War and the Depression Era. However, the right to health would not maintain its prominence in the decades that followed. The right to health was downplayed – even ignored for some decades within WHO – as an essential part of the international human rights framework even as it developed into binding international law and state obligations during the 1950s, 1960s, and 1970s.[2] Cold War politics and the changing international structures of state sovereignty and economics would see to this downplaying.

Our current experiences with COVID-19 and the pandemic's profound global impact raises the question about the misguidedness of this approach. We should reconsider whether the right to health should be restored to the earlier understanding as a 'fundamental right'. Something vital was lost along the way which has not been fully recaptured. A historically informed take on epidemics and human rights should therefore not just present a background story but should also question whether contemporary framings are sufficiently advanced in their normative and legal thinking to address our current human rights challenges.

1 Human rights in a time of cholera (and typhus): Rudolf Virchow and the emergence of social medicine in the 1840s

In 1988, the Director of WHO's Global AIDS Program Jonathan Mann explained in an interview the historical significance of the response to the HIV/AIDS pandemic that had developed since the first evidence of the virus was documented in 1981. It had been a race against time to identify the virus, understand its virology, track its spread, initiate testing and public health campaigns, and face the rapidly increasing mortality around the world. These were well-known features of dealing with an emerging global pandemic. However, this time was different. The response to this global health crisis had also required integrating a human rights approach into the response. Stigma and discrimination were so widespread that they exacerbated the HIV epidemic, brought untold suffering and death, and undermined efforts to develop more effective responses (Hildebrand 2009).

Mann had been a driving force behind linking public health and human rights in the global response to HIV/AIDS. He presented this new development in the following manner:

> I would say that there has always been a human rights dimension to malaria, diarrheal disease, immunization and smallpox. But it was never really understood, it was never really seen and yet with AIDS we see perfectly clearly that if we don't protect the rights of those who are infected we endanger us all – that the rights of everyone are protected by ensuring that the rights of some are protected.
>
> *(Hildebrand dir. 2009, min 8:33)*

Over the decades, this approach has helped save millions from HIV infection and from AIDS-related deaths. It has helped transform global health and led to a strengthened focus on malaria, tuberculosis and more robust health systems among others. It has meant that today human rights have become 'a cornerstone of global health governance' (Gostin & Meier 2018, p. 21). There are still many political contestations, underfunded areas, gaps, and unresolved issues. Stigma and discrimination also endure, but the awareness of the pivotal relationship between health and human rights and its institutional anchoring has made giant strides in recent decades. This is a story well-known to organizations, activists, and scholars working in the field of HIV/AIDS.

However, Jonathan Mann's assessment is not fully accurate. It deserves a wider historical berth because there had been earlier influential attempts to understand and explain the human rights dimensions of epidemics. This is where Rudolf Virchow and the birth of social medicine fits into the story. Virchow is renowned within medicine and public health. Among his numerous contributions, he is widely recognized as a founder of social medicine and pathology. One medical scholar wrote that 'it is no exaggeration to herald Virchow as the principal architect of the foundations of scientific medicine' (Eisenberg 1984, p. 524). He is by no means an insignificant historical actor.

Despite all of this, Virchow has not been fully acknowledged as a critical character in the larger human rights story, even though he has provided inspiration for some contemporary actors. Virchow shows us that social rights have a much longer and deeper history than they are usually assigned by human rights scholars and practitioners. Furthermore, as new scholarship by Stephen J. Sawyer and William J. Novak (forthcoming) argues, we need to be attuned to how such rights language was linked to nineteenth-century historical discussions where issues of statecraft and politics were at the heart of the matter. This includes highlighting the technologies of public action through which socio-economic needs were acted upon. Virchow also shows us that the historical roots of social and economic rights were more broadly grounded and not limited to the social-democratic or socialist movements to which they are often connected. Virchow represents an example showing that liberalism could be a source or even a driver of social and economic rights promotion and protection acting well beyond traditional notions of its laissez-faire nature. This connection is worth keeping in mind when writing or contemplating the history of social and economic rights. As one of his biographers has written, '[a]s early as 1848, Virchow had developed a political philosophy marrying classical liberal principles with a governmental responsibility for social well-being. He then applied this ideological synthesis to health reform activities for the rest of his life' (McNeely 2002, p. 64).

In 1848, Virchow was a young doctor based in Berlin. At the beginning of the year, he had been appointed as medical officer to a commission investigating a typhus epidemic in Upper Silesia (in south-eastern Poland today). The experience informed his medical and political perspectives on society for the remainder of his life (Gaffney 2018, p. 63). Virchow was greatly concerned with the devastating social and economic conditions among the poorest strata of society that the typhus and repeated cholera epidemics exposed. He was in opposition to the conservatism of both the political culture and the medical profession of the time. He therefore launched a new journal *Medicinische Reform* ('Medical Reform') in July 1848 with a far-reaching agenda for public health. He had created his own pulpit for his public health and rights campaigning.

Now, 1848 was not just any year in European history. It was a year of political revolutions, constitutionalism, the fall of monarchies, and counterreaction. These events have often been seen through the lens of societal groups calling for democratic reform and civil and political rights. Rudolf Virchow, fully aware of this and of his own position on the barricades in Berlin, would ensure that the debates also included a strong social rights component through an emphasis on the right to health. He called out unaccountable and useless rulers with their antiquated perceptions of justice in the *Medicinische Reform* journal (Virchow 1848a, p. 4). Writing in July 1848, Virchow evoked the dramatic days in March of that year in a way that almost programmatically informed his agenda for public health reform: 'Finally came the days of March. The great struggle of critical thinking against authoritarian rule, of natural history against dogma, of eternal human rights against human arbitrariness…' (Virchow 1848b, p. 9).

Virchow was adamant that the state had a responsibility to do more and to mitigate the deadly social conditions that epidemics dramatically exposed and that revealed a deeper pattern of social injustices. He laid out an argument for the state as a duty-bearer responsible for creating a public health system that could sustain an individual's right to health. The state, he wrote, 'must help everyone to live a healthy life. This simply follows from the conception of the state as the moral unity of all individuals composing it, and from the obligation of universal solidarity' (Virchow 1848c, p. 15).

Virchow wanted to mobilize the medical profession and medical science for the cause and in the process, he described doctors in legal terminology declaring that 'doctors are the natural advocates of the poor and the social question falls to a large extent within their jurisdiction' (McNeely 2002, p. 25; Farmer 2003, p. 234). He was also explicit in his use of rights language. It was not just an implied meaning we can distil with historical hindsight. He spoke to real political, economic, and social transformations taking place surrounding the role of the state in the nineteenth century in language we can recognize in the twenty-first century:

> [T]he concept of all having equal rights to healthful existence follows from the definition of the state as the moral unity of its members, i.e. of individuals enjoying equal rights and obligated to act in solidarity. The endeavour of the state to implement these rights mainly falls to the Public Health Services.
>
> *(Virchow 1848c, p. 16)*

Virchow did not just argue that poverty was a primary determinant of the outbreaks of epidemics such as typhus and cholera. He also argued that poverty was – at least in part – made by the powerful. His interest in social determinants led him to call for wider political solutions to the problems. Virchow championed political liberation and a democracy where people were equal before the law. He brought the whole social domain into the political equation and in the process defined a right to health alongside the need for educating people and providing other social support (Virchow 1848c, p. 36). We can see aspects of what would become part of social rights – such as the right to food and the right to an adequate standard of living – in the way he argued his case for public health and social medicine. Writing in 1848, he explained that:

> [M]easures must be taken to protect the poor, who have no soft bread, no good meat, no warm clothes, no bed, who cannot carry out their work on a diet of rice soup and camomile infusion; to protect the poor, who are most affected by the disease, through an improvement of their situation.
>
> *(Virchow 1848c, p. 24)*

Virchow was keenly aware of the disproportionate impacts on certain parts of the population caused by disease and poverty. His focus was on social class, but his lens could also be applied to gender, race, and ethnicity – as it would be in the twentieth century when the field of social medicine had developed further.

Rudolf Virchow did not just have a profound influence on the evolution of public health and social medicine. He remained a prominent political representative in Berlin and national German politics for most of the second half of the nineteenth century, as well as being a leading liberal opponent to Bismarck in the 1860s. This took place in parallel with his continued scientific endeavors. He also had a surprising influence on the way the right to health entered the international legal human rights framework a century later. The lessons from the typhus and cholera epidemics of this time show us that the 1840s speak to present-day realities. Virchow has continued to be a point of reference into the twenty-first century when it comes to human rights-based approaches to health in the global domain, e.g., in the context of the HIV/AIDS pandemic (Farmer 2001).

2 Health, racial discrimination and social rights constitutionalism after the First World War

If the First World War itself had not already wrought enough devastation, a global pandemic emerged targeting countries and populations weakened by the war. The 'Spanish flu' pandemic ravaged the world in 1918 and 1919, ending only in 1920. It is widely regarded as the worst pandemic of the twentieth century, causing perhaps as many as 50 million deaths. The pandemic has not – despite its enormous toll – left many traces such as public memorials and has not occupied much space in cultural memory. It was perhaps overshadowed by the First World War, which saw empires fall and new nation-states emerge from their ruins. The 2018 centenary did see a number of new books published telling the story and re-inscribing the influenza of 1918 in time to become something of a reference when COVID-19 emerged in 2020. These works tell the story of how it spread, how it affected people and societies, and how a public health response was mobilized. These books did not explore a link to rights.

The interwar period does not normally feature in human rights histories. However, we should not ignore this moment in history because the post-First World War period did witness a noticeable advance in health and human rights thinking in two important ways. The first way was social rights constitutionalism of which health was a part. The second way was in human rights declarations drafted by civil society movements that brought together racial discrimination, human rights and public health with rights claims made on the relevant political systems.

It is unclear if the influenza of 1918 played a specific role in these developments because diseases and epidemics remained a significant part of peoples' lives – tuberculosis being another deadly example – despite some advances in medicine and public health responses. Both strands, constitutionalism and the civil society perspective on health as a human right, deserve historical attention.

In his 1848 report on the typhus epidemic in Upper Silesia, Rudolf Virchow made the case for the right to health constitutionalism. He wrote: 'A sound constitution must affirm beyond any doubt the right of the individual to a healthy life' (Taylor & Rieger 1985, p. 553). This call was not really met at the time of writing. However, by the end of the First World War health would feature in a number of constitutions. The main 'social rights constitutions' during this period were from Mexico (1917), Weimar Germany (1919), and the Soviet Union (1936). These constitutions originated from very different political systems, came into existence for different reasons and reflected very different rights philosophies that were not necessarily exemplary versions of right to health constitutionalism. However, together they illustrate an emerging trend. Health was beginning to feature in this context as a natural component of social provisioning and policy.

The Weimar Constitution is an undervalued example of twentieth-century social rights constitutionalism probably because the Weimar Republic collapsed into a Nazi takeover. The political ambitions underpinning the Republic – which included a social-democratic and liberal compromise over its Constitution – failed in ways that have overshadowed the significance of the social rights provisions of the 1919 Constitution (Eichenhofer 2019, p. 5). One could almost speak of a bill of social rights inserted into it. The Weimar Constitution's Article 161 was not as fully articulated a right to health as would emerge internationally after 1945 but it did address the plight and misery of the population by obligating the state to establish a system for health insurance. The Article read as follows:

> The Reich shall, with the controlling participation of the insured, establish a comprehensive scheme of insurance for the conservation of health and of the capacity to work, for the protection of maternity, and for the amelioration of the economic consequences of old age, infirmity, and the changing circumstances of life.
>
> *(McBain & Rogers 1922, p. 207)*

This was of course not merely about dealing with epidemics. It was a more holistic approach to disease and public health, but the experience of epidemics certainly factored into the mindset that developed this social rights-oriented approach. The same can be said about the way health featured in the 1936 Soviet Constitution. Epidemics were one aspect of a larger disease landscape that led the Communist regime to include in the Constitution a guarantee to provide comprehensive medical services to, in principle, the entire population through a national health system. It should be noted that this was social rights in a version that did not recognize inherent rights of individuals but framed rights as something that the state gave to its people. (For an elaboration on the peculiarities of social rights in the Soviet Communist system, see Newton forthcoming.)

Health featured in the debates on the 1917 Mexican Constitution, which is also widely recognized as a social rights constitution. The focus here was more on health, hygiene and safety conditions in the workplaces such as factories, mines, and workshops. It also included health protections for women linked to working conditions around childbirth. These were not the strongest protections, but the example helps point to an emerging pattern (Ramos 1967).

This pattern of linking public health and human rights was also clear in two remarkable human rights declarations produced by civil society movements between 1918 and 1945. These deserve a mention because they add further historical depth to the exploration of the health and human rights nexus.

In August 1920, the Universal Negro Improvement Association – founded a few years before by the Jamaican-born activist Marcus Garvey – held their first annual convention in New York. It was a large-scale, month-long event that attracted thousands of people to attend the sessions in Liberty Hall in Harlem. For one convention event, attendees filled Madison Square Garden with more than

20,000 people in attendance. Participants came from all over the United States, the Caribbean, and Africa.

One of the convention's main ambitions was to produce a bill of rights that would form the basis of the movement's claims for black freedom and justice around the world. Black people had fought in Europe during the First World War and were now facing a dramatic increase in the number of lynchings in the United States as the war ended (Ward 2016, pp. 55–56). In the colonies, Africans were suffering multiple forms of discrimination and violent abuses. The bill of rights was to be a powerful response to this. Or as Marcus Garvey explained:

> We are here because we are tired of being a suffering people. We are here because we desire our liberty. We believe that all those human rights that are common to the rest of mankind should also be enjoyed by us and for that purpose we assemble ourselves in this great international convention to discuss the ways and means through which we will get that liberty that we have been deprived for the last five hundred years.
>
> *(Hill 1983, p. 481)*

Marcus Garvey and his movement have become known as the greatest mobilizers of black opinion in the twentieth century, as the Universal Negro Improvement Association would mobilize millions of supporters across several continents (Ewing 2014). It is therefore a sad irony that the human rights document that the 1920 convention drafted and adopted – *The Declaration of Rights of the Negro Peoples of the World* – is largely ignored in international human rights scholarship (Jensen 2020). It has received a few references in the scholarship on Marcus Garvey and the UNIA. In 2006 the historian Robert Trent Vinson wrote, 'The "Declaration of Rights of the Negro Peoples of the World" articulated the grievances, aims, objectives and guiding philosophy of the UNIA as an anti-white supremacist movement' (Vinson 2006, p. 290). It merits greater attention.

The vision of the 1920 Declaration shows that well before the 1948 Universal Declaration of Human Rights, the linking of the broad categories of rights (civil, political, economic, social and cultural rights) was vital for political projects concerned with liberty, justice, equality, dignity, and non-discrimination. The articles on social rights covered education, work, and health. The content reflected the experiences that delegates shared about conditions in their own countries or localities. These reports fed directly into the drafting of the Declaration. The participants heard a report from the Caribbean about how male and female agricultural workers faced tuberculosis, malnutrition, diminished powers of resistance against diseases, skin diseases, and so on because of low remuneration and poor working and living conditions. A delegate from New Haven, Connecticut described how people of color were discriminated against (treated 'with indifference and injustice') in the public hospitals. The conditions described spoke to an unreasonable and disproportionate disease burden placed on black people because of racial discrimination exacerbated by poverty (Hill 1983, pp. 530 & 534).

The 1920 Declaration of Rights of the Negro Peoples of the World could not ignore this reality. It therefore included an article on health both in its preamble and in the main section. The latter article on health contained a community and health care practitioner perspective by declaring it was

> an injustice to our people and a serious impediment to the health of the race to deny to competent licensed Negro physicians the right to practice in the public hospitals of the communities in which they reside for no other reason than their race and colour.
>
> *(Hill 1983, p. 576)*

This may not match the formula for the right to health that we know today but it spoke directly to the issue of access to health care and discrimination, which remains key to human rights thinking in the health domain. It is worth remembering that this was inserted into something that was presented as a bill of rights and a demand for liberty worldwide. The delegates of the UNIA convention believed that health belonged in this context.

This thinking was elaborated further in a prominent civil society human rights declaration presented two decades later. In December 1943, the African National Congress (ANC) in South Africa adopted the so-called 'African Claims in South Africa'. It has been described as a landmark in the human rights tradition of the ANC (Asmal 2005, p. 1). It sits in a lineage that includes the 1955 ANC Freedom Charter and South Africa's Constitution from 1996.

'African Claims' was drafted in the context of the Second World War. It was a direct response to the Atlantic Charter that US President Franklin D. Roosevelt and Britain's Prime Minister Winston Churchill had agreed upon in August 1941 and to which other allied nations had subsequently subscribed. 'African Claims' was both global and domestic in its outlook and committed to fighting tyranny worldwide and in South Africa. The ANC leadership argued that 'the only alternative to force, violence and oppression was a new order of human rights' (Asmal 2005, p. 4). The contents of 'African Claims in South Africa' should be viewed from this perspective.

The 'African Claims' document had three main sections. The first two sections were entitled 'We fight for world democracy' and 'The Atlantic Charter and Africans'. The third section carried the heading 'Bill of Rights: Full Citizen Rights and Demands' and shows again how civil, political, social, economic, and cultural rights were readily bridged in human rights documents before the 1948 Universal Declaration. The health-related human rights were not just one article but a whole sub-section under the label of 'Public Health and Medical Services' that described the rights and demands in some detail, including duties of the state. It called among other things for the establishment of free medical and health services for all sections of the population:

> We regard it as the duty of the state to provide adequate medical and health facilities for the entire population of the country. We deplore and deprecate

> the fact that the state has not carried out its duty to the African in this regard … As a result of this neglect, the general health of the entire African population has deteriorated to an alarming extent.
>
> *(Asmal 2005, p. 20)*

It was a strong call against discrimination and inequalities in health that caused gross malnutrition, higher mortality and morbidity rates among the African population. Interestingly, it also made a call to 'remedy this state of affairs,' namely through 'a drastic overhauling and reorganization of the health services of the country with due emphasis on preventive medicine with all that implies in the modern public health sense' (Asmal 2005, p. 20).

It is worth noting how the health section of this bill of rights combined rights, duties, obligations, and remedies in the same text. It was insightful and imaginative – an aspect which was also reflected when ANC urged the adoption of 'a proper system of vital statistics for the whole population including Africans' (Asmal 2005, p. 21). This would be an important measure to meet the health needs of the country's African population and deal with the disproportionate impact of the range of diseases affecting the population – a recurring public health theme we can notice going back to Rudolf Virchow in the 1840s. The rather expansive health section in this bill of rights appeared just before the section demanding the repeal of all discriminatory laws in South Africa.

The above examples illustrate that there were noteworthy developments in the health and human rights domain between 1918 and 1945. After the Second World War, the United Nations would be the main forum for the internationalization of human rights. It did not necessarily offer much progress for the health and human rights nexus during its early years despite a promising start in 1946.

3 From 'fundamental right' to a new pandemic turning point: the right to health after 1945

The 1946 World Health Organization (WHO) Constitution was the opening act in the post-war history of the right to health. It began with an expansive definition stating that 'health is a state of complete physical, mental and social well-being and not merely the absence of disease or infirmity'. This was followed by a definition of the right to health stipulating that: 'The enjoyment of the highest attainable standard of health is one of the fundamental rights of every human being without distinction of race, religion, political belief, economic or social condition' (WHO 1946). The UN Member States that founded WHO had made health a 'fundamental right'. It was a noteworthy starting point.

The debate changed as the negotiations shifted to the UN Commission on Human Rights over the next decade until the draft Covenant on Economic, Social and Cultural Rights was transferred to the UN General Assembly in 1954. The 1948 Universal Declaration did not contain a separate article on health, but health was part of a broader Article 25 that also mentioned medical care.

The negotiations related to the Covenant were more interesting than Article 25 of the UDHR for the purpose here. It was decided to include a specific article on the right to health and in 1951, draft texts were put forward. WHO and Egypt argued for a more elaborate, substantive article, and each submitted proposals. The debate went back and forth over these drafts, focused on whether a more detailed article or a short and simple version was preferable. The sub-text for this was a debate over the nature of state obligations in the field of public health. For some reason, Egypt withdrew their relatively elaborate proposal. Chile decided to intervene and formally take over the Egyptian proposal. The debate continued but Chile, now with WHO's backing, drove the negotiations to a conclusion in which their proposal prevailed against resistance from a number of states. The 1951 draft article on the right to health was adopted by the UN Commission on Human Rights as follows:

> The States parties to this Covenant recognize the right of everyone to the enjoyment of the highest standard of health obtainable. With a view to implementing and safeguarding this right, each State party hereto undertakes to provide legislative measures to promote and protect health and in particular:
>
> 1. To reduce infant mortality and to provide for healthy development of the child;
> 2. To improve nutrition, housing and, sanitation, recreation, economic and working conditions and other aspects of environmental hygiene;
> 3. To control epidemic, endemic and other diseases;
> 4. To provide conditions which would assure the right of all its nationals to a medical service and medical attention in the event of sickness.
>
> *(UN Commission on Human Rights 1951, p. 18)*

We can study this as legal standard-setting. We should, however, also recognize this as reflecting the history of epidemics inserting itself in the international human rights framework. Each sub-point reflected long-standing global public health realities or conditions that epidemics had affected and that lived experience made relevant for rights protection.

This deeper history can be made more concrete and specific. The drafting history should not be limited to UN committee meetings. A reasonable argument can be made that the relevant context is broader and involves the birth of human rights-oriented social medicine with Rudolf Virchow in the 1840s. It was no coincidence that it was Chile that delivered a successful more detailed draft article. The country was at this point in time introducing a national health system aiming to offer universal health care. The groundwork had been laid by a young Chilean doctor turned Minister of Health from 1939 who had studied with one of Rudolf Virchow's German students Max Westenhofer. Westenhofer had migrated to Chile and had become Director of the Department of Pathology at the University of Chile. He influenced the young Chilean doctor who became a strong champion of social medicine and as Minister of Health drove public health reform towards the creation of a national health system (Gaffney 2018, pp. 67, 138–139). The Minister's name was Salvador Allende.

The influence of social medicine on the UN human rights negotiations in 1951 were visible in the arguments presented by Chile. In response to states that wanted a minimalist formula for the right to health, the Chilean representative Hernán Santa Cruz – a co-drafter of the Universal Declaration – argued that 'it was essential … to mention specifically the responsibility incumbent on the State for taking preventive action against diseases and combating it through public health services'. He continued, '[i]t would … be regrettable if an article on the right to health ignored the relationship between health and the standard of living' (UN Commission on Human Rights 1951, p. 15). The Chilean proposal would, with a revision to sub-paragraph 2, be the language adopted in the 1966 International Covenant on Economic, Social, and Cultural Rights. This is the legal basis for modern understandings of the right to health.

The right to health, however, was not framed as a fundamental right in the international human rights legal framework. Furthermore, WHO would from 1953 onwards turn away from the interest in human rights which it had shown in earlier years (Meier 2010). While Cold War politics partly explains this shift, there was also a tension between a more technical versus a more socially oriented approach to medicine and public health. The retreat from the 1946 aims was nonetheless distinct. It left the right to health largely ignored for twenty-five years until WHO started to bring it back into international health diplomacy discussions. This happened with the 1978 Alma Ata Declaration, where WHO secured international agreement on 'Health for All' as a major policy goal under the leadership of its Danish Director-General Halfdan Mahler.

At the 1979 World Health Assembly, Mahler was in a contemplative mood as he delivered his opening speech. In front of the United Nations Member States, he stated: 'Plato said some 2000 years ago: "What is honoured in a country is cultivated there." Do we today honour world health or not?' (Mahler 1979, p. 19). Mahler gave this speech at a time when WHO was preparing to declare smallpox eradicated globally – still one of the greatest successes in the organization's history. This was, however, no reason for WHO or the international community to rest on its laurels. What smallpox eradication meant – in Mahler's mind – was that funds were now freed up for the international community to address a whole range of other diseases and massive health problems around the world. Mahler was adamant that to be successful the international community needed to 'honour' and 'cultivate' the right to health and that WHO itself needed to revive its early human rights commitment. This meant resurrecting the question of obligations held by states. Mahler argued that developed countries had a double responsibility:

> to their own people and to the peoples of the developing countries struggling to extricate themselves from historical injustice and from the vicious circle

> of poverty and disease – there is a very close relationship between what a country does within its own boundaries and what it is able to do for other countries.
>
> *(Mahler 1979, p. 19)*

This represented an internationalization ofVirchow's thinking. Mahler was speaking to an evolving global reality aware of the political obstacles to achieving the ambitious human rights-oriented health goals for primary health care established by the Alma Ata Declaration the previous year. Mahler had earlier referred to Rudolf Virchow's statement that 'Medicine is a social science, and politics is nothing more than medicine on a large scale' in a speech to the World Health Assembly (Mahler 1976, p. 53). The renewed emphasis on the right to health in the late 1970s still owed an intellectual debt to the German doctor who had faced typhus and cholera epidemics more than a century earlier.

The Alma Ata Declaration and its agenda faced many political challenges and obstacles. The health and human rights agenda did not secure sufficient traction from this process. It would require the emergence of a new pandemic to change this. HIV/AIDS became the turning point. This brings us back to Jonathan Mann, the Director of WHO's Global Program for AIDS. He was certainly right about the contemporary health and human rights story owing much to the global HIV/AIDS response.

The human rights approach to HIV offered a powerful lens through which to expose stigma, discrimination, prejudice, and other violations, and link these to the international legal obligations of states. This helped to define actions to address them, with activism being the energizing factor. In the HIV/AIDS response, this was done with a continued focus on affected communities and key populations, such as LGBTQ+ persons, sex workers, drug users, people in detention, and others because the disproportionate impacts of the virus on these populations were so blatant. Many hard battles have been fought over the years just to have these groups recognized in internationally-agreed decisions and declarations. These battles were fought to allow public health evidence to prevail over discrimination and criminalization. It is a fight that continues because health remains a human rights battlefield.

It is widely recognized that the global HIV/AIDS response transformed global health. The global health changes were political, institutional, medical, financial, legal and social. The right to health was an important entry point to mobilize the international legal framework but the lesson was also that the human rights approach to HIV/AIDS engaged with the broad spectrum of human rights, proving their deep interrelatedness. It may well be that the right to health was not seen as a 'fundamental right' as per the 1946 WHO Constitution, but it had proven to be a foundational human right in tackling one of the major global crises of our time. It is also proving to be foundational in the age of COVID-19.

4 Conclusion

As we define our responses to and recovery from the COVID-19 pandemic, it is important to keep in mind that the right to health has a long history. It is a history shaped by the experience of epidemics (as well as other diseases). It is not merely a normative standard that can be applied. Virchow's example shows that human rights were foundational for the birth of social medicine and thereby for modern public health thinking. It is a story that places the right to health within a much larger story about the transformations of the modern state from the nineteenth century to the twenty-first century in a dynamic relationship between norms, values, and experience. The historical connection manifested itself at important post-1945 moments when the health and human rights nexus progressed. It is therefore timely to reconsider this longer story in the midst of the COVID-19 pandemic and explore what lessons it offers because in important ways COVID-19 is a new chapter in an old story about epidemics, health, human rights, and humanity.

Notes

1 Formerly and incorrectly referred to as 'the Spanish flu'.
2 A substantive body of academic scholarship on the right to health has emerged during the 2010s. See John Tobin (2012), *The Right to Health in International Law*. Oxford University Press, Oxford; Jonathan Wolff (2012), *The Human Rights to Health*. Norton & Company, New York; José M. Zúñiga, Stephen P. Marks and Lawrence O. Gostin eds. (2013), *Advancing the Human Rights to Health*. Oxford University Press, Oxford; Audrey Chapman (2016), *Global Health, Human Rights and the Challenge of Neoliberal Policies*. Cambridge University Press, Cambridge; Alicia Ely Yamin (2016), *Power, Suffering and the Struggle for Dignity. Human Rights Frameworks for Health and Why They Matter.* University of Pennsylvania Press; Adam Gaffney (2018), *To Heal Humankind. The Right to Health in History*. Routledge, London; Benjamin Mason Meier and Lawrence O. Gostin (2018), *Human Rights in Global Health. Rights-Based Governance for A Globalizing World*. Oxford University Press, Oxford. Earlier works on the right to health do exist but the number of books in the last decade speak to the prominence that the right to health has now achieved.

References

Asmal, K (ed.) 2005, *Legacy of Freedom. The ANC's Human Rights Tradition*, Jonathan Ball Publishers, Johannesburg.

Chapman, AR 2016, *Global Health, Human Rights, and the Challenge of Neoliberal Policies*, Cambridge University Press, Cambridge.

Eichenhofer, E 2019 '100 Jahre soziale Grundrechte in der deutschen Verfassungsordnung – historische Entwicklung und Zukunftsperspektiven', *Arbeit und Recht*, vol. 5 .

Eisenberg, L 1984, 'Rudolf Ludwig Karl Virchow, Where Are You Now That We Need You?', *The American Journal of Medicine*, vol. 77, no. 3, pp. 524–532.

Ewing, A 2014, *The Age of Garvey: How a Jamaican Activist Created a Mass Movement and Changed Global Black Politics*, Princeton University Press, Princeton.

Farmer, P 2001, *Infections and Inequalities: The Modern Plagues*, University of California Press, Los Angeles.

Farmer, P 2003, *Pathologies of Power: Health, Human Rights and the New War on the Poor*, University of California Press, Los Angeles.
Gaffney, A 2018, *To Heal Humankind: The Right to Health in History*, Routledge, London.
Gostin, LO & Meier, BM 2018, 'The Origins of Human Rights in Global Health', in LO Gostin & BM Meier (eds.), *Human Rights in Global Health: Rights-based Governance for a Globalizing World*, Oxford University Press, Oxford, pp. 21–42.
Hildebrand, S (ed.) 2009, *Jonathan Mann – The Legacy of a Human Rights Advocate*, short documentary, UNAIDS, Geneva, www.youtube.com/watch?v=kNp5bB10MSc
Hill, RA (ed.) 1983, *The Marcus Garvey and Universal Negro Improvement Association Papers*, vol. 2, University of California Press, Berkeley.
Jensen, SLB 2020, '"Our Rightful Place in the Sun": Marcus Garvey and the 1920 Declaration of Rights of the Negro Peoples of the World', *The Daily Maverick (SA)*, 13 August.
Mahler, H 1976, 'Review of the Annual Report of the Director-General on the Work of WHO in 1975', in *Part II Verbatim Record of Plenary Meetings, Summary Records and Reports of Committees: Twenty-Ninth World Health Assembly*, 3–21 May, Geneva, World Health Organization, Geneva, pp. 51–56.
Mahler, H 1979, 'Review of the Report of the Director-General on the Work of WHO in 1978' in *Verbatim Records of Plenary Meetings, Reports of Committees: Thirty-Second World Health Assembly*, 7–25 May, World Health Organization, Geneva, pp. 19–24.
McBain, HL & Rogers, L 1922, *The New Constitutions of Europe*, Doubleday, Page & Company, Garden City.
McNeely, IF 2002, *"Medicine on a Grand Scale": Rudolf Virchow, Liberalism, and the Public Health*, Wellcome Trust Centre for the History of Medicine, London.
Meier, BM 2010, 'Global Health Governance and the Contentious Politics of Human Rights', *Stanford Journal of International Law*, vol. 46, no. 1, pp. 1–50.
Meier, BM & Gostin, LO (eds.) 2018, *Human Rights in Global Health. Rights-Based Governance for A Globalizing World*, Oxford University Press, Oxford.
Newton, S (forthcoming), 'The Soviet Social: Rights and Welfare Reimagined', in SLB Jensen & C Walton (eds.), *Social Rights and the Politics of Obligation in History*, Cambridge University Press, Cambridge.
Ramos, FY 1967, 'The Social Rights Enshrined in the Mexican Constitution of 1967', *International Labour Review*, vol. 96, no. 6, pp. 590–608.
Sawyer, SW & Novak WJ (forthcoming), 'Of Rights and Regulation: Technologies of Democratic Governance in the Eighteenth and Nineteenth Centuries', in SLB Jensen & C Walton (eds.), *Social Rights and the Politics of Obligation in History*, Cambridge University Press, Cambridge.
Taylor, R & Rieger, A 1985, 'Medicine as Social Science: Rudolf Virchow on the Typhus Epidemic in Upper Silesia', *International Journal of Health Services*, vol. 15, no. 4, pp. 547–559.
Tobin, J 2012, *The Right to Health in International Law*, Oxford University Press, Oxford.
UN Commission on Human Rights 1951, *Seventh Session: Summary Record of the Two Hundred and Twenty Third Meeting, E/CN.4/SR.223*.
Vinson, RT 2006, '"Sea Kaffirs": "American Negroes" and the Gospel of Garveyism in Early Twentieth-Century Cape Town', *Journal of African History*, vol. 47, no. 2, pp. 281–303.
Virchow, R 1848a, 'The Aims of the Journal "Medical Reform"', in LJ Rather (ed.), *Collected Essays on Public Health and Epidemiology*, vol. 1, Amerind Publishing, New York, pp. 3–5.
Virchow, R 1848b, 'The Ministry of Health', in LJ Rather (ed.), *Collected Essays on Public Health and Epidemiology*, vol. 1, Amerind Publishing, New York, pp. 6–13.
Virchow, R 1848c, 'Public Health Services', in LJ Rather (ed.), *Collected Essays on Public Health and Epidemiology*, vol. 1, Amerind Publishing, New York, pp. 14–29.

Ward, JM 2016, *Hanging Bridge. Racial Violence and America's Civil Rights Century*, Oxford University Press, Oxford.

World Health Organization (WHO) Constitution (1948) opened for signature 22 July 1946, 14 UNTS 185.

Witt, JF 2020, *American Contagions: Epidemics and the Law from Smallpox to COVID-19*, Yale University Press, New Haven.

Wolff, J 2012, *The Human Rights to Health*, Norton & Company, New York.

Yamin, AE 2016, *Power, Suffering and the Struggle for Dignity: Human Rights Frameworks for Health and Why They Matter*, Pennsylvania Studies in Human Rights, University of Pennsylvania Press, Philadelphia.

Zúñiga, JM, Marks, SP & Gostin, LO (eds.) 2013, *Advancing the Human Rights to Health*, Oxford University Press, Oxford.

2

HUMAN RIGHTS-BASED VERSUS POPULIST RESPONSES TO THE PANDEMIC

Martin Scheinin and Helga Molbæk-Steensig

Populism traditionally thrives on crisis. So much so that the construction or exasperation of crises through securitizing language is a cornerstone of the populist rhetorical style that is central to authoritarian legitimacy building. Crises can provide legitimacy to extraordinary politics, which consistently have proved to be the antithesis to human rights compliance. In the context of the crisis brought on by the COVID-19 pandemic, there has been a need for extraordinary policies, which increases the risk of populist opportunism.

There is, however, a way to design and put in place the necessary and extraordinary policies needed in the COVID-19 pandemic based in human rights law and with a view to respecting, protecting, and fulfilling the human rights of every person. Before presenting an outline for such human rights-based strategies against COVID-19 as the main section of this chapter, we will first address what defines such strategies by contrasting them with populist or authoritarian responses to the pandemic. The first defining characteristic of human rights-based responses to COVID-19 is the recognition of the equal value and rights of every human being. Here, one needs to be aware that traditional, ancient, or medieval approaches to epidemics may have been based on prioritizing the collective, the privileged regime, or the wealth and security of the nation. Lessons drawn from pre-human rights times may still permeate playbooks of epidemiologists, which means that technocratic responses to the pandemic call for human rights scrutiny. The second defining characteristic is that human-rights-based responses are inclusive, democratic, and evidence-based, and they pay particular attention to protecting vulnerable individuals and groups.

Populism, on the other hand, works in the opposite way. Leaders use rhetorical devices to divide the population into 'the people' and 'the other' where only the welfare and the opinions of the first group is of interest (Müller 2015). In connection with the COVID-19 emergency this division is a recipe for disaster and a poor guide in political decision making. Those disregarded by the regime are just as much, if not more, at risk for infections. Recognizing populist responses as such is therefore important, even if the populists themselves have good reason and often significant resources to attack scholarship labeling them as such. Recognizing populist responses can help in predicting how the use of certain rhetorical tools useful for both the 'left' and the 'right' lead to policies aimed at reducing the checks on state power and dismantling of the rule of law while opening the backdoor for corruption and kleptocracy (Sandbu 2020).

To render the term populism useful, scholars have struggled to establish objective indicators of it. Some rely on overall analyses of party programs conducted or reviewed by country experts and verified through peer review, grading parties by their populist tendencies (Eiermann, Mounk, & Gultchin 2017; Rooduijn et al. 2019); others rely mainly on rhetoric (Hawkins et al. 2019). Generally, these mappings represent academic consensus and may function as decent shorthand for most purposes, but they may lack the necessary traceability to dispel critique from the populists themselves. After all, a key aspect of populist platforms, in addition to the othering of individuals belonging to certain social or minority groups, is the rejection of experts and elites (Mudde & Kaltwasser 2017). The likes of Hungary's Prime Minister Victor Orbán or Poland's president of the Law and Justice Party Jarosław Kaczyński may be unimpressed with the consensus upon which thirty-five country experts or the wider community of social scientists have agreed. Another issue is that even these aggregated studies are not in full agreement. For example, the study led by Roodujin includes the Italian Five Stars movement as populist (Lewis et al. 2018) whereas Eiermann, Mounk, and Gultchin (2017) do not.

A way of getting around these issues is by using proxies. The proxy of studying securitizing rhetoric holds some promise. The main reason why the concept of populism is of interest to scholars is that it is conceived as an intention to groom popular sentiment in preparation for the dismantling of constitutional safeguards and divisions of power. Securitization is the speech act of rendering a political topic into a security threat – a danger to the life of the nation, the necessity of a decisive response to which is not up for debate and which in turn can be used to justify extraordinary politics (Buzan et al. 1998). This includes the use of emergency powers or the less structured allowance of human rights interferences with a wider margin of discretion afforded to the executive. Such speech acts can take the shape of using war, weapon, or disease metaphors. Classics include the 'war on terror', 'war on drugs', the references to the influx of refugees or migrants as 'an invasion', or to domestic minorities as 'a cancer', or indeed, to carriers of COVID-19 as 'invisible enemies'.

In relation to the COVID-19 pandemic, these markers of populism (divisive rhetoric, anti-science, and securitization) are readily applicable, but the situation is also doubly complex. Due to the nature of this crisis, governments have had to make decisions on the basis of incomplete medical and epidemiological information. It has also become clear that not acting to contain the virus or to alleviate suffering caused by it is neither normatively neutral nor human rights-wise acceptable. As a result we have seen democratic leaders legitimately using the language of emergency and interfering with, or even derogating from, human rights, whereas some rulers that generally score high on the populism-scales have downplayed the emergency and blocked or reversed evidence-based measures to contain it (Scheppele 2020). Jair Bolsonaro of Brazil and Donald Trump of the United States, for instance, not only aggravated the situations in their own countries but also bear responsibility for catastrophic consequences of COVID-19 in wider South America, frustrating the declarations of states of emergency in many of these countries (Kirkpatrick & Cabrera 2020). Does this mean that these leaders are not in fact populists? Hardly. In fact, their anti-elite, anti-expertise, and anti-immigrant rhetoric, and the built-in tendency of the virus to hit disadvantaged communities hardest, fit in well with the populist othering of specific minority or socioeconomic groups. In this sense, downplaying the severity of the COVID-19 pandemic bears some resemblance to the denial of the climate crisis that has permeated populist sentiments in the United States for years. For a human rights-compliant response to the COVID-19 pandemic, the government's positive obligations to take effective measures to protect the population against adverse effects on human rights caused by the virus are central.

The academic community has not remained silent on this topic. With remarkable speed and from their various stages of lockdowns, this community has compiled several comparative collections of country reports on government responses to COVID-19. For instance, OpinioJuris collected a series of thematic blog posts on COVID, constitutionalism and rights (Bates 2020; Hodgson & Seiderman 2020; Istrefi 2020; Scheinin, 2020b). Verfassungsblog gathered a large collection of country reports on constitutional challenges arising from COVID-19 worldwide (Grogan 2020 lists them). Democracy Reporting International compiled reports from all twenty-seven EU member states on rule of law and human rights compliance of state measures against COVID-19 (Fournier and Meyer-Resende 2020). Furthermore, the UN Special Rapporteur on the promotion and protection of human rights while countering terrorism released a tracker of responses in cooperation with the ICNL (Ní Aoláin 2020), as did Oxford University (2020). What this chapter will contribute is a guide to what a human rights-based approach to managing a pandemic looks like. This is based on existing international legislation and practice, and as will be evident, it differs widely from populist/authoritarian approaches but also rebuts the claim that human rights would prevent governments from effectively battling the pandemic.

1 Human rights-based responses to COVID-19

Even in societies not following the populist-authoritarian approach outlined above, there is a grave risk that an evidence-based approach to COVID-19 is seen as a balancing act between information generated by the two epistemic communities of epidemiologists and economists, the latter not only referring to academics but also to many powerful policy actors. It would then be for the elected politicians to 'strike a balance'. Decisions need, however, to be informed also by other epistemic communities, including human rights experts and social scientists who can assess how people actually behave and why. A human-rights-conforming strategy must protect the human rights of the population, understood holistically as interdependent and indivisible. The right to life deserves primacy but other human rights also require careful analysis. What follows below is a twenty-point outline for national strategies to combat COVID-19. This list differs from for example Human Rights Watch's checklist (2020) in that it deals with both the emergency phases and the long-term measures that are proving necessary for living with the virus. The list is illustrated by both positive and negative examples since one country may have in some respect acted in accordance with human rights and may also have been insensitive or even ignorant to human rights elsewhere.

1. When empirical (epidemiological and other) information is incomplete, it is permissible, and from a human rights law perspective even obligatory for States to make strategic decisions based on assumptions. Doing nothing is not a normatively neutral or normatively acceptable approach. Human rights, including the right to life and the right to health come with significant positive obligations to protect and ensure their enjoyment (e.g., International Covenant on Civil and Political Rights (ICCPR) Article 2 and General Comment (GC) No. 31; International Covenant on Economic, Social and Cultural Rights ((ICESCR) Article 2 and GC No. 3). The Government Response Stringency Index (Ritchie et al. 2020) and the timeline it presents for different countries demonstrate that early responses have had lasting but not necessarily eternal positive results in containing the epidemic (e.g. Germany or South Korea), while countries that acted late are often suffering both from continued high levels of transmission and deaths and from more far-reaching restrictions upon liberty such as in Brazil and the United States.
2. When making decisions based on assumptions, international human rights law prescribes that responsible governments should err on the side of human rights compliance. Other things being equal, the option should be chosen that is in best conformity with human rights, understood holistically, in line with the principle of interdependence and indivisibility of all human rights: political, civil, economic, and social (UN resolution 48/121, Vienna Declaration, para I.5). In practice this is a complex exercise. Human rights will many times be on both sides of the equation, calling for a nuanced and comprehensive assessment. Compliance with one right may often provide a legitimate aim that justifies limitations upon another. China and Italy, for instance, were two countries that acted early to restrict public gatherings (Ritchie et al. 2020). This is of course a measure that could violate human rights, but also one which when accompanied by human rights-protective considerations can be a permissible interference when balanced against the potential impact on the rights to life and health of not restricting public gatherings. Procedural safeguards, temporal limitations of any restrictions, or facilitation of alternative safer ways for

assemblies to take place are all modalities for reconciling the implementation of economic, social, and cultural rights and other human rights.

3. Human rights assessment cannot be replaced by proxies. For instance, giving a boost to the economy by easing restrictions that will prevent contagion cannot be justified simply by saying that liberty should prevail. Furthermore, exclusive focus on intensive care (ICU) capacity proved a bad proxy for the right to life – for instance, people in nursing homes for the elderly will often not be transferred to the ICU. This is where the technocratic epidemiological strategy of Sweden failed. The Swedish strategy was based on the notion of 'flattening the curve' with the assumption that as long as citizens did not get sick at the same time, Sweden would have enough ICU space to avoid excess deaths. By 15 December 2020 Sweden had 760 deaths per million inhabitants while in the other Nordic countries that number was between 73 and 166 (Ritchie et al. 2020).

   Human rights assessment should be based on international human rights treaties and their institutionalized practices of interpretation as to what is normatively required under them. This means being guided by the ICESCR and ICCPR from 1966, and the institutionalized interpretive practice under them, including but not limited to General Comments issued by the respective treaty bodies, as well as by the added value of other human rights treaties such as the Convention on the Elimination of All Forms of Discrimination Against Women, Convention on the Rights of the Child, Convention on the Rights of Persons with Disabilities, and International Convention on the Elimination of All Forms of Racial Discrimination.

4. When, as will many times be the case, human rights appear to collide, the essential or minimum core of one human right (ICCPR GC No. 27, para. 13; EU Charter Article 52 (1); ICESCR GC No. 14, para. 43) should be presumed to have priority over non-core dimensions of other, colliding human rights. Any proposed restrictive measures must undergo a structured assessment for their permissibility. The essential core of every human right needs to remain protected; restrictions must be proven necessary, which translates to both being effective towards the proclaimed legitimate aim and being minimally intrusive in respect of human rights. The resulting human rights intrusion must remain proportionate to the effect delivered. In practice, the right to life (e.g., ICCPR Article 6 and GC No. 36) should always receive extra careful consideration in the assessment of proposed measures or available options. This does not, however, mean that simply stating the aim of saving lives would relieve a state from its other human rights obligations so that it could, for instance, disregard the essential core of freedom of expression (ICCPR Article 19 and General Comment No. 34; OHCHR 2020b) or freedom of movement (ICCPR Article 12 and General Comment No. 27). Some restrictions upon these and other rights may very well be justified, others not. For instance, the temporary sealing off of the capital region of Finland, including one third of the whole country's population, emulated the Italian experience in Lombardy. It seems

however, that in Finland it was ill-designed as a blunt measure to protect the right to life, especially for the population within the capital region, since it was not accompanied by effective measures of support and protection to vulnerable groups (Scheinin 2020a).

5. In the context of a deadly pandemic, the right to life has a very close relationship with the right to health (ICESCR Article 12 and General Comment No. 14; OHCHR 2020d) and other economic, social or cultural (ESC) rights. Therefore, States cannot ignore these when designing a human-rights-based strategy against COVID-19. For instance, the right to an adequate standard of living (ICESCR Article 11 and General Comments Nos. 4, 7, 12 and 15), or the right to education (ICESCR Article 13 and General Comment No. 13), remain applicable during a pandemic and need to be included in a comprehensive human rights assessment. Just like civil and political rights, ESC rights may appear on both sides of the equation when deciding on concrete steps to take. Emerging studies suggest that the right to health and the right to education may be best optimized by keeping preschools and primary schools open with safety measures, while at the same time adopting hybrid models of onsite and online education for adolescents, with a particular focus on meeting special educational needs (Michaud & Kates 2020).
6. States have an obligation to counter any discrimination, by public or private actors, in the fight against the pandemic, and also any discriminatory impact of the pandemic itself (ICESCR Article 2 and General Comment No. 20; ICCPR Article 26 and General Comment No. 18; CEDAW; CERD; CRPD). Potential situations of discrimination that require particular attention include: nursing homes for the elderly (ICESCR General Comment No. 6; OHCHR 2020e), many persons with disabilities (CRPD; ICESCR General Comment No. 5), prisons and other places of detention (ICCPR Article 10 and General Comment No. 21; IASC 2020), migrant workers housed in close quarters (e.g., workers in construction or seasonal agriculture), people doing precarious work, and underprivileged immigrant or ethnic communities (ICESCR Article 7 and General Comment No. 23; OHCHR 2020a; OHCHR 2020c; Council of Europe 2020b). The COVID-19 outbreak within the meatpacking industry and in the surrounding community in Gütersloh, Germany, provides an illustrative case of (i) the role of precarious and exploitative working conditions in the spread of the virus, (ii) targeted and local, rather than blunt and nationwide, measures in addressing contagion, and (iii) the role of the law and courts in reviewing the proportionality of the restrictions resulting from such measures (Oberverwaltungsgericht Nordrhein-Westfalen 13 B 940/20.NE).
7. All measures must have proper constitutional basis and safeguards (ICCPR General Comment No. 27, paras. 11–18; Council of Europe 2020a). The controversial Hungarian declaration of a 'state of danger' on the basis of vague constitutional provisions and the subsequent adoption of the so-called Enabling Act, which allows the government to rule by decree without a sunset clause,

are examples of how the lack of a proper legal basis and procedural safeguards impact the intrusiveness of restrictive measures.

8. Many measures to combat the pandemic can be introduced as voluntary, in the form of evidence-based recommendations. Where a culture of protecting oneself and strangers does not take hold, human rights law will permit the introduction of obligatory and enforced restrictions that meet the permissible limitations test. They should be secondary to voluntary measures, backed by evidence as to their effect of preventing or reducing contagion. Measures should also be targeted, temporary, and minimally intrusive so as to comply with the requirement of being necessary in a democratic society, and the resulting intrusion should remain proportionate to the evidence-proven benefit obtained (ICCPR General Comment No. 37, para. 40). Mandatory measures must lapse after their prescribed time of temporary validity, unless renewed based on a new assessment of their necessity.
9. One instance where mandatory measures appear justified as human rights compliant even without a preceding effort to rely on mere recommendations is in the prevention of super-spreading events in the form of public gatherings. Mass events (such as concerts or mass sports events) may need either to be made safe or prohibited for a defined period. The same applies also to smaller gatherings when they represent contagion-risky activities (e.g., team sports practices, nightclubs, and discotheques). The policies and the resulting legal instruments must be evidence-based rather than compromises resulting from lobbying by business actors. The State of New York, which has been severely affected by COVID-19, issued a series of regulations that seek to address the role of restaurants and bars in contagion (New York State Executive Order 2020).
10. Where restrictions are imposed upon those public gatherings that represent the exercise of human rights, authorities must provide and facilitate safe options for the meaningful exercise of freedom of assembly, including demonstrations (ICCPR Article 21), freedom of association (ICCPR Article 22), and freedom of religion (ICCPR Article 18 and General Comment No. 22), as well as the right to family life, which includes the right to arrange important events such as weddings or funerals (ICCPR Articles 17 and 23 and General Comments Nos. 16 and 19). Such arrangements and requirements must be evidence-based and may include, for instance, a combination of online and offline activities, an obligation to wear face masks, or the compartmentalization of a single event into smaller safe ones. The Human Rights Committee's recent General Comment No. 37 on freedom of assembly and the discussions around it (Scheinin 2020c) provide best practice guidance.
11. While human rights law allows for temporary lockdowns and curfews, such measures should always have a proper legal basis and should be evidence-based, geographically targeted, and temporary (ICCPR Article 12 and General Comment No. 27). This requires a strong preference for micro-lockdowns rather than nationwide measures and transparent indicators on what constitutes compelling evidence that such a lockdown is necessary. Evidence could for

example be a predefined absolute number of new cases, the local or regional value for the effective reproductive number (R) of the virus, and its change from the previous monitoring period.

12. The aim of strategies adopted by governments should be to protect the life and human rights of all members of the population. This entails remaining vigilant with respect to COVID-19 and determined to stop any new occurrence of exponential growth at the relatively flat bottom of the curve. Regular monitoring and publication of R at the national and regional level should be a key indicator in applying this strategy. Following its first crisis phase, Italy provides a promising example of transparent weekly national and regional monitoring reports (Ministero della Salute 2020), which however did not prevent a new crisis phase in late October 2020 when rising regional R values were insufficiently acted upon.
13. Special attention must be given to protecting members of vulnerable segments of society, including but not limited to the elderly, with full respect of their dignity and human rights. Instead of isolation, they must be offered attention, support, activities, and regular meetings with their close ones, while at the same time minimizing the risk of contagion. Germany's overall relative success in preventing COVID-19 deaths is in large part attributed to managing longer than others to limit transmission in long-term care facilities (Wieler, Rexroth, & Gottschalk 2020).
14. Human rights are not only legal obligations of States but also have an interpersonal ethical dimension. There is a need to promote a culture of people protecting both themselves and strangers, through routine hygienic measures such as frequent washing of hands with soap and avoiding all contact with others when sick. The wearing of a face mask to protect others should be promoted as routine in defined situations, such as when using public transport, in intergenerational contact, in shops, and when providing or receiving services. While obligatory mandates will often be justified under human rights law, cultural adaptation may best be served through evidence-based recommendations. The modest level of inconvenience of face masks during an epidemic, including during the potentially long phase when the virus remains dormant in society or keeps reappearing as outbreaks, is the 'new normal'. Facemasks have a role both in stopping the exponential growth of the epidemic and in suppressing contagion where R has already been pressed down but new cases nevertheless keep emerging. Probably these elements of COVID-19 strategies will continue also beyond this pandemic as a cultural adaptation in the West, following the example of many Asian countries where the same happened before the emergence of COVID-19. Vietnam is referred to as a success story in the containment of COVID-19, and its continuing imposition of an obligation to wear facemasks is a part of that story (Pollack et al. 2020).
15. Carriers of COVID-19 need to be found through constant vigilance and testing. They and their families must be afforded support, whether arriving from abroad or infected within the country. Quick and reliable tests must be

available on request, including a follow-up test after an optimal number of days if the first one turned out negative. Testing only symptomatic cases will discover only the tip of the iceberg and needs to be complemented by access to testing by asymptomatic persons, screening amongst potentially exposed categories of persons, and, if need be, pooling of tests where systems become overburdened. In Europe for instance, Denmark, Germany, Iceland, and Norway tested extensively early on in proportion to the number of cases found (Ritchie et al. 2020). Highly restrictive measures, such as enforced quarantine or detention (ICCPR Article 9 and General Comment No. 35) should be applied individually and with caution even where the law provides for that option, in order not to engage in arbitrary detention or demotivate people from seeking to be tested.

16. Where smartphone apps alerting for potential risk of contagion are introduced, their success relies on their accordance with the right to privacy (ICCPR Article 17 and General Comment No. 16; Abeler et al. 2020). They require a high number of downloads and use in order to be successful, and therefore cannot work without the cooperation of the broad population. Special care must be taken not to miss parts of the population that do not have access to a smartphone. In practice, this means that public trust is central to their success. COVID-19 must not act as an excuse for a new wave of mass surveillance, nor can it appear as doing this. To this end, exposure alerting apps must be truly voluntary, and they must not collect identifiable personal data. As an example, using the proxy of the number of downloads as a success-rate, Iceland has 40 percent population coverage with its voluntary app whereas India has less than 10 percent with their mandatory app (Gardner 2020). Whenever an app user is diagnosed with the virus, he or she should be free to decide whether a generic alert is sent to other app users who were in the proximity of the person during the possibly contagious phase. They should then have a right to get tested and be guaranteed quick and easy access. As such, apps should not be used in traditional contact-tracing of contagious illnesses; in fact, they should not be called contact-tracing apps. Their only function should be alerting app users who were in the vicinity of a person who has tested positive. By October 2020 very few countries had succeeded in establishing high enough download rates for the apps to live up to their potential. This includes countries where the privacy parameters have been designed to be in accordance with human rights standards such as Germany (Wieler, Rexroth, & Gottschalk 2020), Ireland (Irish Government 2020), and Finland (Finnish Institute for Health and Welfare 2020).
17. While wide testing both for COVID-19 and for antibodies showing a past infection will be necessary in the fine-tuning of a human-rights-based strategy, such testing should be based on representative randomized samples of the population and used for epidemiological monitoring and forecasting. So-called 'immunity passports' to segregate between two categories of people whose rights and obligations may be differentiated should be rejected (ICCPR Article 26 and General Comment No. 18; ICESCR Article 7 and General Comment

No. 23; Privacy International 2020). Seropositive status should therefore be excluded as a criterion for employment recruitment. That said, it would be permissible to offer active employees a test in order to assess what protective equipment a person will need to wear. Seropositive status is a matter of sensitive personal data which can be discussed in confidence with the employer's doctor but must not be available to the employer or line manager.

18. Labor law and social security law should be amended to guarantee people's income, so that it can be made a legal requirement and promoted as a cultural adaptation that nobody will go to school or to work or use public transport with the slightest symptoms of a respiratory infection. Wearing a mask should be only a secondary solution. In all instances of quarantine or of staying at home because of any respiratory infection symptoms, the law must secure a salary or adequate social security benefit and prohibit dismissal because of such absence (ICCPR Article 26 and General Comment No. 18; ICESCR Articles 6, 7, and 9 and General Comments Nos. 18, 19, and 23). During the first half of 2020, many countries provided some form of income support to citizens under lockdowns and quarantines (Ritchie et al. 2020), but many job retention schemes only benefit those in regularized employment, excluding the precariously employed and the underemployed, not to mention irregular workers. Direct money transfers as used, for instance, in Japan, the United States, and Serbia are a heavy drain on the economy without necessarily reaching the people most in need (OECD 2020). Similarly, measures against the virus may isolate irregular workers from their employers. Italy experienced this when the agricultural sector found itself without access to its workforce, necessitating an unprecedented regularization of irregular workers (Testore 2020).
19. In order to reconcile freedom of movement with the protection of the right to life and the right to health, means of transport must be made safe. An analogy can be sought from the nuisance, design changes, technology, and money put into making air travel safe against the threat of terrorism. In all means of public transport (buses, trains, boats, airplanes etc.), physical distancing must be systematically secured between passengers, attention must be paid to contagion risk because of air-conditioning or airflows, and any queueing and other congestion before departure and upon arrival must be eliminated. Travel time may become longer, and airline prices may rise, which are parts of the process of cultural adaptation. If cruise ships cannot be made safe, the world may need to be without them. In early August 2020 multiple clusters of contagion emerged in relation to cruise ships in Norway, including the famous cruise line Hurtigruten (Sjøfartsdirektoratet 2020). In response, a regulation was issued to cap the number of passengers at one hundred (Helsedepartementet COVID-19 forskriften 2020).
20. Travel bans based on country of nationality or departure, or the closing of borders, are usually not human-rights-compliant measures. It is a danger also to public health to promote the populist myth that the foreigner is the carrier of the virus. COVID-19 will remain dormant in many societies, and therefore

any clusters of contagion need to be found early. Instead of travel bans and restrictions, countries should facilitate general but primarily voluntary testing before or during travel or upon arrival, and provide easy access to a second test after an optimal number of days. Any mandatory tests must be administered by health professionals in compliance with medical ethics, which requires individual assessment of the person having either contracted the virus or been exposed to contagion. Non-discriminatory individual quarantine orders based on objective medical criteria, including the likelihood of the person having been exposed to contagion, are compatible with human rights. Advance information about these measures will reduce travel without impeding it. Actual measures by governments have been very different and uncoordinated (Ritchie et al. 2020). Human rights considerations have usually played a small role in designing the measures.

2 Conclusion: the choice between populism and human rights

The unprecedented and still accumulating experience of the COVID-19 pandemic demonstrates the urgent need for human rights-based strategies for epidemics. There cannot be a single human rights strategy for all countries and all epidemics because of differences between viruses, rates, and means of contagion, probability of population immunity, the proportion of infections resulting in death or permanent disability, the impact on national health services, and availability of vaccination and medication. COVID-19 is a 'perfect storm' of a virus with a combination of natural characteristics that resulted in a global pandemic and a death toll that, within its first nine months, had exceeded a million persons and is likely to reach two million only four months later.

It is, however, also readily evident that in several cases the policies enacted by incumbent politicians and rhetoric furthered by certain opposition politicians are in direct contradiction to international human rights law and best practice. In terms of rhetoric, US President Donald Trump was quick to insist on calling COVID-19 the 'Chinese virus', sparking a surge in Sinophobia, discrimination, and hate crimes against people of Asian descent (Haynes 2020). Similarly, the leader of the right-wing populist Lega in Italy, Matteo Salvini, quickly and falsely linked the spreading of COVID-19 with the disembarkation of refugees in Italian harbors (Dire.it 2020). Although the government led by Giuseppe Conte did not take part in the same inflammatory rhetoric, it did bow under pressure by closing Italian harbors to disembarkation of refugees rescued at sea, declaring that Italy was no longer a place of safety in accordance with the UN Convention on the Law of the Sea (Italian Ministries of Foreign Affairs, Interior and Health 2020).

In terms of anti-expert sentiments, President Trump was particularly vocal, ignoring or suppressing expert advice, denouncing recommendations from the World Health Organization, and preposterously suggesting injections of bleach as a cure for COVID-19 (BBC 2020). He was also particularly ready to question potential results of elections taking place during the pandemic, but he was not alone in using this crisis to meddle with the democratic process (Panetta 2020). The Polish presidential election was contentious for taking place with short deadlines and strict rules for participation whilst much of Europe was under lockdown, which disenfranchised much of Poland's PIS-critical diaspora. In other places elections have been postponed. In Hungary the Enabling Act has given the prime minister the power to decide when, if ever, it will be safe to conduct new elections (Kovács 2020). The International Foundation for Electoral Systems found that 116 elections worldwide were postponed due to COVID-19 (IFES 2020). While certainly not all of these are delayed for sinister purposes, a pandemic increases those risks, especially in less established democracies.

Experiences in different parts of the world with human rights-based responses to COVID-19 will be a major contribution with lasting impacts on global preparedness for new epidemics and pandemics. The pathogens will be different, and the set of measures that meet the requirements of being both effective and human rights-conforming will be different. But the role of the normative framework of international human rights law should be the same, and therefore some or many of the elements of adequate human rights strategies adopted during, or in the aftermath of COVID-19 will be essential in combating future pandemics.

Similarly, the pandemic has also shown how incompetently populists and authoritarians are likely to react to real crises, whether opportunistically extending emergency powers like Hungary's Victor Orbán or by first downplaying the crisis like Jair Bolsonaro of Brazil or Donald Trump in the United States and then, as the situation gets worse, redirecting public funding earmarked for anti-pandemic measures into private corporations (Gregg et al. 2020). The benefit of contrasting populist-authoritarian political choices with the human rights-based approach, is that such an analysis makes it obvious that populist-authoritarian regimes are not in compliance with international law and best practices. The human rights-based approach, in which all human rights are considered, and are continuously present on both sides of the equation can both act as a guide and leave States ample room to address and combat a deadly pandemic with better results.

References

Abeler, J, Bäker, M, Buermeyer, U & Zillessen, H 2020, 'COVID-19 Contact Tracing and Data Protection Can Go Together', *JMIR mHealth and uHealth*, no. 8, vol. 4.

Bates, E 2020, 'COVID-19 Symposium: Article 2 ECHR's Positive Obligations–How Can Human Rights Law Inform the Protection of Health Care Personnel and Vulnerable Patients in the COVID-19 Pandemic?', *OpinioJuris*, 1 April, viewed 30 December 2020, http://opiniojuris.org/2020/04/01/covid-19-symposium-article-2-echrs-positive-obligations-how-can-human-rights-law-inform-the-protection-of-health-care-personnel-and-vulnerable-patients-in-the-covid-19-pandemic/

BBC News 2020, 'Coronavirus: Outcry after Trump Suggests Injecting Disinfectant as Treatment', 24 April, viewed 30 December 2020, www.bbc.com/news/world-us-canada-52407177

Buzan, B, Wæver, O, & De Wilde, J 1998, *Security: A New Framework for Analysis*, Lynne Rienner Publishers, London.

Convention on the Elimination of All Forms of Discrimination against Women (CEDAW) 1979.

Convention on the Rights of Persons with Disabilities (CPRD) 2006, UN Doc. A/RES/61/106.

Convention on the Rights of the Child (CRD) 1989.

Council of Europe 2020a, 'COVID-19: Toolkit for Member States', viewed 30 December 2020, www.coe.int/en/web/congress/covid-19-toolkits

Council of Europe 2020b, 'Governments Must Ensure Equal Protection and Care for Roma and Travellers during the COVID-19 crisis', 7 April, viewed 30 December 2020, www.coe.int/en/web/commissioner/-/governments-must-ensure-equal-protection-and-care-for-roma-and-travellers-during-the-covid-19-crisis

Cunha, L & Machado, M 2019, 'Under Pressure but Crucial: The Brazilian Supreme Court under Bolsonaro', *Blog of the International Journal of Constitutional Law*, viewed 30 December 2020, www.iconnectblog.com/2019/06/symposium-the-brazilian-supreme-court-and-the-protection-of-democracy-in-the-age-of-populism-under-pressure-but-crucial-the-brazilian-supreme-court-under-bolsonaro/

DIRE.IT, 'Coronavirus, Salvini: 'Migranti l'unico problema, il governo ha morti sulla coscienza', 13 August, viewed 30 December 2020, www.dire.it/13-08-2020/493844-coronavirus-salvini-migranti-lunico-problema-il-governo-ha-morti-sulla-coscienza/

Eiermann, M, Mounk, Y & Gultchin, L 2017, 'European Populism: Trends, Threats and Future Prospects', *Tony Blair Institute for Global Change*, 29 December, viewed 30 December 2020, https://institute.global/insight/renewing-centre/european-populism-trends-threats-and-future-prospects

Finnish Institute for Health and Welfare 2020, 'Koronavilkku the Finnish COVID Tracking app', viewed 30 December 2020, https://koronavilkku.fi/en/

Fournier, T & Meyer-Resende, M 2020, 'Phase Two of Covid-19 Responses Across the EU – The Rule of Law Stress Test Continued', *Democracy Reporting International*, 27 July, viewed 30 December 2020, https://democracy-reporting.org/dri_publications/phase-two-of-covid-19-responses-across-the-eu-the-rule-of-law-stress-test-continued/

Gardner, A 2020, 'Contact-tracing Apps: There's No Evidence They're Helping Stop COVID-19', *The Conversation*, 21 October, viewed 30 December 2020, https://theconversation.com/contact-tracing-apps-theres-no-evidence-theyre-helping-stop-covid-19-148397

Gregg, A & Torbati Y 2020, 'Pentagon Used Taxpayer Money Meant for Masks and Swabs to Make Jet Engine Parts and Body Armor', *The Washington Post*, 22 September, viewed 30 December 2020, www.washingtonpost.com/business/2020/09/22/covid-funds-pentagon

Grogan, J 2020, 'Introduction and List of Country Reports', *Verfassungsblog: On Matters Constitutional*, 6 April, viewed 30 December 2020, https://verfassungsblog.de/introduction-list-of-country-reports/

Hawkins, K, Aguilar, R, Silva, B, Jenne, E, Bojana, K & Cristobal, K, 2019, 'Global Populism Database, v1', *Harvard Dataverse*, viewed 30 December 2020.

Haynes, S 2020, 'As Coronavirus Spreads, So Does Xenophobia and Anti-Asian Racism', *TIME*, 6 March, viewed 30 December 2020, https://time.com/5797836/coronavirus-racism-stereotypes-attacks/

Helse-Og Omsorgsdepartmentet, 'Endr. i covid-19-forskriften', 8 March 2020, viewed 30 December 2020, https://lovdata.no/dokument/LTI/forskrift/2020-08-03-1609

Hodgson, T & Siederman, I 2020, 'COVID-19 Symposium: COVID-19 Responses and State Obligations Concerning the Right to Health', *OpinioJuris*, 1 April, 30 December 2020, http://opiniojuris.org/2020/04/01/covid-19-symposium-covid-19-responses-and-state-obligations-concerning-the-right-to-health-part-1/

Human Rights Watch 2020, 'COVID-19: A Human Rights Checklist', viewed 30 December 2020, www.hrw.org/sites/default/files/supporting_resources/202004_northamerica_us_covid19_checklist2.pdf

Inter Agency Standing Committee of OHCHR and WHO (IASC) 2020, 'Interim Guidance COVID-19: Focus on Persons Deprived ofTheir Liberty', 27 March, viewed 30 December 2020, https://interagencystandingcommittee.org/other/iasc-interim-guidance-covid-19-focus-persons-deprived-their-liberty-developed-ohchr-and-who

International Convention on the Elimination of All Forms of Racial Discrimination 1966.

International Covenant on Civil and Political Rights 1966.

International Covenant on Civil and Political Rights General Comment No. 37 on Article *21* 2020.

International Covenant on Economic, Social and Cultural Rights 1966.

International Foundation for Electoral Systems (IFES) 2020, *Elections Postponed Due to COVID-19 – As of December 15, 2020*, viewed 31 December 2020, www.ifes.org/sites/default/files/elections_postponed_due_to_covid-19.pdf

Irish Government 2020, 'COVID Tracker App', viewed 30 December 2020, https://covidtracker.gov.ie/privacy-and-data/

Istrefi, K 2020, 'To Notify or Not to Notify: Derogations from Human Rights Treaties', *OpinioJuris*, 18 April, viewed 30 December 2020, http://opiniojuris.org/2020/04/18/to-notify-or-not-to-notify-derogations-from-human-rights-treaties/

Italian Ministeries of Foreign Affairs, Interior and Health, *Decree on Italy as a Place of Safety*, 7 April, viewed 30 December 2020, www.integrazionemigranti.gov.it/Attualita/Notizie/Documents/M_INFR.GABINETTO.REG_DECRETI(R).0000150.07-04-2020%20(3).pdf

Kirkpatrick, D & Cabrera, J 2020, 'How Trump and Bolsonaro Broke Latin America's COVID-19 Defenses', *New York Times*, 27 October, viewed 30 December 2020, www.nytimes.com/2020/10/27/world/trump-bolsonaro-coronavirus-latin-america.html

Kovács, K 2020, 'Hungary's Orbánistan: A Complete Arsenal of Emergency Powers', *Verfassungsblog: On Matters Constitutional*, 6 April, 30 December 2020, https://verfassungsblog.de/hungarys-orbanistan-a-complete-arsenal-of-emergency-powers/

Lewis, P, Clarke, S, Barr, C, Holder, J & Kommenda, N 2018, 'Revealed: One in Four Europeans Vote Populist', *The Guardian*, 20 November, viewed 30 December 2020, www.theguardian.com/world/ng-interactive/2018/nov/20/revealed-one-in-four-europeans-vote-populist

Michaud, J & Kates, J 2020, 'What Do We Know About Children and Coronavirus Transmission', *USA: Kaiser Family Foundation*, 29 July, viewed 30 December 2020, www.kff.org/coronavirus-covid-19/issue-brief/what-do-we-know-about-children-and-coronavirus-transmission/

Ministero della Salute, 'Report monitoraggio settimanale Covid-19: bassa criticità, ma in alcune aree casi in aumento', 26 June, viewed 30 December 2020, www.salute.gov.it/portale/nuovocoronavirus/dettaglioNotizieNuovoCoronavirus.jsp?lingua=italiano&id=4941

Mudde, C & Kaltwasser, CR 2017, *Populism: A Very Short Introduction*, Oxford University Press, Oxford.

Müller, J-W 2015, 'Parsing Populism: Who Is and Who Is Not a Populist These Days?', *Juncture*, vol. 22, pp. 80–89.

New York State Executive Order No. 202.45, *Continuing Temporary Suspension and Modification of Law Relating to the Disaster Emergency*, 15 June, viewed 30 December 2020, www.governor.ny.gov/news/no-20245-continuing-temporary-suspension-and-modification-laws-relating-disaster-emergency

Ní Aoláin, F, 2020, 'COVID-19 Civic Freedom Tracker: Keep Civic Space Healthy', *International Center For Not-For-Profit Law*, viewed 30 December 2020, www.icnl.org/covid19tracker/?location=61&issue=&date=&type=

Oberverwaltungsgericht Nordrhein-Westfalen, 13 B 940/20.NE 2020, viewed 30 December 2020, www.justiz.nrw.de/nrwe/ovgs/ovg_nrw/j2020/13_B_940_20_NE_Beschluss_20200706.html

OECD 2020, 'Supporting Livelihoods During the COVID-19 Crisis: Closing the Gaps in Safety Nets', 20 May, viewed 30 December 2020, www.oecd.org/coronavirus/policy-responses/supporting-livelihoods-during-the-covid-19-crisis-closing-the-gaps-in-safety-nets-17cbb92d/

OHCHR 2020a, 'Covid-19 and Minority Rights: Overview and Promising Practices', viewed 20 December 2020, www.ohchr.org/Documents/Issues/Minorities/OHCHRGuidance_COVID19_MinoritiesRights.pdf

OHCHR 2020b, 'Disease Pandemics and the Freedom of Opinion and Expression', UN Doc. A/HRC/44/49, viewed 30 December 2020, www.undocs.org/A/HRC/44/49

OHCHR 2020c, 'Racial Discrimination in the Context ofThe Covid-19 Crisis', viewed 30 December 2020, www.ohchr.org/Documents/Issues/Racism/COVID-19_and_Racial_Discrimination.pdf

OHCHR 2020d, 'Special Rapporteur Dainius Pūras: COVID-19 Measures Must Be Grounded First and Foremost on the Right to Health', viewed 30 December 2020, www.ohchr.org/EN/NewsEvents/Pages/DisplayNews.aspx?NewsID=25945&LangID=E

OHCHR 2020e, 'Virtual Debate "Human Rights of Older Persons in the Age of COVID-19 and Beyond" with the High Commissioner for Human Rights and the new Independent Expert on the Enjoyment of all Human Rights by Older Persons', 12 May, viewed 30 December 2020, www.ohchr.org/EN/NewsEvents/Pages/DisplayNews.aspx?NewsID=25879&LangID=E

Oxford University 2020, 'Coronavirus Government Response Tracker (OxCGRT)', viewed 30 December 2020, www.bsg.ox.ac.uk/research/research-projects/coronavirus-government-response-tracker

Panetta, G 2020, 'Trump Hints that He Could Refuse to Accept the Results of the 2020 Election if He Loses', *Business Insider*, 19 July, viewed 30 December 2020, www.businessinsider.com/trump-suggests-that-he-wont-accept-the-2020-election-results-if-he-loses-2020-7

Pollack, T, Thwaites, G & Rabaa, M 2020, 'Emerging COVID-19 Success Story: Vietnam's Commitment to Containment', *Our World in Data*, Exemplars in Global Health, 30 June, viewed 31 December 2020, https://ourworldindata.org/covid-exemplar-vietnam

Privacy International 2020, 'The Looming Disaster of Immunity Passports and Digital Identity', viewed 30 December 2020, https://privacyinternational.org/long-read/4074/looming-disaster-immunity-passports-and-digital-identity

Ritchie, H, Ortiz-Ospina, E, Beltekin, D, Mathieu, E, Hasell, J, Macdonald, B, Giattino, C & Roser, M 2020, 'Policy Responses to the Coronavirus Pandemic', *Our World in Data*, viewed 30 December 2020, https://ourworldindata.org/policy-responses-covid

Rooduijn, M et al. 2019, 'The PopuList: An Overview of Populist, Far Right, Far Left and Eurosceptic Parties in Europe', viewed 30 December 2020, https://standinggroups.ecpr.eu/extremismanddemocracy/the-populist/

Sandbu, M 2020, 'Populists and Kleptocrats are a Perfect Match', *Financial Times*, 22 September, viewed 30 December 2020, www.ft.com/content/ef4111a6-8ac8-419e-8747-8ce1b887cb61

Scheinin, M 2020a, 'The COVID-19 Emergency in Finland: Best Practice and Problems', *Verfassungsblog: On Matters Constitutional*, 16 April, viewed 30 December 2020, https://verfassungsblog.de/the-covid-19-emergency-in-finland-best-practice-and-problems/

Scheinin, M 2020b, 'COVID-19 Symposium: To Derogate or Not to Derogate?', *OpinioJuris*, 6 April, viewed 30 December 2020, http://opiniojuris.org/2020/04/06/covid-19-symposium-to-derogate-or-not-to-derogate/

Scheinin, M 2020c, 'U.N. Human Rights Committee General Comment No. 37 on Freedom of Assembly: An Excellent and Timely Contribution', *Just Security*, 30 July, viewed 30

December 2020, www.justsecurity.org/71754/u-n-human-rights-committee-general-comment-no-37-on-freedom-of-assembly-an-excellent-and-timely-contribution/

Scheppele, K 2020, 'Underreaction in a Time of Emergency: America as a Nearly Failed State', *Verfassungsblog: On Matters Constitutional*, 9 April, 30 December 2020, https://verfassungsblog.de/underreaction-in-a-time-of-emergency-america-as-a-nearly-failed-state/

Sjøfartsdirektoratet (Norwegian Maritime Authority) 2020, 'Rapport fra revisjon av sikkerhetsstyringssystemet', 24 August, viewed 30 December 2020, www.mynewsdesk.com/material/document/99525/download?resource_type=resource_document

Testore, G 2020, 'Italian Government Adopts Targeted Regularisation for Migrant Workers', *European Commission*, 18 May, viewed 30 December 2020, https://ec.europa.eu/migrant-integration/news/italian-government-adopts-targeted-regularisation-for-migrant-workers

Wieler, L, Rexroth, U & Gottschalk, R 2020, 'Emerging Covid-19 Success Story: Germany's Strong Enabling Environment', *Our World in Data*, viewed 30 December 2020, https://ourworldindata.org/covid-exemplar-germany

3

HUMAN RIGHTS IN TIMES OF PANDEMICS

Necessity and proportionality

Katharina Ó Cathaoir

Faced with a global pandemic, parliaments that previously agreed on little, unanimously and rapidly breathed new life into antiquated health laws in the first half of 2020.[1] This unflinching recognition of states' obligations to protect public health from an immediate threat is in stark contrast to the usual meandering pace and adversarial nature of public health regulation. However, adopting legislation is a means but not the end; legislation must conform with human rights obligations.

Human rights-based governance is crucial in a pandemic as, beyond the immediate impacts, pandemics can also trigger 'epidemics of fear' with those infected viewed as outsiders or 'invaders' (Annas 2016, pp. 342–343). Meanwhile, those worst affected by infectious diseases are often groups for whom stigma can have catastrophic effects: the historically vulnerable and the poor, who lack the means and resources to isolate themselves from disease. COVID-19 reproduces this pattern, with emerging evidence suggesting that racial and ethnic minorities and persons with disabilities are disproportionately impacted by both the virus and restrictions (Tai et al. 2020; Kirby 2020).

The aim of this chapter is to contribute a health and human rights analysis to the growing body of literature on COVID-19. This contribution therefore argues for a human rights approach that is driven by solidarity, trust, and transparency, not coercion and fear. Human rights underscore the responsibilities of states, in contrast to individualizing and responsibilizing disease, which we have observed during COVID-19 and other pandemics.

This chapter[2] first outlines states' obligations under international human rights law and the International Health Regulations (IHR) to protect the population from infectious diseases, drawing on general comments and relevant case law. Second, it introduces the human rights-based approach to infectious disease developed in response to HIV/AIDS, which proscribes stigma and discrimination as public health tools. Third, this chapter analyzes stay-at-home orders adopted in European states from the perspective of health and human rights, making three core arguments: (1) states have adopted limitations on rights that run contrary to scientific evidence, which is not in line with the IHR; (2) states have not adequately considered whether the public health aim could be achieved by less restrictive measures, again in contrast with the IHR and human rights, and (3) finally, COVID-19 has led to a worrying recourse to criminal law to secure compliance, instead of building trust.

This chapter focuses on European restrictions on movement, in particular lockdowns and stay-at-home orders. While it does not claim to be a comprehensive review, it reflects on core human rights principles, which are applicable in all jurisdictions, including non-discrimination, necessity, proportionality, and positive obligations under the rights to life and health.

1 States' obligations to protect life and health

Preventing and responding to pandemics is a state obligation under international human rights law and international health law. The Human Rights Committee (HRC) and the European Court of Human Rights (ECtHR) recognize states' *positive obligations* to safeguard the right to life under their respective instruments, the International Covenant on Civil and Political Rights (ICCPR) and the ECHR. In its General Comment on the Right to Life, the Human Rights Committee noted states' obligation to 'adopt any appropriate laws or other measures in order to protect life from all reasonably foreseeable threats' (GC No. 36, para. 18). ECtHR jurisprudence also holds that states must 'take appropriate steps to safeguard the life of those within its jurisdiction' (*Lambert and Others v. France*, para. 117).

The Human Rights Committee has emphasized that states must address the underlying conditions in society that cause threats to life, including infectious disease, by ensuring essential goods and services and adequate general conditions (GC No. 36, para. 26). States should also take special measures to protect 'persons in situation of vulnerability whose lives have been placed at particular risk because of specific threats', such as, persons with disabilities and persons deprived of their liberty (GC No. 36, para. 26–30). The ECtHR has taken a more limited approach but increasingly recognizes the state's obligations to ensure a functioning healthcare system, such as adopting regulations to compel hospitals to take appropriate measures to protect patients' lives (*Lambert and Others v. France*, para. 105), and a public health system that provides for adequate emergency medical care (*Asiye Genç v. Turkey*). A deficient regulatory system is however, not sufficient to find a violation of Article 2; rather, 'it must be shown to have operated to the patient's detriment' (*Lambert and Others v. France*, para. 107). States are further under an obligation to determine the cause of death of patients and ensure an adequate investigation (*Šilih v. Slovenia,* para. 192). In some cases, where the fault goes beyond 'mere error or medical negligence', this must include criminal investigation (*Asiye Genç v. Turkey*, para. 73).

In light of these obligations, states' failure to take positive measures to protect the population from COVID-19, or ensure that hospitals can meet the burden, could amount to a violation of their positive obligations under the right to life. Furthermore, failing to take account of the 'special needs' of a disadvantaged class, like elders, women, or persons with disabilities, could amount to discrimination under Article 14 ECHR (*DH and others v. The Czech Republic*, para. 207). Yet, the ECtHR holds that:

> the choice of means for ensuring the positive obligations under Article 2 is in principle a matter that falls within the Contracting State's margin of appreciation. There are different avenues for ensuring Convention rights, and even if the State has failed to apply one particular measure provided by domestic law, it may still fulfil its positive duty by other means ... However, for this obligation to be satisfied, such proceedings must not only exist in theory but also operate effectively in practice.
>
> *(Lopes De Sousa Fernandes v. Portugal, para. 216)*

Therefore, it appears that states have discretion in deciding which measures are most suitable to discharge their obligations under the right to life, although this discretion is not unfettered.

The International Covenant on Economic, Social and Cultural Rights (ICESCR) places obligations on state parties to take steps to achieve the full realization of the right to the highest attainable standard of health, including through 'the prevention, treatment and control of epidemic, endemic, occupational and other diseases' and 'the creation of conditions which would assure to all medical service and medical attention in the event of sickness' (Article 12). Likewise, under Article 11.3 of the European Social Charter, states are under an obligation to 'prevent as far as possible epidemic, endemic and other diseases'. While the right to life and health are inherently interconnected, the right to health imposes a more detailed list of positive obligations.

The Committee on Economic, Social and Cultural Rights' (CESCR) General Comment on the Right to Health introduces a non-binding but authoritative interpretation of states' obligations. Several aspects can inform our understanding of states' obligations to protect the population's health during the COVID-19 pandemic. Firstly, the AAAQ framework calls on states to ensure availability, accessibility, acceptability and quality (AAAQ) in health and healthcare (GC No. 14, para. 12). This includes ensuring sufficient health personnel, access to health facilities without discrimination, and affordable healthcare that is respectful and of good quality (GC No. 14, para. 12). The General Comment furthermore emphasizes protection of vulnerable groups, non-discrimination, and provision of adequate information. The right to health encompasses a 'margin of discretion' in choosing which measures are suitable (para. 53). However, participation is central to the right to health and requires states to engage with the affected populations in determining priorities. While the European Social Committee's interpretation of states' obligations has been limited in the field of infectious disease, it has found France in violation of the European Social Charter for failing to adopt special measures to address tuberculosis and other infectious diseases among Roma migrants (*Médecins du Monde International v. France*, para. 163).

Alongside states' obligations under human rights law, all states are bound by the World Health Organization's International Health Regulations (IHR). The purpose of the IHR is to 'prevent, protect against, control and provide a public health response' to infectious diseases of international concern with 'full respect for the dignity, human rights and fundamental freedoms of persons'. States' obligations include developing minimum core public health capacities, such as surveillance capacities, and an implementation plan. However, many states have consistently failed to meet their obligations in the field of pandemic preparedness, the consequences of which are now being felt (Oppenheim et al. 2019).

In summary, human rights and international health law underscore that states must create conditions to prevent disease and build an adequate public health infrastructure. The right to life and the right to health impose obligations on states parties to take steps to control COVID-19 and protect all members of society, with special focus on the most vulnerable. The state holds special responsibilities to those deprived of their liberty (i.e., prisoners, children in care, persons in residential care, and persons with disabilities). Under the right to health, state obligations include providing access to affordable, safe healthcare without discrimination and informing the population on effective means of prevention. Under the right to life, the question of whether a State has failed to meet its obligations will rest on the facts of the individual case. Generally, states must ensure emergency healthcare and investigate unexpected deaths. While states have latitude in choosing which measures to adopt to meet their obligations under the right to health and life, this is restricted by other rights (e.g., liberty and freedom of movement) (see section 3).

Finally, the pandemic has raised important questions about rationing in healthcare. Concerns have been raised that persons were denied treatment for COVID-19 on an equal footing with others on the basis of protected characteristics, such as disability or age (Chen & McNamara 2020). At the early stages, public concern focused on the possible need to ration ventilators. Who should live and who should die in the case of medical rationing? Human rights law makes an important contribution to addressing this complex legal and moral problem by prohibiting determinations based on a protected characteristic, such as race, gender, age, and disability. For example, assuming that elders or persons with disabilities are not strong enough to be offered the same treatment opportunities as those similarly situated runs contrary to a human rights-based approach.

Furthermore, states can breach their obligations toward the public's health by myopically addressing COVID-19. For example, in response to the pandemic, states suspended preventative and curative healthcare. While this may have been necessary in some instances, it may also result in devastating health consequences: in Ireland, an extra 50,000 people were added to the national outpatient waiting list (Cullen 2020); in Denmark, hospitals operated on 75,000 fewer patients than the previous year (Hansen et al. 2020). These figures highlight the pre-existing healthcare challenges, the need for adequate investment in healthcare and to ensure that restrictions on the right to health are proportionate.

Having established the state's obligation to protect life and health, the next section highlights the contribution of a human rights approach to public health crises.

2 Coercion, stigma, and human rights

Public health laws can stigmatize the poor and vulnerable, while criminalization can obstruct the public health response. A human rights approach offers a shift from law as a means of coercion, stigma, and discrimination to empowerment and participation. Yet, while a human rights approach emerged in response to the HIV/AIDS pandemic, subsequent disease outbreaks have shown that human rights are often sidelined in emergencies.

Over the last twenty years, public health communities have moved toward a strategy of de-stigmatization of HIV, while UN agencies, human rights organizations, and experts have campaigned for a human rights response to HIV/AIDS. Governments' initial responses were rife with discrimination and stigma, for example, criminalizing sex between men and instituting penalties for transmission of HIV. It became clear that discrimination and stigma are not effective tools of public health. There is no credible evidence that HIV criminalization protects individuals or society; instead it drives fear and isolation, which can lead individuals to avoid testing and treatment (Burris & Cameron 2008). By stigmatizing those affected by a disease we lose sight of the surrounding structures which regulate and exacerbate transmission: poverty, inadequate housing, and unsafe food and water. At an individual level, stigma can disincentivize testing for fear of negative consequences including social stigma and the risk of losing financial, housing, or work opportunities. Furthermore, those worst affected by infectious disease are often the poor or persons belonging to historically discriminated groups, who do not have the same resources as the wealthy to insulate themselves from disease. As Murphy highlights, 'quarantine, surveillance and the like have historically been targeted at the most disadvantaged – the poor and at immigrants, for example' (Murphy 2013, p. 80).

Through removing discriminatory laws and policies that are not evidence based, disease status can be destigmatized and trust developed with the affected community to ensure an effective public health response. Furthermore, focusing on the structural causes of disease, like poverty and poor living conditions, is in line with states' human rights obligations under the right to life and health.

However, a human rights approach has not been consistently applied to disease outbreaks. During the 2003 SARS outbreak, several affected countries implemented quarantine and isolation measures to limited public health benefit (Jacobs 2007). The leading expert in international law and infectious disease noted that such measures were not per se incompatible with human rights, but must be justified (Fidler 2003). During the West African Ebola outbreak, governments ordered the military to cordon off areas of infection – prohibiting entry and exit. At the time,

Donald G. McNeil Jr., writing for the *New York Times*, warned that such approaches can be 'brutal and inhumane' if positive measures are not taken and trust built with the affected community (McNeil 2014). Similarly, stigmatization and discrimination of persons with tuberculosis (the top infectious disease killer worldwide), as well as inappropriate quarantine and isolation, remains dominant (Citro et al. 2016). The UN Special Rapporteur on the elimination of discrimination against persons affected by leprosy noted that 'stigmatization remains institutionalized in the States' architecture and functioning'; over fifty states have discriminatory laws against those affected by leprosy (OHCHR 2020).

While stay-at-home orders and closed borders are novel for most European citizens, there are recent examples of these techniques being used as public health responses. The response to HIV/AIDS underlines the contribution of a human rights approach and urges states to govern with solidarity, not force. However, COVID-19's long incubation period has confounded states and led to draconian restrictions. Such measures must be scrutinized in light of international and regional obligations. The next section reflects on these measures, employing a health and human rights approach.

3 Restrictions, restrictions everywhere

At the height of the 'first wave' of the COVID-19 pandemic, all European states adopted legislation to compel their populations to reduce social contact. The most prescriptive restrictions ordered residents to stay at home unless they had a specified 'necessary' purpose, such as work or buying essential groceries. Furthermore, gatherings were restricted in all EU states, ranging from complete prohibitions to allowing gatherings of 100 people. Some governments required individuals to fill out a pass to leave their residence. Other states took less direct measures, not requiring individuals to justify movements but regulating their behavior in other ways, for instance, through encouraging or mandating work from home and recommendations on distancing. This approach was popular in the Scandinavian and Baltic states, while the former approach dominated most of Europe to varying degrees.[3]

Stay-at-home orders amount to limitations on numerous human rights, including private and family life, freedom of assembly, freedom of religion, the right to liberty, and freedom of movement, and must therefore be justified. Stay-at-home orders may be viewed as legitimate public health measures because they reduce social contact, which spreads the virus; however, to conclude (as some commentators have) that such measures are per se proportionate is problematic in light of the disproportionate burdens imposed. As quickly became clear, stay-at-home orders have disproportionate impacts on certain persons and groups.

As described in section 1, states have obligations to analyze the impacts of restrictions on all of society and adopt positive measures to protect the public, especially the most vulnerable. Notably, individuals living in a violent environment were placed at increased risk when forced to stay at home with an abuser in a situation of heightened stress (Bradbury-Jones & Isham 2020). Introducing stay-at-home orders but failing to protect women and children from domestic violence may violate the Istanbul Convention and states' positive obligations under Article 14 ECHR (*Opuz v. Turkey*). Likewise, stay-at-home orders may limit individuals' ability to access adequate food, water, and healthcare, which can result in violations of rights to health, food, and social security. This can have serious implications for the most vulnerable. For example, directives requiring elders or persons with compromised immune systems to remain home placed those without social support at risk. For persons in institutional care, self-isolation at home is illusory. Similarly, essential workers, often underpaid and without the option of working from home, must instead face the pandemic as carers, cleaners, and shop assistants.

In this section I examine the proportionality of a selection of these often-disjointed measures. Although states have obligations to prevent loss of life and protect the public's health from COVID-19, proportionality limits states' freedom to restrict rights. Proportionality is a legal device common to international human rights and health law that seeks to ensure that states do not adopt unnecessary or unjustifiably restrictive measures. I identify several characteristics that are problematic from a human rights perspective: the failure to advance less restrictive measures, the creep of criminalization into public health laws, and states' willingness to ignore scientific evidence. I argue that the failure to engage with these principles has led to disproportionate burdens on certain groups and individuals.

3.1 Restrictive measures lacking evidence

Under international health and human rights law, states should adopt less restrictive measures when equally effective. However, the ECtHR often imposes a lighter standard of review, depending on which right is engaged. Here I explore four examples from different European countries where states appear to have taken more restrictive measures than necessary, which may run counter to the public's health and civil liberties.

First, in some countries or regions, outdoor exercise was strictly curtailed in a bid to reduce social interactions and stop congregation. These restrictions have particularly severe impacts on the poor, especially those living in cramped accommodations without access to a garden or balcony. Furthermore, as lockdowns were loosened, countries imposed arbitrary limits devoid of scientific evidence, like only permitting exercise within a specific kilometer radius of one's residence, which seems unnecessary for those living in rural areas or impractical for many in cities. Conversely, other countries permitted visiting nature or parks (Prague Ministry of Health 2020) and some, like Belgium, encouraged outdoor exercise (with other household members or one friend) (Belgian Federal Government 2020).

Second, a small number of countries introduced regulations that imposed specific restrictions on elders when less restrictive approaches may have been equally effective. For example, in Hungary:

> For their own and their families' interest, persons who have attained the age of 65 years shall be allowed to visit a grocery store, drugstore, market or pharmacy only between 9 a.m. and 12 a.m.
>
> *(Hungary Ministry of Justice 2020)*

This provision can, on the one hand, be welcomed as a special measure to protect elders from transmission and ensure that the health system does not become overloaded. But is it proportionate to limit entry of a specific group based on age (a protected category)? Furthermore, that only those over sixty-five, not all persons vulnerable to COVID-19 (see below) are included is not in line with scientific evidence. Directly discriminating against people based on age, which is often associated with appearance, can also lead to stigma or discrimination based on perceived age. The decree states that it will be enforced by police with the possibility of fine, subject to the principles of proportionality and necessity. Fining an elder for shopping outside this three-hour window is difficult to justify as proportionate or a legitimate public health measure. In examples like this, less restrictive measures seem to have been overlooked. A less restrictive approach could be to set aside specific times for persons at risk and to encourage them to shop at designated times but not prohibit entry at other times, given that the measure is intended to be protective, not prohibitive. Equally, the state should take positive measures to ensure that those who cannot shop will have access to adequate food.

Similarly, Malta issued an order that directed vulnerable persons to stay at home unless such persons 'need to leave their residence to attend medical appointments, obtain medical care or treatment, acquire food, medicine, other daily necessities, or to attend to any other essential or urgent personal matter' (Malta Superintendent of Public Health 2020). In this instance, vulnerable persons are framed broadly to include 'pregnant women' and other categories, including persons who have suffered cardiac arrest in the last six months. These groups seem to be approached from a precautionary standpoint that is not based on scientific evidence. The blanket inclusion of pregnant women is reminiscent of the neglect of women in scientific research, based on a desire to protect the fetus rather than the health of the woman (Liu & Mager 2016). Furthermore, the fact that daily exercise is not included as a legitimate purpose can be questioned as scientifically justified (exercise is an important predictor of good health) and disproportionate.

In Spain, children were placed under 'house arrest' for six weeks, after which, in response to criticism, children under fourteen were permitted to go outside for one hour with their parents (EU Agency for Fundamental Rights 2020, pp. 3–4). A study found that parents reported changes in their children's emotional state and behavior including difficulty concentrating, boredom, and irritability (Orgilés et al. 2020). While the study found that both Italian and Spanish children were impacted, the latter, who had no opportunities for outdoor physical activity, experienced more severe impacts. Save the Children Spain found that half of the children interviewed reported negative effects and anxiety (Save the Children 2020). Blanket restrictions based on age are direct discrimination and must have an 'objective and reasonable justification'. While the ECtHR has been sympathetic towards 'protective regime[s]' (*D.G. v. Ireland*, para. 115) of detention of children, the regime imposed by the Spanish government – although with children's protection in mind – is contrary to their best interests under the Convention on the Rights of the Child.

Given that women continue to take responsibility for most of the care giving, such restrictions, lacking in scientific justification, can have a disproportionate impact on mothers of young children. It is particularly jarring that in some jurisdictions, like Spain, exceptions were permitted for individuals to walk their dog, but not their baby.

The question should therefore be asked, whether states can and should impose less restrictive measures, for example, allowing for exercise subject to distancing or at specific times, avoiding restrictions on vulnerable persons, and relying on guidance. This legal standard is enshrined in the revised International Health Regulations, which underscore that public health measures 'shall not be more restrictive of international traffic and not more invasive or intrusive to persons than reasonably available alternatives that would achieve the appropriate level of health protection'. In determining whether to implement restrictions, states should have regard to scientific principles, scientific evidence, and specific guidance or advice from the WHO (Article 43). States should implement the IHR 'with full respect for the dignity, human rights and fundamental freedoms of persons'. The IHR should be given weight given that they are *lex specialis* in the field of infectious disease.

The requirement to consider less restrictive measures is also supported in international human rights doctrine. For example, the Human Rights Committee states that limitations on movement:

> must be appropriate to achieve their protective function; they must be the least intrusive instrument amongst those which might achieve the desired result; and they must be proportionate to the interest to be protected.
>
> *(GC No. 27, para. 14)*

In General Comment No. 37, the Human Rights Committee explained that proportionality (in the context of freedom of assembly) requires:

> a value assessment, weighing the nature and detrimental impact of the interference on the exercise of the right against the resultant benefit to one of the grounds for interfering. If the detriment outweighs the benefit, the restriction is disproportionate and thus not permissible.
>
> *(GC No. 37, para. 40)*

CESCR General Comment No. 14 also holds in relation to the right to health that the 'least restrictive alternative must be adopted where several types of limitations are available'. Limitations on grounds of protecting public health should be of limited duration and subject to review (para. 29). Thus, with growing scientific evidence on COVID-19, state actors should review the limitations imposed on rights.

However, the standard imposed by the ECtHR varies depending on whether a measure amounts to deprivation of liberty or a restriction of movement. When Article 5 is engaged, given the seriousness of deprivation of liberty, the Court normally expects that less restrictive measures have been considered but found inappropriate (*Saadi v. the United Kingdom*, para. 70). In a seminal public health judgment, the Court found that

> the essential criteria when assessing the 'lawfulness' of the detention of a person 'for the prevention of the spreading of infectious diseases' are whether the spreading of the infectious disease is dangerous to public health or safety, and whether detention of the person infected is the last resort in order to prevent the spreading of the disease, because less severe measures have been considered and found to be insufficient to safeguard the public interest.
>
> *(Enhorn v. Sweden, para. 44)*

Yet, when assessing violations of other rights, the Court has often declined to examine whether the state could have adopted less restrictive measures. In a case on whether a statutory ban on secondary industrial action violated freedom of association, the Court held that:

> the question is not whether less restrictive rules should have been adopted or whether the State can establish that, without the prohibition, the legitimate aim would not be achieved. It is rather whether, in adopting the general measure it did, the legislature acted within the margin of appreciation afforded to it.
>
> *(National Union of Rail, Maritime and Transport Workers v. UK, para. 103)*

Similarly, when assessing the right to private and family life, the Court often examines whether a 'fair balance' has been struck between different interests (*Hatton and Others v. UK*, para. 123). However, the Court has concluded that the 'blanket and indiscriminate nature' of a law was disproportionate, which implicitly suggests that less restrictive measures would have been more appropriate (*S. and Marper v. UK*). In a case on freedom of movement, the ECtHR simply held that 'restrictive measures should be *appropriate* to achieve their protective function' (*Bartik v. Russia*, para. 46).

While stay-at-home orders will always amount to restrictions on freedom of movement, the most restrictive approaches may rise to the level of restrictions on liberty under Article 5 ECHR. The ECtHR has repeatedly held that when distinguishing between the right to liberty and freedom of movement the

> starting-point must be his or her specific situation and account must be taken of a whole range of factors such as the type, duration, effects and manner of implementation of the measure in question. The difference between

> deprivation and restriction of liberty is one of degree or intensity, and not one of nature or substance.
>
> *(De Tommaso v. Italy, para. 80)*

The Court should also take the type and manner of implementation into account (para. 81). In *Guzzardi v. Italy*, the applicant was forced to live on an island of only 2.5 square meters with permanent surveillance, which was found to engage Article 5. However, in *De Tommaso* not being able to leave home at night except in case of necessity (but being permitted to leave during the day) did not amount to deprivation of liberty (but instead a restriction on freedom of movement). Considering that the ECtHR has found that 'house arrest' (an order to stay at home for 90 days) is deprivation of liberty under Article 5 (not only restriction of movement) (*Buzadji v. The Republic of Moldova*), then requiring children and vulnerable persons to stay at home for several weeks (as described above) should be viewed as a restriction of liberty that requires states to demonstrate that they have considered whether the public health aim could be met by less restrictive measures.

Thus, states should give greater consideration to whether the public health aims of certain COVID-19 restrictions can be achieved by less restrictive means. There are compelling health reasons to argue that prohibitions on exercise are disproportionate. Exercise is an important determinant of health, yet, emerging research shows a fall in physical activity during the most restrictive periods in Tirol, Austria and Croatia (Schnitzer et al. 2020). Similarly, strict limits, such as requirements to remain within a specific radius, could be more appropriate as guidelines instead of hard law, given the diversity of living circumstances. Should COVID-19 restrictions come before the ECtHR, the Court, following the IHR and international human rights instruments, should adopt the less restrictive measures test, regardless of whether the restriction is found to fall under Article 5.

3.2 COVID-19 criminals

In the pursuit of compliance, states appear to frequently rely on police as enforcers. Police have been given far reaching powers to fine and, in rare circumstances, imprison those who do not comply with public health guidance. This is in opposition to the human rights approach and ignores the advice of UNAIDS which called on states to avoid using criminal law to mitigate the spread of COVID-19 and instead build trust (UNAIDS 2020).

As discussed in section 2, the imposition of criminal sanctions in public health crises can have troubling side effects. Trust is central to any successful public health response and imposing criminal sanctions for non-compliance may undermine trust and lead citizens to view COVID-19 regulations as adversarial or imposed, instead of fostering collective responsibility necessary for a successful public health response. Excessive punishments, like severe fines or imprisonment, will have disproportionate impacts on the poor or persons with dependents. Such population groups may also lack the time and resources to appeal against illegitimate fines. Criminalization is a poor substitute for tackling the structural causes of transmission.

Criminal law under the guise of public health can also be misused to target outsiders and push political agendas. In Denmark, an amendment to the immigration act was included in a bill to introduce stricter punishments for those who commit crimes connected to COVID-19. Although a strict immigration regime already allows for the expulsion of foreigners who commit crimes, the law now specifies 'an unconditional custodial term connected to COVID-19' as a ground for deportation (Denmark Ministry of Justice 2020). This must be seen in the light of the already established – and criticized – so-called 'ghetto'-laws and policies where the same crime may be punished more severely if committed in specific areas with high immigrant populations perceived as particularly 'troubled'. While the COVID-19 provision probably has little practical consequences given that foreigners could already be deported if they had committed a crime punishable by one year's imprisonment, it is a reminder of how pandemics can be used to capitalize on xenophobia and distrust of minorities.

In Ireland, COVID-19 legislation gave police a central role in enforcing restrictions between April and June 2020, enshrining powers to direct persons to comply with the rules and to arrest individuals for failure to comply. The police became more visible: 50,977 police checkpoints were set up between 8 April and 20 June 2020 to monitor compliance with restrictions on movement (Policing Authority 2020, p. 6). Police also began using 'anti-spit hoods' (a device placed over the head of a suspect) as a means of protecting officers from transmission, despite evidence of physical and mental impacts (Policing Authority 2020, p. 18). Concerns have been raised regarding this form of restraint, in particular its use on vulnerable persons with mental illness and minors. Similarly, minors reported feeling targeted by police when outside, particularly if living in areas dominated by social housing, and they reported a lack of understanding for the minors' need to, for example, take a walk due to cramped accommodations or a difficult family situation (Policing Authority 2020, p. 11). Although overall criminal activity reduced in Ireland, reports of domestic violence increased by 25 percent and notifications to the child protection agency increased by 18 percent (Policing Authority 2020, p. 5). This suggests that more resources must be invested in investigating and preventing interpersonal violence.

Fines have been widely used in some states. In England, police used fixed penalty notices (FPN) to enforce breaches of COVID-19 regulations on movement and gatherings. It has been reported that approximately 142,000 of such fines were imposed during the height of the first lockdown. In Spain, fines have been applied more aggressively; in the first seventy-five days of the lockdown over 1 million fines were issued (López-Fonseca 2020). The College of Policing guidance on policing the lockdown in England and Wales advised that fines should be the last resort. It is particularly problematic that Black and Asian persons were found to be 1.8 times more likely to receive an FPN (Currenti & Flatley 2020). In Scotland, a third of FPNs were issued to persons living in the 10 percent most deprived areas (McVie

2020). Furthermore, there is a poverty dimension: those who pay the fines avoid prosecution and fines are halved if paid within two weeks. This approach favors those with means and allows them to avoid consequences, while those with limited means do not have the same luxury. In Denmark, three fines were appealed against and struck down by a city court that held that the police had not proven that the defendants could or should have known that they were acting contrary to the law (Copenhagen City Court 2020).

In conclusion, it should be questioned whether police are best positioned to enforce public health legislation, especially without adequate training and support in a high stress situation. These examples highlight the risks of stigma and discrimination, in particular, in communities that do not enjoy good relations with law enforcement. Using fines as a public health tool can undermine trust and impose disproportionate burdens on the poor.

4 Conclusions

Governments have enacted far reaching restrictions, previously unknown to European democracies, in response to COVID-19. While the pandemic has caught many by surprise, experts have long warned that a severe disease outbreak was looming due to deforestation, rising sea levels, and urbanization (Gates 2015). Yet governments, often driven by short-sighted political goals, have failed to meet their obligations to shore up health security in line with human rights and the International Health Regulations (Gostin & Ó Cathaoir 2018). Now faced with an emergency, states must not neglect human rights obligations and principles in their response. To do so would set a dangerous precedent, likely to be replicated in later outbreaks. COVID-19 is not the last pandemic we will face.

This chapter has highlighted the human rights implications of stay-at-home orders and criticized four aspects of state responses. First, following the IHR and human rights, the resort to restrictive measures when viable alternatives exist should be reconsidered. It is suggested, for example, that bans on outdoor exercise should be avoided given the positive impact of exercise on health and the negative impacts of sedentary life. Instead, less restrictive measures should be pursued, such as prohibiting exercising in groups. This connects with the second issue highlighted in this analysis: for the wealthy and those living in safe environments, stay-at-home orders may provide a response proportionate to the scope of the challenge, while for other groups impacts may be disproportionate and sometimes discriminatory. Third, while scientific certainty is impossible with a novel virus, measures that run contrary to scientific evidence should be avoided. In particular, measures that covertly pursue other aims, such as targeting minorities, are illegitimate. Finally, policy makers must learn from past epidemics, in particular HIV/AIDS, which established that widespread use of criminal sanctions runs contrary to human rights and public health.

Instead, government responses should be based on trust. The principles of transparency and solidarity are particularly important. Transparency underscores that states must adequately inform and include all segments of the population in decision-making, including minorities. The necessity of public outreach is heightened in an emergency due to the collective vulnerability of the population. Adequate access to the reasons underlining law-making is particularly important given that states are choosing to enact such different measures. Furthermore, accountability is unachievable if citizens lack the information needed to evaluate and criticize decision-making. Yet, during the COVID-19 outbreak, the basis for government decisions have been unclear or unknown.

Solidarity within and beyond borders is vital to ensure a human rights response to COVID-19. It requires that governments protect the health of all segments of the population and do not neglect the most vulnerable. Alarming reports reveal that persons in the care of the state, including persons in residential care, asylum seekers, refugees, and prisoners, are dangerously exposed and increasingly isolated from the outside world. At an international level, global solidarity mandates that governments look for common solutions to shared challenges, such as shortages in personal protective equipment. Under the right to health, states have a 'collective responsibility' to address disease outbreaks (GC No. 14, para. 40). Countries with resources must support those that are hardest hit and ensure equitable distribution of COVID vaccines.

Notes

1 For example, the first 'COVID' amendment to the Danish Communicable Disease Act 1979 was presented on 26 March and adopted on 31 March 2020 (Folketinget, L 158 Forslag til lov om ændring af lov om foranstaltninger mod smitsomme og andre overførbare sygdomme og forskellige andre love). An amendment to the Irish Health Act 1947 was introduced on 16 March and signed into law on 20 March 2020 (Oireachtas, Health (Preservation and Protection and other Emergency Measures in the Public Interest) Bill 2020, No. 3 of 2020).

2 The chapter draws on data gathered by myself and postdoctoral researcher Ida Gundersby Rognlien for Legislating Corona: Proportionality, Non-Discrimination and Transparency (PRONTO) funded by Independent Research Fund Denmark (Grant number: 0213-00025B), available here: https://jura.ku.dk/english/welma/research/legislating-corona-proportionality-non-discrimination-and-transparency-pronto/.

3 Information on the restrictions discussed in this paragraph can be found on the PRONTO website https://jura.ku.dk/english/welma/research/legislating-corona-proportionality-non-discrimination-and-transparency-pronto.

References

Annas, GJ 2016, 'Ebola and Human Rights: Post-9/11 Public Health and Safety in Epidemics', *American Journal of Law & Medicine*, vol. 42, no. 2–3, pp. 333–355.

Asiye Genç v. Turkey 2015, no. 24109/07.

Bartik v. Russia 2006, no. 55565/00.

Belgian Federal Government 2020, *Coronavirus: Reinforced Measures*, viewed 24 March 2020, www.belgium.be/en/news/2020/coronavirus_reinforced_measures

Bradbury-Jones, C & Isham, L 2020, 'The Pandemic Paradox: The Consequences of COVID-19 on Domestic Violence', *Journal of Clinical Nursing*, vol. 29, no. 13–14, pp. 2047–2049.

Burris, S & Cameron, E 2008, 'The Case Against Criminalization of HIV Transmission', *The Journal of the American Medical Association*, vol. 300, no. 5, pp. 578–81.

Buzadji v. The Republic of Moldova 2014, no. 23755/07.

Chen, B & McNamara, DM 2020, 'Disability Discrimination, Medical Rationing and COVID-19', *Asian Bioethics Review*, vol. 12, pp. 511–518.

Citro, B, Lyon, E, Mankad, M, Panday, KR & Gianella, C 2016, 'Developing a Human Rights-Based Approach to Tuberculosis', *Health & Human Rights*, vol. 18, no. 1, pp. 1–8.

Committee on Economic, Social and Cultural Rights 2000, *General Comment No. 14: The Right to the Highest Attainable Standard of Health (Art. 12 of the Covenant) E/C.12/2000/4*.

Copenhagen City Court, SS 80-17775/2020, 80-17778/2020, 80-17780/2020, 14 September 2020.

Council of Europe 1996, *European Social Charter (Revised)*.

Cullen, P 2020, 'COVID-19: Almost 50,000 More People Waiting for Outpatient Appointments Since Start of Year', *The Irish Times*, 15 August, www.irishtimes.com/news/ireland/irish-news/COVID-19-almost-50-000-more-people-waiting-for-outpatient-appointments-since-start-of-year-1.4330702

Currenti, R & Flatley, J (National Police Chiefs' Council) 2020, 'Policing The Pandemic: Detailed Analysis on Police Enforcement of the Public Health Regulations and an Assessment on Disproportionality Across Ethnic Groups', *National Police Chiefs' Council*, https://news.npcc.police.uk/resources/policing-the-pandemic-4

De Tommaso v. Italy (2017), no. 43395/09.

Denmark Ministry of Justice 2020, *Lov om ændring af straffeloven, retsplejeloven og udlændingeloven L 157*, 2 April 2020.

D.G. v. Ireland 2002, no. 39474/98.

DH and others v. The Czech Republic (2007), no. 57325/00.

Enhorn v. Sweden (2005), no. 56529/00.

EU Agency for Fundamental Rights 2020, 'Protect Human Rights and Public Health in Fighting COVID-19', viewed 4 May 2020, https://fra.europa.eu/sites/default/files/fra_uploads/es_report_on_coronavirus_pandemic-_may_2020.pdf

European Convention for the Protection of Human Rights and Fundamental Freedoms, as amended by Protocols Nos. 11 and 14, 4 November 1950, ETS 5, Council of Europe.

Fidler, DP 2003, 'SARS and International Law', *American Society of International Law*, vol. 8, no. 7.

Forslag til lov om ændring af lov om foranstaltninger mod smitsomme og andre overførbare sygdomme og forskellige andre love, 31 March 2020, No. 158, Ministry of Health, Denmark.

Garda Síochána (Policing Authority) 2020, 'Policing Performance by the Garda Síochána in Relation to COVID-19 Regulations', www.policingauthority.ie/assets/uploads/documents/Report_on_the_Policing_Performance_by_the_Garda_S%C3%ADoch%C3%A1na_in_relation_to_COVID-19_regulations_20_May_2020.pdf

Gates, B 2015, 'The Next Outbreak? We Are Not Ready', www.ted.com/talks/bill_gates_the_next_outbreak_we_re_not_ready?language=dz

Gostin, L.O. & Ó Cathaoir, K 2018, 'Lurching from Complacency to Panic in the Fight Against Dangerous Microbes: A Blueprint for a Common Secure Future', *Emory Law Journal,* vol. 67, no. 3.

Guzzardi v. Italy 1980, no. 7367/76.

Hansen, MV, Ottosen, J, & Nielsen, F 2020, 'Hospitalerne har nået 75.000 færre operationer i år', *Danmarks Radio*, 9 September, www.dr.dk/nyheder/regionale/oestjylland/hospitalerne-har-naaet-75000-faerre-operationer-i-aar-lisas-liv-er-sat

Hatton and Others v. the United Kingdom 2003, no. 36022/97.

Human Rights Committee 1999, *General Comment 27, Freedom of Movement (Art. 12)*, U.N. Doc CCPR/C/21/Rev.1/Add.9.

Human Rights Committee 2018, *General Comment No. 36 (2018) on Article 6 of the International Covenant on Civil and Political Rights, on the Right to Life CCPR/C/GC/36 (30 October 2018)*, para. 18.

Hungary Ministry of Justice 2020, *Government Decree on restricting movement*, as in force 10 April 2020, No. 71/2020, section 6(1).

I.B. v. Greece 2013, no. 552/10.

Jacobs, L.A. 2007, 'Rights and Quarantine During the SARS Global Health Crisis: Differentiated Legal Consciousness in Hong Kong, Shanghai, and Toronto', *Law & Society Review*, vol. 41, no. 3.

Kirby, T 2020, 'Evidence Mounts on the Disproportionate Effect of COVID-19 on Ethnic Minorities', *The Lancet*, vol. 8, no. 6, pp. 547–548.

Lambert and Others v. France 2015, no. 46043/14.

Liu, K. & Mager, N.A.D. 2016, 'Women's Involvement in Clinical Trials: Historical Perspective and Future Implications', *Pharmacy Practice*, vol. 14, no. 1, pp. 708.

Lopes De Sousa Fernandes v. Portugal 2017, no. 56080/13.

López-Fonseca, O 2020, 'Spain Resorted to 'Gag Law' More Than Ever Before During Coronavirus Lockdown', *El País*, 30 June, https://english.elpais.com/politics/2020-06-30/spain-resorted-to-gag-law-more-than-ever-during-coronavirus-lockdown.html

Malta Superintendent of Public Health 2020, *Public Health Act: Protection of Vulnerable Persons Order*, L.N. 111 of 2020, No. 761, cap. 465.

McNeil, D.G. 2014, 'Using a Tactic Unseen in a Century, Countries Cordon Off Ebola-Racked Areas', *New York Times*, 12 August, www.nytimes.com/2014/08/13/science/using-a-tactic-unseen-in-a-century-countries-cordon-off-ebola-racked-areas.html

McVie, S 2020, 'Data Report on Police Use of Fixed Penalty Notices under the Coronavirus Regulations in Scotland', *Scottish Centre for Administrative Data Research*.

Médecins du Monde International v. France (2011), no. 67/2011

Murphy, T 2013, *Health and Human Rights*, Hart Publishing, Oxford.

National Union of Rail, Maritime and Transport Workers v. the United Kingdom 2014, no. 31045/10.

Oppenheim, B, Gallivan, M, Madhav, NK & Brown, N 2019, 'Assessing Global Preparedness for the Next Pandemic: Development and Application of an Epidemic Preparedness Index', *British Medical Journal Global Health*, vol. 4, no. 1.

Opuz v. Turkey 2009, no. 33401/02.

Orgilés, M, Morales, A, Delvecchio, E, Mazzeschi, C & Espada, JP 2020, 'Immediate Psychological Effects of the COVID-19 Quarantine in Youth from Italy and Spain', *Frontiers in Psychology*, vol. 11.

Prague Ministry of Health 2020, *Extraordinary Measure*, No. MZDR 12745/2020-4/MIN/KAN, section 1(h).

S. and Marper v. the United Kingdom 2008, nos. 30562/04, 30566/04.

Saadi v. the United Kingdom 2008, no. 13229/03.

Save the Children (Spain) 2020, 'A tu lado qué Nos cuentan las familias', www.savethechildren.es/sites/default/files/2020-03/informesavethechildrenatulado.pdf

Schnitzer, M, Schöttl, SE. Kopp, M & Barth M 2020, 'COVID-19 Stay-at-home Order in Tyrol, Austria: Sport and Exercise Behaviour in Change?', *Public Health*, vol. 185, pp. 218–220.

Šilih v. Slovenia (2009), no. 71463/01.

Tai, DBG, Shah, A, Doubeni, CA, Sia, IG, & Wieland, ML 2021, 'The Disproportionate Impact of COVID-19 on Racial and Ethnic Minorities in the United States', *Clinical Infectious Diseases*, vol. 72, no. 4.

United Nations 2020, 'We Are All in this Together: Human Rights and COVID-19 Response and Recovery', viewed 23 April 2020, www.un.org/en/un-coronavirus-communications-team/we-are-all-together-human-rights-and-covid-19-response-and

UNAIDS Geneva 2020, 'Rights in the Time of COVID-19 — Lessons from HIV for an Effective, Community-led Response', *UNAIDS*, www.unaids.org/sites/default/files/media_asset/human-rights-and-covid-19_en.pdf

UN Commission on Human Rights 1984, *The Siracusa Principles on the Limitation and Derogation Provisions in the International Covenant on Civil and Political Rights*, E/CN.4/1985/4.

UN General Assembly 1989, *Convention on the Rights of the Child.*

UN General Assembly 1966, *International Covenant on Civil and Political Rights.*

UN General Assembly 1966, *International Covenant on Economic, Social and Cultural Rights.*

United Nations Human Rights Office of the High Commissioner (OHCHR) 2020, 'World Leprosy Day: UN Expert Calls on States to end Discrimination against Affected Women and Children', viewed 24 January 2020, www.ohchr.org/EN/NewsEvents/Pages/DisplayNews.aspx?NewsID=25495&LangID=E#:~:text=Alice%20Cruz%20is%20the%20first,by%20the%20Human%20Rights%20Council

World Health Organization (WHO) 2005, *International Health Regulations.*

4

COVID-19 RISK COMMUNICATION

The right to information and participation

Tove H. Malloy

Do you speak COVID-19? This intriguing question was asked by the non-profit organization Translators without Borders in March 2020. In a policy brief aimed at governments and authorities, the organization asserted that, if it is to enable people to make informed decisions, effective risk communication involves not only language but also format, relevant content, and choosing the right channels (TwB 2020). Other expert networks on communication argued that risk communication must be community-centered rather than message-centered (Di Carlo 2020), while interest organizations representing people with disabilities, including the blind and deaf communities, called attention to the difficulty for their members to access and understand COVID-19 risk communication (APIAHF 2020). Communication experts and interest groups began this outreach once the World Health Organization (WHO) declared COVID-19 a pandemic. There was a genuine concern that lives were at risk because information about how to avoid the coronavirus and what to do if infected was not reaching all members of society.

Information about risks and recommended actions in relation to COVID-19 became a major part of everyday life across the globe and was rolled out at all levels, from heads of states to local community leaders. Access to that information was a major concern from the beginning. Authorities around the world scrambled to reach out to far corners of states and territories. The ability of all members of society to make informed decisions regarding the precautions they should take to protect themselves from the virus was of utmost importance. Yet, it soon became clear that some people did not act according to instructions. The virus spread more rapidly among some groups in society, even as they believed they were following guidance and instructions. Soon, it became clear communication gaps were leading to these disparate outcomes. Even where authorities were keen to ensure access to the right to information of all members of society, they were not able to ensure that the information was effectively comprehended.

What appears to be a communication dilemma is, in fact, also a human rights concern. For this reason communications experts were not alone in their pleas for better risk communication. Human rights actors also spotted the problem. The United Nations (UN) Secretary General has issued numerous statements on COVID-19, some of which refer to specific groups such as people with disabilities (UNSG 2020b) or elderly persons (UNSG 2020a). The WHO has issued a special guide to risk communication and community engagement (RCCE) to assist authorities in making sure they reach all segments of society (WHO 2020). The UN High Commissioner for Human Rights has been explicit in her call for ensuring effective risk communication. 'Relevant information on the COVID-19 pandemic and response', she asserts, 'should reach all people, without exception'. This requires:

> making information available in readily understandable formats and languages, including indigenous languages and those of national, ethnic and religious minorities, and adapting information for people with specific needs, including the visually- and hearing-impaired, and reaching those with limited or no ability to read or with no internet access.
>
> *(UN OHCHR 2020)*

The High Commissioner further emphasizes that:

> [p]eople have a right to participate in decision-making that affects their lives. Being open and transparent, and involving those affected in decision-making is key to ensuring people participate in measures designed to protect their own health and that of the wider population, and that those measures also reflect their specific situations and needs.
>
> *(UN OHCHR 2020)*

The message is clear. The right to information requires interpretation and participation.

At the regional level, the Council of Europe and the Organization of Security and Co-operation in Europe (OSCE) have both voiced similar concerns. The Chair of the Committee of Experts of the European Charter on Regional or Minority Languages has observed that countries have not systematically shared information, instructions, guidelines, or recommendations in languages other than the official language of the country. This also concerns the traditional regional or minority languages spoken in the respective countries. 'The communication of relevant recommendations in these languages is of utmost importance for the wellbeing of the speakers of regional or minority languages', the Chair noted (Council of Europe 2020).

The OSCE's High Commissioner on National Minorities has also pleaded for governments to be sensitive to language needs:

> States should provide basic services in the languages used by various communities as far as possible, especially in healthcare and in communications about the health crisis and official responses. People with limited knowledge of the official language(s) can become particularly vulnerable if they cannot understand what is expected from them.
>
> *(OSCE 2020)*

The concerns of these human rights actors seem to indicate that there is an increasing consensus about the dilemma between access to information and comprehending it. This raises a number of questions about the right to information. What is the right to information, and how is it applied? In particular, '*how is it applied during a pandemic?*'

This chapter begins with a short theoretical discussion about the right to information. Next, it will trace the right to information in international human rights law to show how it has developed and whether it possesses the tools to support risk communication in times of pandemics. It will do so through a broad examination of international conventions and selected jurisprudence as well as soft law tools. This includes a short discussion of language and translations rights in law. It will then turn to a key aspect of the argument, that is, what is needed to ensure that risk communication is effectively comprehended and allows for individuals and all groups in society to make informed and autonomous decisions. This entails examining aspects of how to frame the messages and develop dialogue with communities to secure their participation and trust in decisions about their own lives. The research questions whether government authorities have taken sufficient and adequate steps to enable people to make informed decisions about COVID-19 risks.

While the communication gap is mostly seen in relation to its impact on vulnerable groups and members of structurally unequal minorities, the concern in this chapter is policy communication as opposed to policy delivery, which will be the focus of Part 2 of this volume. Hence, in concluding, it will be suggested that international human rights experts and international organizations should revisit the interpretation of the right to information and develop a more enlightened definition that ensures effective comprehension and provides the foundation for informed decision-making.

1 What is the right to information?

Several aspects of the right to information may illustrate its place in the moral landscape of human rights. First, the right to information is a derivative right, meaning that it draws morally on other fundamental human rights values. Specifically, the right to information is a derivative of the so-called speech rights, the freedom of opinion and the freedom of expression. This means that the right to information is not an intrinsic human right but is rather more likely to be an instrumental right (McDonagh 2013). An instrumental right helps human beings in achieving fundamental rights, such as the right to life. Instrumental rights are thus utilitarian in that they focus on maximizing something of high value and importance in life. The technical difference between intrinsic and instrumental rights is that intrinsic rights protect the rights-holder directly, whereas the instrumental right protects the interests of the rights-holder. In other words, the right to information is not a stand-alone right (McDonagh 2013) and the right to COVID-19 information is an instrumental right. On the other hand, one could argue that the right to know about COVID-19 and to understand what to do to avoid COVID-19 are closely linked not only to the right to health but also to the right to life. Comprehending how to avoid contracting a virus that kills many people is perhaps more than an instrumental need.

Second, by virtue of being derived from the speech rights, the right to information is intricately linked to democracy and democratic ideals, such as transparency and participatory decision-making. When former South African President Nelson Mandela was drafting the new democratic constitution of South Africa, he made certain that the right to information was one of the first rights included in the instrument (Mandela 1996). Mandela understood that it is a lack of information and a lack of knowledge that allows illiberal systems to thrive. With information and knowledge, citizens can better secure their democratic rights. Access to and understanding of information is one of the keys to democracy. Guaranteeing people's right to seek and receive public information serves as a critical tool for fighting corruption, enabling citizens to participate more fully in public life, making governments more efficient, and helping persons exercise their fundamental human rights. Moreover, it allows citizens to participate in setting priorities in decision-making, holding their government accountable, and ensuring equal treatment and equal justice. It therefore provides citizens with the ability to become good citizens.

Third, the right to information implies that the recipient of the information will be put in a position of being able to make informed decisions. The question is: what does being able to make informed decisions entail? First of all, the decision-maker must have *physical* access to the information. This can involve diverse types of media, including digital broadcasting, printed and social media, as well as tools to read and hear these, if the decision-maker is disabled. However, it is also relevant that the decision-maker has *cognitive* access to the information. In order to have cognitive access, the decision-maker must be literate and able to understand the language of the communication; she must have some skills to transform the information into her own situation. This means that the information may have to be translated into other languages and interpreted into different cultural settings. Interpretation is needed if people are illiterate and only understand pictures or pictograms, if people have a disability that prevents them from hearing or seeing the information/pictures, if people do not understand the language of the message, or if the directives in the information are not transferrable into people's culture and traditions. There can be many reasons why a piece of information may be very difficult both to comprehend and understand. Therefore, there are numerous reasons why a person may not be able to make an informed decision about her actions.

2 The right to information in international human rights law

The right to information has retained a specific interpretation in international human rights law and been in focus since the UN's inception. The right was firmly established as a derivative of the speech rights in Article 19 of the Universal Declaration of Human Rights (UDHR) in 1948. By the time the International Covenant on Civil and Political Rights (ICCPR) was being drafted, the UN had further expanded the right to information to include information across frontiers and the free choice of medium. This was elaborated mainly with a view to define the responsibilities of the provider of information to secure that modern mass media was open and unbiased (CCPR 1983). The Human Rights Committee (HRC), which monitors the ICCPR, soon established its interpretation of the right to information in its jurisprudence. However, it focused entirely on the right to *access* information (e.g. *Gauthier v. Canada* (1999); *S.B. v. Kyrgyzstan* (2009); *Toktakunov v. Kyrgyzstan* (2011)). This path has also been followed in the Committee's General Comment 34 (CCPR 2011), by the successive Special Rapporteurs on freedom of opinion and expression, as well as the Convention on Access to Information, Public Participation in Decision-Making and Access to Justice in Environmental Matters, the so-called Aarhus Convention (2001) and the Council of Europe Convention on Access to Official Documents (2009). At a regional level, the jurisprudence of the European Court of Human Rights (ECtHR) has also focused mainly on access (e.g., *Sunday Times v. UK* (1979); *Guerra v. Italy* (1998); *Tarsasag a Szabadsag v. Hungary* (2009); *Kenedi v. Hungary* (2009)). Therefore, *physical* access became the main understanding of and approach to the right to information.

This is not to say that access is not important. For instance, the Aarhus Convention provides for the right to know about environmental issues that may affect the lives of individuals especially when their lives are in danger. Several events have put this in an acute perspective. The lack of access to and understanding of environmental information has in fact jeopardized the right to life of many. This is the case of the people living near the Bhopal plant in India in 1983, in what is considered among the world's worst industrial disasters. Over 500,000 people were exposed to methyl isocyanate gas. In *Oneryldiz v. Turkey* (2004), the ECtHR established that the responsible local Turkish authorities were informed about the build-up of methane in a refuse dump near a shanty town but had taken no action. As a result of a methane explosion and a subsequent landslide, thirty-nine people died. The ECtHR held that the authorities had not provided the inhabitants with information enabling them to assess the risks of remaining in the shanty town (McDonagh 2013). This obligation of governments to inform the population or specific groups that there are reasons to believe that their lives could be at risk has also been established in other cases like *Osman v. United Kingdom* (*Osman v. United Kingdom* 1998; McDonagh 2013). Access is indeed an important dimension of the right to information. The responsibility to provide information proactively in times of eminent dangers illustrates this.

With the 2006 UN Convention on the Rights of Persons with Disabilities (CRPD), the UN developed a more enlightened approach to the right to information that involves translation and interpretation. Article 2 of CRPD provides a set of definitions that are useful in interpreting the right to information in a broader perspective. With regards to communication, it declares that

> 'Communication' includes languages, display of text, Braille, tactile communication, large print, accessible multimedia as well as written, audio, plain-language, human-reader and augmentative and alternative modes, means and formats of communication, including accessible information and communication technology.

This indicates that communication entails much more than the individuals' physical access to information; it may require interpretation tools, such as audio and other formats. With regards to language, the Convention is also helpful. 'Language' it holds, 'includes spoken and signed languages and other forms of non-spoken languages'. (Art 2). This general change of approach from seeing the right to information in terms of access to promoting it in terms of interpretation was followed up by UNESCO a few years later.

In 2010, UNESCO connected the right to information to human rights and democracy in a new way. At a conference on the freedom information organized in Brisbane, Australia, UNESCO recognized the link of the right to information to informed decision-making, to participation, to equality, and to empowerment. The final statement of the conference, the Declaration on Freedom of Information: The Right to Know, also known as the Brisbane Declaration, declares in its Preamble that 'the right to information is critical for informed decision-making, for participation in democratic life, for monitoring of public actions, and for enhancing transparency and accountability' (UNESCO 2010). The Preamble also highlights that the right to information is instrumental for the realization of people's empowerment. Furthermore, the right to information should strengthen civic trust and promote equality of all groups in society, including women and indigenous peoples. It emphasizes that comprehension is a component of the right to information and suggests that governments bridge the digital and knowledge divide by overcoming low literacy levels and poor internet connectivity. Finally, the Preamble asserts that by 'making information available in local languages and in a form that is easily understandable by diverse audiences' the right to information will contribute to empowerment (UNESCO 2010). Unfortunately, the Brisbane Declaration is not legally binding, but the message seems clear. The right to information involves language rights and translation.

3 Language and translation rights

Indeed, a key to effective comprehension and understanding of risk communication is language and translation. As noted above, when the COVID-19 pandemic broke out, some European human rights actors called attention to this, and many national governments have been providing sign language interpretation as well as translations into majority and minority languages (Nunez 2013, p. 407). However, in international human rights law translation is usually only addressed as a right in the judicial realm in connection with criminal and other proceedings, the rights of prisoners of war and other types of prisoners as well as in connection with seeking asylum (Nunez 2013; ECHR 1950, Art 6; ICCPR 1966, Art 4). In a few cases it is also recognized in connection with social rights, such as labor rights (ILO Convention No. 169 1989, Articles 12 and 30; the International Convention on the Protection of the Rights of all Migrant Workers 1990, Articles 16 and 18; European Economic Community 1968 & 1972). At the regional level, language rights have become a core part of the European human rights protection regime through a number of treaties as well as soft law instruments. The Council of Europe's European Charter on Regional or Minority Languages (1992) and European Framework Convention on the Protection of National Minorities (1995) are both legally binding, and they provide for the right to access information and authorities in minority languages as well as translation free of charge in situations of interaction with public authorities (European Charter for Regional or Minority Languages, Art 10(4)). The OSCE Oslo Recommendations regarding the linguistic rights of national minorities (1998, recommendation 20) and Thematic Commentary No. 3 on the Language Rights of Persons Belonging to National Minorities under the Framework Convention (2012) are soft law instruments that provide guidance to governments and authorities regarding these matters.

The UN Special Rapporteur on Indigenous Peoples is concerned about language rights and comprehension of risk communication in his 2020 report to the UN General Assembly. In this report, he addresses the issue of how information about COVID-19 and prevention measures is disseminated in indigenous communities (UNSR 2020a). In the Special Rapporteur's view, the problem is that:

> COVID-19 prevention guidelines and advisories are not always translated into indigenous languages, may not be culturally relevant in content or presentation or may be disseminated only via television, online or in other formats inaccessible to certain indigenous peoples. Information for indigenous persons with visual, hearing or intellectual impairment is also rarely available.

He further notes that communication platforms, such as local radio, phone calls, texting and social networks, should be used, depending on the medium most accessible by the communities, to 'convey information in accessible and culturally appropriate formats' (UNSR 2020a, p. 10). He goes as far as to assert that there are indigenous communities that appear to be unaware of the pandemic. Thus, he recommends that with regards to communities living outside the range of communication platforms, measures should be taken to facilitate the visit of outreach persons. In other words, language and translation rights and direct interaction with communities are the tools that he considers relevant in terms of making risk communication comprehensible. There seems to be a growing consensus that the right to information is more than physical access. It requires tools that enable people to effectively comprehend the issues at stake. These tools had, in fact, been identified before the outbreak of the COVID-19 pandemic.

4 What is required from COVID-19 risk communication?

In 2018, the WHO issued a guide to risk communication on the occasion of the 100th anniversary of the so-called Spanish Flu (WHO 2018). The guide draws on experience with virus elimination across the globe in the twenty-first century, including the Ebola epidemic, and focuses on three areas: risk communication, community engagement, and medical advice. With regard to risk communication, the guide argues that the 'ultimate goal is that everyone at risk is able to take informed decisions to mitigate the effects of a disease outbreak and take protective and preventive action' (WHO 2018, p. 42). Effective risk communication not only saves lives and reduces illness (by informing people on how to protect their health), but it also enables countries and communities to preserve their social, economic, and political stability in the face of emergencies. The guide defines risk communication as 'the real-time exchange of information, advice and opinions between health experts or officials and people who face a threat (hazard) to their survival, health or economic or social well-being' (WHO 2018, p. 42).

However, the guide cautions that there has been a shift in the twenty-first century in how risk communication is received. It argues that experts and authorities are less trusted, that people now seek health advice mostly from public online sources and through their trusted social networks. The fact that people search online is problematic because there has been an increase of 'citizen journalism' on social media, which may not provide accurate information. The phenomenon of 'infodemics' or the rapid spread of information, including rumors, gossip, and unreliable information is a worrying trend. Thus, trust has become a major issue in risk communication. Without trust, people are unlikely to follow the advice given. The latest and most accurate information must be conveyed frequently, and uncertainties related to an epidemic must be acknowledged in order to maintain credibility and public trust (WHO 2018, p. 26). Effective risk communication depends, therefore, on the credibility of those giving advice; their expressions of caring and empathy; and their ability to identify with people at risk (WHO 2018, p. 44).

With regards to community engagement, the guide recalls that people live in unique social-cultural contexts, each with their own relationship dynamics, perception of risks, and trusted sources of advice. These all influence whether people will accept health advice or not. Experience has shown that 'merely telling people what to do, however scientific, does not always work. Engaging them is more effective' (WHO 2018, p. 38). The guide further emphasizes that 'people have a right to information that could protect their health and save lives, social fabric and economic wellbeing', and communities are the frontline in detecting and managing epidemics. Most importantly, it explains that communities are able to implement mitigation measures through a change of individual and family practices and by implementing community measures that enable changes at the systems level. The tools recommended include establishing dialogue, building trust, and empowering communities (WHO 2018, pp. 38–39).

In his 2020 report to the Human Rights Council, the Special Rapporteur on the promotion and protection of the right to freedom of opinion and expression draws on the WHO guide to caution governments that COVID-19 risk communication must involve transparent and understandable communication; it must create trusted and dynamic relationships, and it must scope the risk in lay language (UNSR 2020b, p. 7). Although the Special Rapporteur's report was submitted early in the pandemic, it underscores that there is no excuse for delivering unprofessional risk communication.

One could draw an analogy to the human right to education. Effective delivery of education entails more than nominal schooling. The first UN Special Rapporteur on Education, Katarina Tomasevski, very appropriately pointed governments to four requirements for effective delivery of education, the so-called 4-A framework: availability, accessibility, acceptability, and adaptability (Tomasevski 2003, 2006). Availability centers on the obligation to provide free and compulsory primary schooling, whereas accessibility requires equal access including ensuring affordability. Acceptability requires governments to ensure that education is of a guaranteed quality, including providing education in indigenous and minority languages, and ensured through oversight as well as that standards of health and safety are maintained. Finally, Tomasevski advocated that education be adapted to what is in the best interest of the child. In fact, she argued that standardization of education often leads to children of diverse backgrounds failing due to difference in starting points. (Tomasevski 2003, 2006). These observations and arguments are very relevant for COVID-19 risk communication and our understanding of the right to information in spite of being framed as the right to education.

As noted above, a number of NGOs have been instrumental in highlighting that risk communication must be effective. Translators without Borders argue that global response plans for COVID-19 must identify risk communication and community engagement as priorities. Such plans must require 'all responders to communicate effectively with communities, counter misinformation, and make sure that people can hold them accountable' (TwB 2020). Specifically, they identify aspects of format and how information is presented because it affects how well it is understood. Anything from pictorial, audio, and video content to larger fonts and good contrasts for older people are mentioned. They also note that two-way information is vital, and it must flow using locally preferred and trusted communication channels. When face-to-face communication is not possible, it is important to make sure that all members of communities have access to other communication tools, including women who are often left to rely on their male relatives as only source of knowledge. Finally, Translators without Borders also address misinformation and mistrust.

Risk communication must be tailored to the intended audience, and it must respond to people's concerns, not just give them instructions. Concepts are vital. 'Social distancing' is very difficult to translate from one language to another, and just as difficult to transpose into cultures which are not able to or familiar with keeping a physical distance. Another aspect is the actions that people should take to avoid the virus or if they catch the virus. Speaking in the context of Ebola, Translators without Borders found that a simple message, 'You have to go early to the Ebola treatment center to be cured' may only frustrate people who do not understand what early entails. Having a message that complies with the grammar and the lexicon of a given language is only the start of a translation work.

Focusing on the community in addition to the message is another important aspect that governments need to learn. Experts argue that we do have experience in this from the Ebola epidemic (Di Carlo 2020). For instance, research has shown that without a clear understanding of the specific cultural situation where communication about risk takes place, translation efforts may be in vain, if not counterproductive. Experts argue that it may be necessary to clarify the disease's relation to colonial and postcolonial medical practices. They also suggest that it is important to understand the prevailing social imaginaries, such as culture-specific ways of interpreting the world in order to understand vernacular rationalizations involving culturally and socially formed expectations. It can be relevant when a pandemic intersects with political events, such as elections, or social events entailing close human interaction, such as funerals. Moreover, the aspect of who carries the message is important. Here experts recommend that community leaders be involved in framing the messages from the beginning. The messenger and/or interpreter must be trusted.

The primary goal of risk communication is that people change their behavior based on the new information they receive. The message must be understood and accepted by as many people as possible. For this to happen, one must keep many aspects in sight in addition to the narrow linguistic ones. The words and metaphors that are chosen matter. The meaning that a message will evoke matters. Which institutions or individuals will deliver the message as well as the use of certain channels and styles are all factors that affect how people will respond to a message. In other words, authorities should adopt an approach that puts the particular community and its socio-cultural context at the center of the translation efforts, rather than the message itself (Di Carlo 2020). This community-centered approach, therefore, empowers the community itself as the producer of messages.

Bringing together insights from the WHO and from communication experts, there seems to be consensus on a number of aspects that will render risk communication more effective. First of all, the message must be community-centered as opposed to message-centered. This is actually the key to setting the strategy for how authorities should plan and disseminate risk communication. Authorities should be proactive in getting the information out early and through the best channels. They should engage directly with community leaders to listen and take feedback so the risk messages become useful to the receivers. Engaging directly will also build trust for the entire process. They should use social media only as appropriate, as not all members of communities have access to it. Thus, they should coordinate with communities regarding pertinent information systems. They should make sure that risk communication is strategic, not an add-on to other parts of pandemic policies. This means allocating adequate resources and building capacity for the next emergency. In other words, there is an aspect of adapting risk communication to community needs that should be taken into consideration when ensuring access to the right to information in times of pandemic.

5 Conclusions

Effective COVID-19 risk communication is key to stopping the spread of the novel coronavirus. Unfortunately, there have been gaps in COVID-19 risk communication in many countries, and it seems that governments have not taken all the necessary and adequate steps in providing effective risk communication. This is in spite of the fact that specialized guidance has existed since 2018, based on previous epidemics. Accordingly, governments should provide access to risk information and proactively ensure that it is disseminated early and reaches all corners of society. They should also seek to make sure that risk information is comprehensible by translating and interpreting messages and by adapting them to community cultures and needs through participation of community leaders. In so doing, risk communication is capable of providing individuals and communities with the option to make informed decisions about their lives.

Since it is predicted that there will be an increasing occurrence of health crises as well as environmental crises in the future, one must ask whether international human rights law has provided governments with an adequate basis for an enlightened understanding of the right to information. Most of the instruments and jurisprudence focus on physical access to information rather than cognitive access, including comprehension and understanding, and very few provision the use of first languages and translation. None speak of adaptation to community cultures and needs. It would seem that the notion of access in the current interpretation of the right to information is not adequate to put responsibility on states to provide effective risk communication. Therefore, international human rights experts and international organizations should develop all the tools needed for governments to live up to the standards required of risk communication. A more enlightened interpretation of the right to information would be a good first step.

References

Asian & Pacific Islander American Health Forum (APIAHF) 2020, *COVID-19 Language Access Legislation Letter to Congressional Leadership*, viewed 19 September 2020, www.apiahf.org/resource/covid19-lep-letter/

CCPR 1983, General Comment No. 10, 'Freedom of Expression (Art. 19)'.

CCPR 2011, General Comment No. 34 'Article 19: Freedoms of Opinion and Expression', CCPR/C/GC/34.

Convention on Access to Information, Public Participation in Decision-making and Access to Justice in Environmental Matters (Aarhus Convention) 2001, opened for signature 25 June 1998, UNTS, vol. 2161, p. 447.

Convention on the Rights of Persons with Disabilities 2006, adopted by the General Assembly 24 January 2007, A/RES/61/106.

Council of Europe Convention on Access to Official Documents 2009, opened for signature 18 June 2009, CETS No. 205.

Council of Europe 2020, 'Communication in RMLs of Utmost Importance in Global Medical Crises', Chair of the Committee of Experts of the European Charter for Regional or Minority Languages, viewed 19 September 2020, https://rm.coe.int/news-statement-covid-education/16809ef4ee

Di Carlo, P 2020, 'Message- vs. Community-centered Models in Risk Communication' *Language on the Move*, 6 August 2020, viewed 19 September 2020, www.languageonthemove.com/message-vs-community-centered-models-in-risk-communication/

European Convention on Human Rights (ECHR) 1950, opened for signature 4 November 1950, ETS No. 005.

European Economic Community 1968, Regulation No. 1612/68 on the Freedom of Movement for Workers within the Community.

European Economic Community 1972, Regulation No. 574/72 Laying down the Procedure for Implementing Regulation No. 1408/71 on the Application of Social Security Schemes to Employed Persons, Self-Employed Persons and their families Moving within the Community.

ILO Convention No. 169, Indigenous and Tribal Peoples Convention 1989, opened for signature 27 June 1989.

International Covenant on Civil and Political Rights (ICCPR) (1966), UNTS, vol. 999, p. 171.

Kenedi v. Hungary 2009, ECtHR 31475/05.

Mandela, N 1996, 'Statement by President Mandela on Human Rights Day 1996', transcript, 20 March, viewed 12 November 2020, http://db.nelsonmandela.org/speeches/pub_view.asp?pg=item&ItemID=NMS782&txtstr=freedom%20of%20information

McDonagh, M 2013, 'The Right to Information in International Human Rights Law', *Human Rights Law Review,* vol. 13, no. 1, pp. 25–55.

Nunez, GG 2013, 'Translating to Communicate with Linguistic Minorities: State Obligations under International Law', *International Journal on Minority and Group Rights,* vol. 20, pp. 406–441.

OSCE 2020, 'High Commissioner on National Minorities Offers Recommendations on Short-term Responses to COVID-19 that Support Social Cohesion', Viewed 19 September 2020, www.osce.org/hcnm/449170

Osman v. United Kingdom (1998) 87/1997/871/1083

Robert W. Gauthier v. Canada 1999, CCPR Communication No 633/1995, U.N. Doc. CCPR/C/65/D/633/1995.

S.B. v. Kyrgyzstan 2009, CCPR Communication No. 1877/2009, U.N. Doc. CCPR/C/96/D/1877/2009.

Sunday Times v. The United Kingdom 1991, ECtHR 50/1990/241/312.

Tarsasag a Szabadsag v. Hungary 2009, ECtHR 618, 37374/05.

Toktakunov v. Kyrgyzstan 2011), CCPR Communication No. 1470/2006, CCPR/C/101/D/1470/2006.

Tomasevski, K 2003, *Education Denied. Costs and Remedies,* New York, Zed Books.

Tomasevski, K 2006, *Human Rights Obligations in Education*, The Netherlands, Wolf Legal Publishers.

Translators without Borders (TwB) 2020, *Do You Speak COVID-19?* Policy Brief, viewed 19 September 2020, https://translatorswithoutborders.org/wp-content/uploads/2020/04/TWB_PolicyBrief-COVID19.pdf

UNESCO (2010) *Declaration on Freedom of Information: The Right to Know*, viewed 19 September 2020, www.unesco.org/new/en/unesco/events/prizes-and-celebrations/celebrations/international-days/world-press-freedom-day/previous-celebrations/2010/brisbane-declaration/

UN OHCHR 2020, *COVID-19 Guidance*, 13 May 2020, viewed 20 December 2020, www.ohchr.org/Documents/Events/COVID-19_Guidance.pdf

UN Secretary General (UNSG) 2020a, *Policy Brief: The Impact of COVID-19 on Older Persons*, viewed 20 December 2020, un_policy_brief_on_covid-19_and_older_persons_1_may_2020.pdf

UN Secretary General (UNSG) 2020b, *Secretary General's Message for 2020*, International Day of Sign Languages 23 September, viewed 20 December 2020, www.un.org/en/observances/sign-languages-day/message

UN Special Rapporteur (UNSR) 2020a, *Report of the Special Rapporteur on the Rights of Indigenous Peoples, José Francisco Calí Tzay*, A/75/185.

UN Special Rapporteur (UNSR) 2020b, *Disease Pandemics and the Freedom of Opinion and Expression, Report of the Special Rapporteur on the Promotion and Protection of the Right to Freedom of Opinion and Expression*, A/HRC/44/49.

World Health Organization (WHO) 2018, *Managing Epidemics: Key facts about Major Deadly Diseases*, viewed 26 September 2020, www.who.int/emergencies/diseases/managing-epidemics/en/

World Health Organization (WHO) 2020, *COVID-19: Risk Communication and Community Engagement: Action Plan Guidance COVID-19 Preparedness and Response*, viewed 19 September 2020, www.who.int/publications/i/item/risk-communication-and-community-engagement-(rcce)-action-plan-guidance

PART 2
Vulnerability and inequality

5

THE HUMAN (RIGHTS) COSTS OF INEQUALITY

Snapshots from a pandemic

Martha F. Davis

Crises have a way of laying bare our society's deep inequalities. The COVID-19 pandemic fits this pattern. Dramatic economic and social gaps preceded the pandemic worldwide. When the virus spread, these pre-existing disparities strengthened COVID-19's hold and deepened its impacts.

A sudden shock such as a pandemic can also set changes in motion, focusing attention and accelerating progress in addressing the structural problems that it illuminates. It should not take a pandemic to inch toward greater economic and social equality, but by the same token, we should not ignore the opportunities for transformative change that such a crisis presents. It remains possible that individuals, communities and governments will emerge from the COVID-19 crisis with a greater awareness of the risks posed by extreme inequality and a more robust commitment to economic and social inclusion and baseline social supports. In the Foreword to this volume, UN Special Rapporteur Olivier de Schutter argues that human rights provide an important framework for such a 'building back' phase – a phase that could include measures such as meaningful resource reallocation, universal social protection floors, and broader constituent participation in policy development.

A threshold issue, however, is the extent to which such efforts should prioritize reduction of inequality. On the one hand, human rights institutions have historically emphasized initiatives to address extreme poverty rather than inequality, seeing poverty as the manifestation of the greatest human need and most serious human rights abuses. Some human rights scholars and activists argue that policies focused on eliminating inequality may ignore those most in need – particularly in developing countries – and can paint an incomplete picture if deprivations are common across populations (UN ECOSOC 2017). On the other hand, those who support greater attention to inequality suggest that initiatives directed at identifying and alleviating extreme poverty are too focused on bright line income measurements without adequate attention to the impacts of larger economic and social contexts. As Philip Alston argues, because '[r]adical inequality inevitably sustains extreme poverty', efforts to address inequality should be a priority for those concerned with poverty reduction (Alston 2015).

Building on Alston's observations, this chapter contends that inequality must be a critical policy focus as states build back and develop pandemic responses. Inequalities chip away at the glue that holds communities together, ultimately implicating the exercise of every human right, whether civil, political, economic, social, or cultural. The persistence of significant economic and social inequalities creates challenges for expanding social inclusion, recognizing collective responsibilities and stimulating active democratic participation – the very factors that enable communities to cooperate in flattening the pandemic curve (UN DESA 2020). Indeed, most poverty activists, scholars, and international institutions also recognize the importance of this relational element; while not rejecting bright line measures, they increasingly assert that understanding poverty in relative terms – incorporating recognition of the role of inequality – yields the most meaningful working definition (Salomon 2011).

This chapter undertakes to review the human rights impacts of the COVID-19 pandemic in situations of significant domestic inequality. It does so by focusing on three areas of inequality that intersect with COVID-19 to undermine human rights and visit devastating impacts on individuals already vulnerable because of factors such as poverty, age, race, disability, or irregular immigration status: (1) digital inequalities; (2) spatial inequalities; and (3) systemic racial inequalities. These three areas embody longstanding issues of global dimension that have taken on even greater significance in the months since the spread of COVID-19. Training a human rights lens on these areas illuminates their interconnections as well as the ways that these particular inequalities exacerbate the insidious impacts of the pandemic.

After surveying these issues both in specific domestic instances and across national boundaries, this chapter concludes by discussing the opportunities for governments to undertake positive, human rights-based responses that could change the landscape of inequality and moderate the impacts of future global disasters. As we can see from the extraordinary pandemic responses that have already been mounted by governments at every level – with examples ranging from eviction moratoria to guaranteed access to household water to widespread virus testing – all that is required is the political will.

1 Digital inequalities and COVID-19

Public health experts worldwide have promoted physical distancing and facemasks as important tools to ward off infection in the absence of a vaccine. With person-to-person interactions made more difficult and even dangerous, digital technology – already in wide use – has now become a critically important platform for work, education, and personal interactions. Because the internet is playing a major role in connecting people and sharing ideas, inequalities in access to the tools of digital technology take on major significance and serve to undermine a range of human rights. Activities from dating to schooling to voting may now be done completely online by digital 'haves' who are being cautious during the pandemic. Importantly, access to digital technology, ubiquitous but nowhere universal, is uneven in the Global North as well as the Global South.

The educational system in the United States is a case in point. A 2019 analysis of forty-two countries engaged with the Organization of Economic Co-operation and Development ranked the United States in the top ten in terms of the gaps between rich and poor (Suneson & Stebbins 2019). When the pandemic reached the United States in early 2020 and public gatherings of all kinds were discouraged or even banned, pre-existing inequalities often derailed efforts to secure students' continued access to education, a microcosm of similar – and in many cases more dire – situations faced by families and communities globally.

Public school systems across the United States closed their classrooms beginning in mid-March of 2020. In many places, online instruction began shortly thereafter and continued for many months, depending on the level of COVID-19's penetration into the local community and among students and school staff. Notably private schools charging hefty tuition and typically serving higher income families, were much more likely to maintain in-person instruction (Miller 2020).

For some students, the transition to remote instruction was virtually seamless, and the change provided benefits by increasing opportunities for personalized instruction and scheduling flexibility (Wexler 2020). However, for those without access to home computers or reliable internet connections (or no connection at all), participation in remote instruction was effectively impossible. Public libraries, which often serve as study centers for low-income students, were closed by the pandemic (Moynihan 2020; Stanley 2020). Educators in urban school districts like Los Angeles, Chicago, New York, and Boston, scrambled to arrange equipment loans and internet hot spots so that students could access classroom content from their homes or common areas in apartment buildings or even school or library parking lots (Camera 2020). Some school districts negotiated arrangements with major internet providers to temporarily extend home wireless service to students during the crisis (Lee 2020). Educators made valiant efforts to reach out to students who would most benefit from personal interactions in order to remain engaged (Strauss 2020). Nevertheless, many students were lost in the course of these transitions. Unable to connect, perhaps without adequate home-based support, they drifted off to other activities.

The pandemic did not create the so-called digital divide. The American educational system had been papering over these technological disparities for some time. In fact, before the pandemic, the Federal Communications Commission (FCC) estimated that twenty-one million Americans had no broadband access; some experts suggest that the FCC's figures represent an undercount, and that the actual number is over 40 million (Poon 2020; Busby & Tanberk 2020). But until lockdowns and physical distancing protocols started, students without access to digital technology at home completed their work on shared computers in libraries, schools, and other community spaces. With those options closed off, experts suggest that for many students, this is a 'lost year' in terms of educational attainment and socialization that will never be made up (Dorn et al. 2020).

If students in the United States, with a strong educational system and a relatively robust technological infrastructure struggled, this was just the tip of the iceberg worldwide. UNICEF reports that 192 countries closed their schools at least temporarily, sending 1.6 billion students home (Vegas 2020). For those learning from home, particularly outside of city centers, internet access is often patchy; for example, UNESCO reports that 43 percent of the world's households lack internet access (UNESCO 2020). In the absence of reliable internet, some countries have relied on radio, television, or phone lessons to reach students and replicate classroom teaching (Asim et al. 2020).

For 463 million students globally, however, there was no remote learning option at all (UNICEF 2020). Child labor skyrocketed, as children – out of school and perceived to be idle – were called on to contribute to family income at a time of increased economic stress (Gettleman & Raj 2020). In India, for example, children ages six to fourteen, who previously attended school, were sent to sift through garbage dumps, barefoot and without any protective gear, in search of recyclable plastic worth a few pennies (Gettleman & Raj 2020). In many places, including Nepal and Kenya, girls who were once in school might be encouraged to marry, giving the struggling family one less mouth to feed (UNFPA 2020). These ripple effects contributed to the conclusion of the UN Special Rapporteur on the Right to Education that 'digitalization of education should never replace onsite schooling with teachers' (UN HRC 2020). For young people whose educational progress is derailed by COVID-19, the impacts of temporary school closures will have implications across generations.

In places where schools have re-opened, economic inequalities continue to exacerbate the negative educational impacts of COVID-19. For example, because low-wage workers are at higher risk of exposure to COVID-19, poor children are more likely to be dealing with COVID-related health issues in their own homes, including requirements that they quarantine or provide care for family members. In addition, in some places local and national policies put children and instructors into harm's way by reopening schools for live instruction without the measures necessary to provide an environment safe from COVID-19 (Felter & Maizland 2020). In such situations, health requirements and repeated surges of COVID-19 cases may once again force school closures and a return to patchy remote learning.

Recognizing that primary education is a human right enshrined in the Universal Declaration of Human Rights, the UN Convention on the Rights of the Child, and other international instruments, some school systems have taken extraordinary steps to provide safe learning environments through costly physical adjustments to schools. For example, UNICEF reports that,

> [in Senegal] schools have spaced-out classroom chairs to keep distance between students. Rwanda is building new classrooms and recruiting more

> teachers. Egypt has created smaller classes and staggered school hours into shifts. Many countries have increased hand washing stations, introduced health checks, and moved sports and other activities outdoors.
>
> *(UNICEF 2020)*

Still, UNICEF projects that twenty-four million students worldwide will drop out of further education as a result of the disruptions triggered by COVID-19 (UNICEF 2020). Most, if not all, of those children will be those who were already vulnerable because of economic inequalities.

Beyond education, digital inequalities during COVID-19 also have significant impacts on individuals' ability to exercise other human rights, affecting their participation in work and community life, and ultimately their health. Telework, telemedicine, remote shopping, participation in virtual events and meetings, and distance learning may all be unavailable to them. Because the daily lives of those without access to digital technology requires physical contact to work, participate in community governance, or obtain daily necessities, their potential exposure to COVID-19 is greater. Thus 'digital inequality' is, especially during the pandemic, a social determinant of health that puts those without digital access directly at risk, with significant implications for their exercise of human rights (Beaunoyer at al. 2020).

2 Spatial inequalities

As noted above, in the absence of a widely available vaccine, physical distancing is a key component of the effort to curtail community spread of COVID-19. But for many people around the world, the ability to maintain a physical distance from others of at least two meters is a luxury enjoyed only by society's economic elite. Those who lack economic and social power, in contrast, are denied the ability to control their space. Especially during a pandemic, this undermines the individuals' and communities' human rights to health, life, and dignity.

In Rio de Janeiro, Brazil, for example, one of the earliest reported COVID-19 deaths was of a black domestic worker, whose low-wage job involved close contact with an employer who contracted COVID-19 on a vacation in Italy (Slattery & Gaier 2020). Working in homes, in the personal spaces of their employers, domestic workers are particularly vulnerable to contracting COVID-19. Likewise, home healthcare aides – a job disproportionately held by low-income immigrant women – are often found caring for the elderly or disabled in close quarters, with no access to personal protective equipment (PHI 2014; Cahan 2020). Despite the risks of such close contacts, these low-wage workers need their jobs to survive and support their families. Yet even when workers are prepared to assume the risks, concerns about the coronavirus may cause employers to cut back on household assistance, resulting in loss of pay for these already-vulnerable workers (ILO 2020).

Prison populations worldwide, where groups marginalized by race or class are often over-represented, generally find physical distancing impossible because they cannot control their own spaces. In Brazil's overcrowded prisons, for instance, healthy prisoners cannot avoid contact with those who have contracted COVID-19 (Teixeira 2020). In China, Uighurs confined to concentration camps likewise lack the freedom to ensure their own safety by physical distancing (Chaudry 2020).

In India, scholars used the lens of a 'Physical Distance Readiness Index' to demonstrate that poorer households were less equipped to physically distance, a limitation that correlated with higher rates of disease (Lingam & Sapkal 2020). The index identified five necessities for physical distancing: '(a) access to safe drinking water; (b) access to clean toilets in the home/within their residential premises; (c) access to electricity; (d) income security … and finally (e) access to mobile phone and Internet' (Lingam & Sapkal 2020). Because many people lacked these basic amenities and had to travel and interact with others to gain access to them, efforts at physical distancing failed, with significant consequences for the nation's public health (Lingam & Sapkal 2020).

Denial of the human right to adequate housing increases individuals' vulnerabilities (Rajogopal 2020). The economic geography that places low-income people in densely settled areas with shared amenities and impediments to physical distancing is typical worldwide. Many urban residents live in informal settlements where cramped living conditions and inadequate public services, especially lack of water and sanitation, can exacerbate risk of contagion. For example, one-fifth of residents of Latin America live in informal settlements (Henderson 2020). Conditions contributing to their disproportionate experience of COVID-19 include 'overcrowding, malnutrition, deficient sewer systems, limited (and often paid) access to drinkable water, overwhelmed or unaffordable health services and indoor air pollution from cooking (with open fires or simple stoves, for example)' (Henderson 2020).

In Europe, Roma communities are often denied spaces needed to physically distance. Instead, Roma are restricted to locations that lack water, sanitation, transportation access, communication infrastructure, and other essentials needed for effective self-isolation during a pandemic. For some Roma communities, these challenges are compounded by an atmosphere in which hate speech and racial targeting further curtail their movements. For example, in Bulgaria, entire Roma communities were summarily quarantined during the pandemic, depriving many residents of work and education opportunities as well as access to health care. This targeting of informal Roma communities is found across Europe, a troubling occurrence rendered even more serious at a time when community members may have special health needs (EU FRA 2020).

A community's population density may not be the sole determining factor in exposure to COVID-19, but the quality of one's place of residence matters (Kadi & Khelfauoi 2020). Residents who lack open space and adequate infrastructure, who share taps and latrines, are more vulnerable to disease, yet this is the status quo in much of the world. In South Africa, for instance, only 73 percent of the population had access to hand-washing facilities on their premises, as of the most recent government survey in 2019 (South Africa 2020). About 30 percent of residents of the Navajo Nation in the United States, a COVID-19 hot spot, lack running water (Dig Deep 2019). Refugee camps are particularly susceptible to the spread of COVID-19 among residents (Alemi et al. 2020). Similarly, Brazil's overcrowded favelas, home to hundreds of thousands of residents, lack water and sewage infrastructure and are ill-equipped to prevent the spread of COVID-19 (Froio 2020). Given the need to share public amenities such as communal toilets and taps, people in such settings can seldom maintain safe physical distances from one another.

In the United States, the Brookings Institution found, unsurprisingly, that more affluent people were more likely to be in a position to avert the threat of disease by maintaining physical distances from others (Reeves & Rothwell 2020). Their distancing advantage – being able to work remotely, to afford home deliveries of food or other necessities, and even to relocate to less densely-populated areas – compounded the health advantages already experienced by the more affluent, such as fewer underlying health conditions (Miranda et al. 2019). In contrast, homeless families sharing crowded living spaces were found to be at substantially higher risk of COVID-19 transmission, with little recourse for avoiding close contact with others (Abrams & Szefler 2020).

Indoor space is not the only space that is at a premium for low-income people. Public health experts indicate that outdoor activities are generally safer than indoor activities in terms of COVID-19 transmission. In fact, the connection between lack of access to public space and heightened disease transmission was well-understood long before the 2020 pandemic (Wang & Lan 2019). Yet lower income people are unlikely to have access to private outdoor space such as a yard, porch, or balcony (Kim 2015). Further, public outdoor spaces such as parks or urban forests are more likely to be found in wealthier neighborhoods (Hays 2019). Access to open space is correlated with race as well as class. For example, a study in South Africa found that suburbs inhabited mainly by whites had the highest area of green space per capita, while low-cost housing occupied by poor black South Africans was 'poorly endowed' with green space relative to other suburban areas (McConnachie & Shackleton 2010). These disparities are compounded when members of marginalized or minority communities are made to feel uncomfortable, unwelcome and threatened in spaces ostensibly denominated as 'public' but that are, in practice, reserved for majority populations (Coda 2020).

No wonder that the WHO Commission on Social Determinants of Health Report in 2008 stated that it is not diseases but social injustice that kills people (Marmot et al. 2008). In that same report, the WHO Commission noted the overlaps, and conceptual and practical connections between the social determinants of health and the norms of human rights (Kenyon et al. 2018). Violations of the human rights to adequate housing and social supports have a causal effect on health vulnerabilities. The unequal impacts of COVID-19 reflect, among other things, the greater opportunities for more affluent people to maintain physical distance and healthy practices, in indoor and outdoor spaces, and at work, home and school. Pre-pandemic inequalities laid the foundation for differential susceptibility to disease. It is no surprise, then, that COVID-19 illness and death disproportionately affect lower income and economically marginalized people in both the Global South and the Global North (Drefahl et al. 2020).

3 Systemic racial inequalities

Inequalities in digital access and personal space are, in theory, vertical inequalities that are not identity-based per se, but that cut across ethnic and racial lines based on income. In contrast, race-based inequalities have historically been identified as classic horizontal inequalities where, either overtly or through systemic biases, benefits have been distributed based on group identity and membership (MacNaughton 2017). As illustrated in the discussion above, however, so-called horizontal inequalities very often contain a (generally covert) vertical element; in particular, access to digital technology and public space is not allocated solely based on happenstance or even economic class, but also on race, ethnicity, gender, and other identities.

Collectively, these covert and overt vertical inequalities have devastating impacts in the context of the COVID-19 pandemic. Around the globe, COVID-19 has had the most serious consequences for marginalized groups within societies, particularly racial minorities. In the United States, African Americans and Latinos are significantly more likely than whites to experience negative impacts from COVID-19 (Gold et al. 2020). Indigenous populations in the United States have also experienced significant outbreaks and disproportionate numbers of deaths (Hatcher 2020). In Europe, where Roma people are marginalized across the continent and often lack access to water and sanitation, Roma are disproportionately affected (EU FRA 2020). In China, members of the Uighur Muslim minority, unable to physically distance and already persecuted by the government authorities in ways that violate human rights, are susceptible to increased health risks from the pandemic (Chaudry 2020). In Brazil, black Brazilians and indigenous workers, often dependent on the informal economy to make a living, are more likely to be exposed to the virus (Baqui et al. 2020).

Since the virus does not itself make distinctions based on race or ethnicity, the explanation for these disparities must lie elsewhere. In fact, the virus, like any disease, seeks out those who are most vulnerable in health terms and those who are in the wrong place at the wrong time, i.e., unprotected and coming into contact with someone carrying the disease. For many, that vulnerability is driven by the multiple ways in which racism is structurally embedded into societies. Human rights violations such as economic distress, lack of access to health care or the means to maintain basic hygiene, inadequate housing, inability to physically distance, hunger, thirst, lack of access to technology, poor educational opportunities, heightened stress – all of these are experienced unequally and more frequently by racial and ethnic minorities than others in any given community. Most of these factors increase the likelihood that an individual will contract COVID-19. Once COVID-19 is contracted, structural racism can lead to serious health and economic consequences, as treatment options and medical decisions may continue to be influenced by racial bias (Hall et al. 2015).

The experience in Brazil offers an example of how a range of race-based inequalities come together to increase the risk of COVID-19. At the beginning of the pandemic, Brazil did not maintain records of death rates based on race (Shenoy 2020). However, as deaths accumulated, the racially disparate impact was increasingly clear. In April 2020, the Brazilian Health Ministry noted high COVID-19 death rates nationwide among Afro-Brazilians (Caldwell & Araújo 2020). Researchers confirmed that hospitalized Afro-Brazilians were significantly more likely to die of COVID-19 than hospitalized whites (Bacqui et al. 2020). According to one report, in the hardest hit state of São Paulo, 'people of color are 62 percent more likely to die from the virus than whites' (Caldwell & Araújo 2020).

Examining this evidence, researchers Kia Lilly Caldwell and Edna Maria de Araújo (2020) concluded that 'structural racism – in the form of high-risk working conditions, unequal access to health and worse housing conditions – is a major factor shaping Brazil's COVID-19 pandemic'. While the pandemic's racially-identified spread in Brazil was not inevitable, they wrote, '[t]he racism that pervades nearly every facet of Brazilian society increases black people's exposure to the virus – then reduces their ability to get to quality care' (Caldwell & Maria de Araújo 2020).

Brazil's story is parallel to that found in other countries and among other racial and ethnic groups like African Americans, indigenous peoples, Uighurs, and Roma. In each of these cases, structures of systemic racism embedded in societal institutions predictably dictate the disparate spread and dire impacts of the pandemic.

4 How we respond: reasons for hope

The inequalities surfaced by COVID-19 are serious and life-threatening for individuals and communities. Their increased visibility during the pandemic may also create opportunities to use a human rights framework to make headway in addressing these issues.

First, as for digital inequalities, it remains to be seen whether COVID-19 will make a permanent dent in the digital divide, but there are some hopeful signs. Certainly, school districts going forward will face pressure to be more fully prepared to provide equitable access to instruction in the event of future pandemics. The Brookings Institution offers a number of suggestions on how to engage the larger community, including corporate citizens, in expanding internet and equipment access to students (Lee 2020). UNICEF argues that governments must 'scale up remote learning opportunities for all children, especially the most marginalized'. The agency admonishes governments to '[f]ind innovative ways – including online, TV and radio – to keep children learning, no matter what' (Miks & McIlwaine 2020). As internet access expands, it will also expand human rights beyond the educational setting – for example, enabling adults to more fully participate in their communities despite physical distancing requirements.

Second, as to spatial inequalities, expanded access to both housing and outdoor space is critical to long-term management of COVID-19 and future pandemics. Investments in achieving the human right to adequate housing by banning forced evictions and providing homes to the homeless, including efforts to address safe access to water and sanitation, would not only moderate social injustice but also fulfill human rights obligations and frustrate the spread of disease. The UN Special Rapporteur on the Right to Adequate Housing's annual report to the UN General Assembly for 2020 takes COVID-19 into account in setting out short- and long-term goals in the area of housing (Rajogopal 2020). It is important, too, that space – not housing alone – be considered. Again, there are hopeful signs, including measured releases of prisoners and efforts to re-purpose vacant hotels and other spaces for those who need adequate, safe shelter – measures that were unimaginable prior to the pandemic. For those employees – including many essential workers – who cannot maintain physical distance while performing their jobs, protective equipment should be mandated and provided by the employer or the State.

Activism around these issues has already made a difference, as many states and local communities adopted short-term moratoria on evictions and utility shut-offs, and offered free COVID-19 testing and distribution of masks. Though positive, these short-term measures must be transitioned into longer term solutions grounded in human rights. Continued pressure is critical to changing the political calculus and encouraging governments to take decisive action – both domestically through social supports and internationally through foreign aid – to address and ameliorate the fundamental spatial inequalities that made COVID-19 so potent.

Third, the challenges of dismantling the systemic racism embedded in both institutional structures and individual decision making are daunting. In the United States, the Black Lives Matter (BLM) Movement has drawn moral authority not only from the horrific and pervasive examples of police violence against black and brown people, but also from the clear evidence that COVID-19 is disproportionately devastating the African-American community. The demands put forward by the BLM movement regarding the pandemic are specific to the United States, but may suggest ways that activists elsewhere could take steps to dismantle systemic racism as well, while increasing accountability at all levels of government decision making. Among these demands are more data collection concerning impacts of COVID-19 on people of color, greater access to COVID-19 testing in black communities, stepped up access to medical care for those affected by the pandemic, and greater controls over medical information (BLM 2020).

For all of these issues, the ultimate question is whether there exists the political will to address the COVID-19-aided inequalities that are diminishing the lives of, and in some cases literally killing, members of marginalized communities. Because preserving public health requires collective commitments and action, this may require politicians and policy makers to look beyond the narrow interests that often drive their decision making.

Rather, if the twentieth century was the era in which *individual* human rights were defined and articulated through the UDHR and other human rights instruments, the twenty-first century demands a wider vision of our shared humanity. To move forward in the face of the existential crises of this century, we must now recognize the ways in which our individual rights and interests are *collectively* intertwined and interdependent. The global challenge of climate change is the obvious example of a crisis that requires a new paradigm. Individual rights are at stake, certainly, but only individuals, communities, and nations working together and in coordination to protect collective rights and interests will be enough to make a difference in the outcome. COVID-19, and the future pandemics that we know will come, pose a similar challenge. Masks, hygienic practices, physical distancing, vaccinations, and other practices designed to promote the public health must be adopted widely in order to effectively combat the deadly contagion; partial or occasional compliance with these measures – or uneven distribution and access – will ensure that the efforts fall short, with repercussions beyond the individual.

This relational perspective is an inherent component of equality. Indeed, the notions of solidarity and linked interests that implicitly underpin equality mark a fundamental difference between the concepts of poverty and inequality. Unlike static definitions of poverty, such as the $1.90/day standard adopted by some international institutions, inequality is a dynamic measure explicitly connected to others in the community. Inequality – and also the concept of relative poverty – exist only in reference to the actions and activities of others. In an important sense, then, addressing inequality is a responsibility that we all bear, because we are all contributors to one degree or another to its creation and persistence. In the context of COVID-19, it is fair to say that the pandemic has exposed both the human rights dangers posed by pervasive inequality and our collective responsibility to use human rights mechanisms to respond to those inequalities.

References

Abrams, E & Szefler, S 2020, 'COVID-19 and the Impact of Social Determinants of Health', *The Lancet*, vol. 8, no. 7, pp. 659–661.

Alemi, Q, Stempel, C, Siddiq, H, & Kim, E 2020, 'Refugees and COVID-19: Achieving a Comprehensive Public Health Response', *Bulletin of the World Health Organization,* vol. 98, No. 8, doi: http://dx.doi.org/10.2471/BLT.20.271080

Alston, P 2015, 'Extreme Inequality as the Antithesis of Human Rights', *OpenGlobalRights*, 27 August, viewed 5 December 2020, www.openglobalrights.org/extreme-inequality-as-the-antithesis-of-human-rights/

Asim, S, Carvalho, S, & Gera R 2020, 'Learning Equity During the Coronavirus: Experiences from Africa', *World Bank Blogs* 3 June 2020, viewed 10 March 2021, https://blogs.worldbank.org/education/learning-equity-during-coronavirus-experiences-africa

Baqui, P, Bica, I, Marra, V, Ercole, A, & van der Schaar, M 2020, 'Ethnic and Regional Variations in Hospital Mortality from COVID-19 in Brazil: a Cross-sectional Observational Study', *The Lancet*, vol. 8, no. 8.

Beaunoyer, E, Dupéré, S, & Guitton, MJ 2020, 'COVID-19 and Digital Inequalities: Reciprocal Impacts and Mitigation Strategies', *Computers in Human Behavior*, vol. 111, 106424, viewed 10 March 2021, doi: https://doi.org/10.1016/j.chb.2020.106424

Black Lives Matter 2020, 'Black Lives Matter Global Network Responses to COVID-19 Ethnicity Data', 9 April, viewed 5 December 2020, https://blacklivesmatter.com/black-lives-matter-global-network-responses-to-covid-19-ethnicity-data/

Busby, J & Tanberk, J 2020, 'FCC Underestimates Americans Unserved by Broadband Internet by 50%', *BroadbandNow*, viewed March 10, 2021, https://broadbandnow.com/research/fcc-underestimates-unserved-by-50-percent.

Cahan, E 2020, 'Most Home Health Aides "Can't Afford Not to Work" – Even When Lacking PPE', *KHN*, 10 Oct., viewed 10 March 2021.

Caldwell, KL & de Araújo, EM 2020, 'In Brazil, Structural Racism Has Made COVID-19 Far Deadlier for Black People', *Foreign Policy in Focus*, viewed 5 December 2020, https://fpif.org/in-brazil-structural-racism-has-made-covid-19-far-deadlier-for-black-people/

Chaudry, V 2020, 'The Impact of COVID-19 on Uighur Muslims: An Ignored Crisis', London School of Economics Human Rights Blog, 23 April, viewed 5 December 2020, https://blogs.lse.ac.uk/humanrights/2020/04/23/the-impact-of-covid-19-on-uighur-muslims-an-ignored-crisis/

Coda, JI 2020, 'Gender-Inclusive Cities: Can Urban Planning Take into Account Women and Minorities', *World Bank*, viewed 5 December 2020, www.worldbank.org/en/news/feature/2020/03/07/ciudades-feministas-diseno-urbano-para-mujeres-y-minorias

DigDeep 2019. 'Closing The Water Access Gap In The United States', viewed 5 December 2020, http://uswateralliance.org/sites/uswateralliance.org/files/Closing%20the%20Water%20Access%20Gap%20in%20the%20United%20States_DIGITAL.pdf

Dorn, E., Hancock, B, Sarakatsannis, J, & Viruleg, E 2020, 'COVID-19 and Student Learning in the United States: The Hurt Could Last a Lifetime', *McKinsey*, 9 June 2020, viewed 10 March 2021, www.mckinsey.com/industries/public-and-social-sector/our-insights/covid-19-and-student-learning-in-the-united-states-the-hurt-could-last-a-lifetime

Drefahl, S, Wallace, M, Messino, E, Aradhya, S, Kolk, M, Brandén, Malmberg, B & Andersson, G 2020, 'A Population-based Cohort Study of Socio-Demographic Risk Factors for COVID-19 Deaths in Sweden'. *Nature Communications*, vol. 11, doi: https://doi.org/10.1038/s41467-020-18926-3

European Union Agency for Fundamental Rights (EU FRA) 2020, 'Coronavirus Pandemic in the EU – Impact on Roma and Travellers', 30 June, viewed 5 December 2020, https://fra.europa.eu/sites/default/files/fra_uploads/fra-2020-coronavirus-pandemic-eu-bulletin-roma_en.pdf

Felter, C & Maizland, L 2020, 'How Countries Are Reopening Schools During the Pandemic', *Council on Foreign Relations*, www.cfr.org/backgrounder/how-countries-are-reopening-schools-during-pandemic

Froio, N 2020, 'Brazil's Vulnerable Left Behind in the Pandemic', *NACLA*, 31 March, viewed 10 March 2021, https://nacla.org/news/2020/03/31/brazil-favelas-covid19

Gettleman, J & Raj, S 2020, 'As Covid-19 Closes Schools, the World's Children Go to Work', *New York Times*, 27 Sept, viewed 5 December 2020, www.nytimes.com/2020/09/27/world/asia/covid-19-india-children-school-education-labor.html?action=click&module=Top%20Stories&pgtype=Homepage

Gold, J, Rossen, L, Ahmad, F, Sutton, P, Zeyu, L, Salvatore, P, Coyle, J, DeCuir, J, Baack, B, Durant, T, Dominiguez, K, Henley, J, Annor, F, Fuld, J, Dee, D, Bhattaraj, A, & Jackson, B 2020, 'Race, Ethnicity and Age Trends in Persons Who Died from COVID-19 – United States, May–August 2020', Morbidity and Mortality Weekly Report, Centers for Disease Control and Prevention, vol. 69, pp. 1517–1521, 23 Oct., viewed 10 March 2021, www.cdc.gov/mmwr/volumes/69/wr/mm6942e1.htm

Hall, W, Chapman, M, Lee, K, Merino, Y, Thomas, T, Payne, B, Eng, E, Day, S & Coyne-Beasley, T 2015, 'Implicit Racial/Ethnic Bias Among Health Care Professionals and Its Influence on Health Care Outcomes: A Systematic Review', *American Journal of Public Health*, vol. 105, no. 12.

Hatcher S, Agnw-Brune, C, Anderson, M, et al. 2020, 'COVID-19 Among American Indian and Alaska Native Persons – 23 States, January 31, July 3, 2020', *Morbidity and Mortality Weekly Report, Centers for Disease Control and Prevention*, vol. 69, pp. 1166–1169, 28 Aug., viewed 10 March 2021, www.cdc.gov/mmwr/volumes/69/wr/mm6934e1.htm

Hays, B, 2019, 'Study: Access to Urban Green Spaces Favor the Rich, Educated', *United Press International*, 17 January, viewed 5 December 2020, www.upi.com/Science_News/2019/01/17/Study-Access-to-urban-green-spaces-favor-the-rich-educated/7741547742967/

Henderson, H, 2020, 'From the COVID-19 Epicentre: Lessons from Latin American Cities' Success and Failures', *The Conversation*, 16 August, viewed 5 December 2020, https://theconversation.com/from-the-covid-19-epicentre-lessons-from-latin-american-cities-successes-and-failures-144000

International Labor Organization 2020, 'Policy Brief: A Gender-Responsive Employment Recovery: Building Back Fairer', ILO, viewed 10 March 2021, www.ilo.org/wcmsp5/groups/public/---ed_emp/documents/publication/wcms_751785.pdf

Kadi, N & Khelfaoui, M 2020, 'Population Density, a Factor in the Spread of COVID-19 in Algeria: Statistic Study', *Bulletin of the National Research Centre*, vol. 44, no. 138.

Kameel, S 2020, 'Libraries are Needed More Than Ever. But Many Aren't Sure How to Reopen Amid the Coronavirus Pandemic', *USA Today*, 11 June, viewed 5 December 2020, www.usatoday.com/story/news/2020/06/11/when-libraries-reopen-after-coronavirus-might-months/5316591002/

Kenyon, K.H., Forman, L, & Brolan, C.E. 2018, 'Deepening the Relationship between Human Rights and the Social Determinants of Health: A Focus on Indivisibility and Power', *Health and Human Rights*, vol. 20, no. 2, pp. 1–10.

Kim, S 2015, 'Public Spaces – Not a "Nice to Have" but a Basic Need for Cities', *World Bank Blogs*, 30 March, viewed 5 December 2020, https://blogs.worldbank.org/endpovertyinsouthasia/public-spaces-not-nice-have-basic-need-cities

Lee, NT 2020, 'How Courageous Schools Partnering with Local Communities Can Overcome Digital Inequalities During COVID-19', *Brookings Institution*, 17 September, viewed 5 December 2020, www.brookings.edu/blog/techtank/2020/09/17/how-courageous-schools-partnering-with-local-communities-can-overcome-digital-inequalities-during-covid-19/

Lingam, L & Sapkal, RS 2020. 'COVID-19, Physical Distancing and Social Inequalities: Are We all Really in this Together?', *International Journal of Community and Social Development*, vol. 2, no. 2, p. 173.

MacNaughton, G 2017, 'Vertical Inequalities: Are the SDGs and Human Rights up to the Challenges?', *The International Journal of Human Rights*, vol. 21, no. 8, pp. 1050–1072.

Marmot, M, Friel, S, Bell R, Houweling, T, & Taylor, S 2008, 'Closing the Gap in a Generation: Health Equity Through Action on the Social Determinants of Health', *The Lancet* vol. 372, pp. 1661–1669, 8 Nov. 2008, viewed 10 March 2021, https://www.thelancet.com/journals/lancet/article/PIIS0140-6736(08)61690-6/fulltext

McConnachie, MM & Shackleton, CM 2010, 'Public Green Space Inequality in Small Towns in South Africa', *Habitat International*, vol. 34, no. 2.

Miks, J & McIlwaine, J 2020, 'Keeping the World's Children Learning through COVID-19', *UNICEF*, 20 April, viewed 5 December 2020, www.unicef.org/coronavirus/keeping-worlds-children-learning-through-covid-19

Miller, C 2020, 'In the Same Towns, Private Schools are Reopening While Public Schools are Not', *New York Times*, 20 July.

Miranda, J, Barrientos-Gutiérrez, T, Corvalan, C, Hyder, A, Lazzo-Porras, M, Oni, T, & Well, J 2019, 'Understanding the Rise of Cardiometabolic Diseases in Low- and Middle-income Countries', *Nat Med* vol. 25, pp. 1667–1679, doi: https://doi.org/10.1038/s41591-019-0644-7

Moynihan, C 2020, 'Most Libraries Are Closed. Some Librarians Still Have to Go In', *New York Times*, 14 April, viewed 5 December 2020, www.nytimes.com/2020/04/14/arts/library-workers-us-coronavirus.html

PHI 2014, 'U.S. Home Care Workers: Key Facts', PHI, viewed 10 March 2021, https://phinational.org/wp-content/uploads/legacy/phi-home-care-workers-key-facts.pdf

Poon, L 2020, 'There are Far More Americans Without Broadband Access Than Previously Thought', *Bloomberg CityLab*, 19 Feb. 2020, viewed 10 March 2020, www.bloomberg.com/news/articles/2020-02-19/where-the-u-s-underestimates-the-digital-divide

Rajagopal, B 2020, 'COVID-19 and the Right to Housing: Impacts and the Way Forward', visited 10 March 2021, www.ohchr.org/Documents/Issues/Housing/COVID19andHousingReportSummary.pdf

Reeves, R & Rothwell, J 2020, 'Class and COVID: How the Less Affluent Face Double Risks', *Brookings Institution*, 27 March, viewed 5 December 2020, www.brookings.edu/blog/up-front/2020/03/27/class-and-covid-how-the-less-affluent-face-double-risks/

Salomon, M. 2011, 'Why Should it Matter that Others Have More? Poverty, Inequality, and the Potential of International Human Rights Law', *Review of International Studies*, vol. 37, no. 5, pp. 2137–2155.

Shenoy, R 2020, 'Advocates Raise Alarm as Countries Fail to Collect Racial Data of Coronavirus Patients', *The World*, 24 April, viewed 5 December 2020, www.pri.org/stories/2020-04-24/advocates-raise-alarm-countries-fail-collect-racial-data-coronavirus-patients

Simmons, KW 1985, 'Equality As A Comparative Right', *Boston University Law Review*, vol. 65, no. 3, pp. 387–482.

Slattery, G & Gaier, R 2000, 'A Brazilian Woman Caught Coronavirus on Vacation. Her Maid Is Now Dead', *Reuters*, 24 March 2020, viewed 10 March 2021, www.reuters.com/article/us-health-coronavirus-rio/a-brazilian-woman-caught-coronavirus-on-vacation-her-maid-is-now-dead-idUSKBN21B1HT

South Africa, 'General Household Survey', p. 39, Table 10.1, www.statssa.gov.za/publications/P0318/P03182019.pdf

Stanley, K 2020, 'Libraries are Needed More than Ever, but Many aren't Sure how to Reopen amid the Coronavirus Pandemic', *USA Today*, 11 June 2020, viewed 10 March 2020, www.usatoday.com/story/news/2020/06/11/when-libraries-reopen-after-coronavirus-might-months/5316591002/

Strauss, V 2020, 'How Relationships between Teachers and Students are Being Tested in COVID-19 Crisis', *Washington Post* 22 April 2020, viewed 10 March 2020, www.washingtonpost.com/education/2020/04/22/how-relationships-between-teachers-students-are-being-tested-covid-19-crisis/

Suneson, G & Stebbins, S 2019, 'These 15 Countries Have the Widest Gaps Between Rich and Poor', *USA Today*, 28 May, viewed 5 December 2020, www.usatoday.com/story/money/2019/05/28/countries-with-the-widest-gaps-between-rich-and-poor/39510157/

Teixeira F 2020, 'In Brazil's Overcrowded Jails, COVID-19 Breeds Fear and Calls for Change', *Reuters* 16 June, viewed 10 March 2021, https://news.trust.org/item/20200616041603-lub3f/

UNESCO 2020, 'Startling Digital Divides in Distance Learning Emerge', *UNESCO*, 4 April 2020, viewed 10 March 2021, https://en.unesco.org/news/startling-digital-divides-distance-learning-emerge

UNICEF 2020, 'UNICEF Executive Director Henrietta Fore remarks at a press Conference on New Updated Guidance on School-related Public Health Measures in the Context of COVID-19', viewed 5 December 2020, www.unicef.org/press-releases/unicef-executive-director-henrietta-fore-remarks-press-conference-new-updated

United Nations Department of Economic and Social Affairs 2020, 'World Social Report 2020: Inequality in a Rapidly Changing World', viewed 5 December 2020, www.un.org/development/desa/dspd/wp-content/uploads/sites/22/2020/01/World-Social-Report-2020-FullReport.pdf

United Nations Economic and Social Council (ECOSOC) 2017, *Extract of the Recommendations on Promoting, Measuring, and Communicating the Value of Official Statistics*, ECE/CES/2017/4.

United Nations Human Rights Council 2020, *Right to Education: Impact of the Coronavirus Disease Crisis on the Right to Education – Concerns, Challenges and Opportunities*, A/HRC/44/39.

United Nations Population Fund 2020, 'Millions More Cases of Violence, Child Marriage, Female Genital Mutilation, Unintended Pregnancy Expected Due to the COVID-19 Pandemic', viewed 5 December 2020, www.unfpa.org/news/millions-more-cases-violence-child-marriage-female-genital-mutilation-unintended-pregnancies

Vegas, E 2020, 'School Closures, Government Responses, and Learning Inequality around the World During COVID-19', *Brookings Institution*, 14 April, viewed 5 December 2020, www.brookings.edu/research/school-closures-government-responses-and-learning-inequality-around-the-world-during-covid-19/

Wang, Q & Lan, Z 2019, 'Park Green Spaces, Public Health and Social Inequalities: Understanding the Interrelationships for Policy Implications', *Land Use Policy*, vol. 83, pp. 66–74.

Wexler, N 2020, 'For Some, Remote Learning Has Surprising Benefits', *Forbes*, 8 May, viewed 5 December 2020, www.forbes.com/sites/nataliewexler/2020/05/08/for-some-remote-learning-has-surprising-benefits/#275cea6d3695

World Bank Group, 2020, *Reversals of Fortune*, The World Bank, Washington DC.

6

RACIAL JUSTICE TO THE FOREFRONT

Do Black lives matter in international law?

Elina Castillo Jiménez

Something clearly shifted in our collective conscience when police killed George Floyd in Minneapolis on 25 May 2020. After months of enduring the challenges of a global public health emergency, watching a man die through our screens catalyzed what many may describe as one of the most notorious manifestations of outrage against anti-Black racism in decades.[1] Mid-2020 will likely be remembered as a pivotal moment for racial justice in the world.

Building on a COVID-19 coping mechanism, people also turned to social media to find solace and join global voices rallying for racial justice (Ramsden 2020). Black Lives Matter was mentioned over 80 million times across Facebook, Twitter, and other social media platforms in the 30 days following the killing of George Floyd (Beckman 2020), and in June 2020, Black Lives Matter was the most frequent search on Google, reaching all-time record levels (Google Trends 2020). People also demonstrated in many cities across the United States and across the globe, demanding a stop to systemic racism.

The leap in public consciousness in 2020 is not a coincidence but the result of years of sustained grassroots work to uplift voices against anti-Black racism. Since the police killings in the United States of Trayvon Martin, Michael Brown, Philando Castille, and many others, the Black Lives Matter movement and others working to achieve racial justice have strengthened their campaigning and organizing capacities, expanding their supporters, developing their tactics, and building alliances across the region, despite many challenges (McFadden 2020). These movements have influenced academia, media, decision-makers, and even other movements to face the layered discrimination that people of African descent endure, consistently calling for effective policies to counteract its effects.

The limitations that systemic racism imposes on the fulfillment and realization of rights of people of African descent are not exclusive to the United States. In Latin America and the Caribbean (LAC), people of African descent, who account for at least 21 percent of the total population of the region, are disproportionately impacted by poverty and extreme poverty (CEPAL 2020a). Furthermore, people of African descent have historically endured structural inequalities that prevent them from fully enjoying their human rights (CEPAL 2020a). Excessive use of force against, and extrajudicial killings of, people of African descent are also important concerns (Amnesty International 2020a).

Since May 2020, a diversity of new voices has joined racial justice demands, including more conservative organizations such as the World Economic Forum, which after pushback from its younger members, is incorporating anti-systemic racism work into their agenda (Schwab & Malleret 2020). Many venture capital investment firms and enterprises have also pledged to invest in Black businesses as a contribution toward alleviating the socioeconomic disadvantages faced by people of African descent. Similarly, in the weeks after the killing of George Floyd, an increased number of non-Black adults in the United States reported having: joined activist efforts in support of racial justice, talked about racial equality with family and friends, and accessed more resources to educate themselves and others on the issue (Parker, Menasce Horowitz, & Anderson 2020).

If structural discrimination and inequalities have been documented for decades, why now has there been a marked increase in individuals, organizations, and institutions not only paying close attention but actively calling for measures to dismantle systemic racism? COVID-19 has surely played a role. In many countries in the Americas, people have been asked or forced to stay home. Among those who can comply with these measures, recent studies show an increase of social media consumption (Koeze & Popper 2020). Watching the social developments described above, I believe it is no longer possible to ignore the inequalities that sustain our systems, nor the calls for transformative measures that can help to address them.

COVID-19 has laid bare the deeply-rooted inequalities in our societies. It is difficult to ignore the multilayered and disproportionate direct impact that this unprecedented global public health challenge has had on marginalized groups, particularly on racialized communities. However, as the reactions to the killings of George Floyd, Breonna Taylor, and others across the globe show, racial justice in the context of COVID-19 has taken on particular characteristics, not only in the way activists and movements are organizing themselves, but also in the way that international and regional human rights mechanisms are responding.

This chapter explores the intersections between racial justice and COVID-19 with two main questions: how have United Nations and regional human rights mechanisms responded to demands to dismantle systemic racism in the context of COVID-19? And, what changes and new insights from those responses can be identified and considered, for the future of the racial justice movement and international human rights law (IHRL)? As I look for answers, I will in section 1 briefly assess the situation of people of African descent and COVID-19 in the Americas. In section 2, I will analyze how UN and Inter-American spaces have approached systemic racism in the context of COVID-19 and whether there is space for developing more effective standards. To conclude, I will provide some insights for campaigning for racial justice within the framework of IHRL.

1 Not a coincidence: disparate impacts of COVID-19 as a reflection of systemic racism

The experience of people of African descent in the Americas demonstrates how COVID-19 has impacted us all but not in the same way. With a legacy of unfulfilled human rights, it is no coincidence that people of African descent are in this disadvantaged position. Poverty, informal work, and police violence, embedded in structural discrimination, are factors that lead to this outcome.

In the United States for example, Black, Indigenous, and Latinx families are losing significantly more loved ones to COVID-19 than Whites. Black individuals are dying at a rate that is double or higher than that of White individuals nationwide (The COVID-19 Tracking Project 2020). Black Americans, who represent less than 15 percent of the national population, are 23–24 percent of the national deaths linked to COVID-19 (AMP Research Lab 2020). COVID-19 itself may not discriminate, but our societies do. And that has translated into a disparate impact on certain communities.

Most available epidemiologic records on COVID-19 from LAC do not disaggregate data by ethnicity (UNFPA 2020). However, the case of Brazil, with one of the largest Afro-descendent populations in the region, shows similar patterns. The Brazilian Ministry of Health flagged higher death rates among Afro-Brazilians early in the pandemic (O Globo 2020). In Rio de Janeiro and São Paulo, historically Afro-Brazilian neighborhoods reported higher death rates due to COVID-19 than White urban areas, with one of every three Afro-Brazilians hospitalized due to COVID-19, compared to one of every 4.4 White Brazilians (Muniz, Fonseca, & Pina 2020). In a review of over 5,500 municipalities, 55 percent of Afro-Brazilians hospitalized due to severe COVID-19 complications died, compared to 34 percent of White Brazilians (Caldwell & Araújo 2020).

Medical studies have found that resilience to COVID-19 is influenced by conditions related to quality of life or social determinants of health (Bambra et al. 2020). Concretely then, marginalized communities, such as people of African descent, face heightened risks to COVID-19 due to historical inequalities and discrimination (CDC 2020; McGonagle et al. 2020). For Afro-descendent communities in the Americas, COVID-19 is a pandemic on top of other long-standing public health challenges.

One challenge is poverty and extreme poverty, which can significantly compromise quality of life, including by limiting access to quality healthcare services, adequate housing, clean water, and social security protection (CIDH 2017). Extreme poverty and poverty levels, as well as the risk of falling into poverty, are significantly higher among people of African descent in LAC in comparison with non-Indigenous and non-Afro-descendent people (CEPAL 2020a). In Brazil and Peru, for example, extreme poverty is almost three times higher among people of African descent, and 41 percent of people living in poverty in Colombia are of African descent (CEPAL 2020a). Gender inequalities put women, girls, and LGBTIQ people of African descent at a heightened risk of poverty (CEPAL 2018).

LAC remains 'the most unequal, not the poorest' region in the world (Noticias ONU 2018). COVID-19 is expected to widen these inequality gaps by disproportionately impacting marginalized communities and increasing their risk of extreme poverty due to income loss and lack of social security protection (CEPAL 2020b). The sustained increase of poverty levels since 2015 sparked several protests across Latin America and the Caribbean through 2019 and well into 2020, despite COVID-19 restrictions, as people demanded better public policies to promote socioeconomic equality and reduce corruption in countries such as Haiti, Chile, and Ecuador (Latin America Risk Report 2020).

For people of African descent in the United States, the situation is not too different. Nationwide, even though the national poverty rate was about 12 percent, over 20 percent of Black people in 2018 were living in poverty (Semega et al. 2019). Black households across the country earn less than 60 percent the income of White households (Luhby 2020). Similar to LAC, people of African descent in the United States are also particularly at risk in terms of job security, health, and COVID-19; with a high prevalence in informal work and front-line industries, many have either fallen into unemployment or they are essential workers, therefore more exposed, together with their families, to COVID-19 (Gould & Wilson 2020).

Another significant public health challenge for people of African descent in the Americas, compounding with COVID-19 and poverty, is violence, particularly by police. In the United States, as of November 2020, Black individuals represent 28 percent of those killed during the year by police officers; 4 percent more than in 2019 (Mapping Police Violence 2020). Police kill Black men at more than twice the rate of White men, yet the population of Black people is less than 15 percent of the total US population (Washington Post 2020). The available data, as well as the heartbreaking public testimonies from victims' relatives, show that many Black families in the United States reasonably fear that one of their members could become one of these statistics (Edwards, Lee, & Esposito 2019).

In Latin America and the Caribbean, disenfranchised Black people face a similar context. People of African descent represented 75 percent of all police killings in 2019 in Rio de Janeiro (Lima, Sims, & Xavier 2020). In Colombia, the killing of taxi driver Javier Ordóñez in September 2020, allegedly under police custody after an encounter with officers in Bogotá, sparked protests that lasted for days, calling for accountability and an end to police abuse (Dickinson 2020). In the Dominican Republic and Jamaica, poor youth and women – often of darker skin – face a higher risk of being arbitrarily detained or tortured by police than any other group (Amnesty International 2016; Amnesty International 2019).

In this context, curfews or lockdowns imposed as a response to COVID-19 across LAC pose a high risk for those who depend on informal work, among whom people of African descent are disproportionately represented (CEPAL 2020a). Between hunger or the risk of the virus and possible criminalization, many are opting for the latter (ILO 2020). Therefore, poor, racialized people are at a high risk of enduring excessive use of force, arbitrary detentions, inhumane treatment, or other potential human rights violations by law enforcement officers (Amnesty International 2020b). This important context shows that people of African descent in the Americas face specific, historical, systemic, and unjustified disadvantages.

Racial discrimination is sanctioned by IHRL. However, as the next section describes, international standards fail to fully grasp the depth and complexity of the systems in which it takes place. But there might be a window of opportunity arising from the developments of 2020 on racial justice, spurred in part by COVID-19.

2 Reacting to systemic racism during COVID-19: a missed opportunity?

Early in the pandemic, the OHCHR and the IACHR issued guidelines on COVID-19 and human rights, including references to the differentiated impact on marginalized communities, such as people of African descent, and the need for states to adopt specific measures for their protection. The OHCHR also expressed concern over data indicating the disproportionate impact of the pandemic on people of African descent (OHCHR 2020b).

Such expressions of concern regarding the situation of people of African descent significantly increased after the killing of George Floyd and the protests that followed. For example, UN experts condemned 'modern-day racial terror lynchings' in the United States (OHCHR 2020c). The CERD urged the United States to 'unequivocally and unconditionally reject and condemn racially motivated killings of African Americans and other minorities' (CERD 2020, p. 1). Over twenty UN Under-Secretaries General of African descent called on the UN to step up and take action to end racial injustice, because 'to merely condemn expressions and acts of racism is not enough' (UN News 2020a).

However, in June–July 2020, a key development on racial justice and COVID-19 took place in the international human rights law community when the Human Rights Council (HRC) convened an urgent debate at the request of the African Group of Countries and civil society organizations, led by the American Civil Liberties Union (UN News 2020b). What insights can be gathered from this debate?

2.1 The debate at the Human Rights Council: an opportunity catalyzed by COVID-19, then missed?

The debate, which began on June 17, was focused on 'current racially inspired human rights violations, systemic racism, police brutality and violence against peaceful protests', in reaction to the urgent demands for racial justice sparked since May 25 (OHCHR 2020a). The main goal was to hold a vote on the establishment of an independent international commission of inquiry regarding systemic racism in law enforcement in the United States, as well as a thematic commission for a more global analysis of the issues (OHCHR 2020a).

As the debate unfolded, the Special Rapporteur on racism and other Special Procedure mandate-holders urged the HRC to establish both a thematic commission and a country-specific commission 'with the necessary authority to investigate systemic racism in law enforcement in the United States' (OHCHR 2020d). The High Commissioner for Human Rights, indicating support for accountability, stated that decisive action was needed to 'address the pervasive racism that corrodes institutions of government, entrenches inequality and underlies so many violations of human rights' (OHCHR 2020e).

During the debate, several speakers of the Western European and Other States Group asserted that because racism is a global problem, focusing on one country would divide, instead of unite in the effort to tackle the problem (UN Web TV 2020). Israel and Australia, for example, implied that 'strong' or 'open, liberal democracies' should not be under this level of scrutiny before the HRC (Parmar 2020). Such positions appear to reinforce the idea that people of African descent killed by law enforcement are a sad occurrence, but not a matter worthy of being analyzed by special mechanisms such as an independent commission of inquiry.

Thus, despite the compelling case made and the attention garnered, the draft resolution originally calling for an international probe on specific facts and circumstances, was diluted to request the OHCHR and relevant Special Procedure mandate-holders to prepare a report on systemic racism, law enforcement, and human rights violations against people of African descent, taking into account the 'incidents' that led to the 'death' of George Floyd and states' responses to 'anti-racist peaceful protests' (UN News 2020b).

Although a report of this nature could be an important step towards improving IHRL responses to systemic racism, an independent commission of inquiry with a specific focus on systemic racism, in a country from the Global North, arguably would have been more transformative, as it could have paved a way for greater accountability on racial discrimination and law enforcement (Parmar 2020). What are we to make of the decision to call for a report instead of an international probe, when adopted against the backdrop of a global groundswell calling for truth, justice, and reparations?

In part, as the Special Rapporteur on racism bravely denounced, 'certain powerful and influential countries' may have used their geopolitical influence to shape the outcome of the debate (OHCHR 2020e). Consequently, a proposal for a novel model to address systemic racism using IHRL standards was blocked and with it, the possibilities of strengthening international accountability mechanisms, at least for the moment.

This debate is an example of a racial justice opportunity being catalyzed by COVID-19. Yet its outcomes also manifest the challenges that arise in response to calls to dismantle systemic racism. Advocates did not achieve the approval of a commission of inquiry in 2020, but perhaps they have achieved something else: they have highlighted some of the limitations and obstacles in fighting systemic racism through the Human Rights Council.

Shortly before the debate, over fifty UN human rights experts openly addressed systemic racism in a joint statement, stating that it 'produces state-sponsored racial violence, and licenses impunity for this violence' and calling on states to 'take this opportunity to address structural forms of racial and ethnic injustice' (OHCHR 2020g). By identifying racism not only as 'systemic' –meaning, spread through the foundations of our societies and permeating all our structures – but also as a cause of specific human rights violations, UN experts in this statement are pointing to a fundamental idea: that racial discrimination does not happen in a vacuum, but thrives within a web of prejudices and stigmas built not only on racial superiority, but on the very existence of races.

Nowadays, the prohibition of racial discrimination is a *jus cogens* norm: all states are required to take positive measures to protect individuals and peoples against it or could otherwise be found in breach of international obligations (ILC 2002). It is also present in a binding treaty, the International Convention on the Elimination of All Forms of Racial Discrimination (ICERD) – ratified by virtually all states – as well as the Durban Declaration, the 2030 Agenda, and the Sustainable Development Goals (SDGs). Discrimination on the basis of race or ethnic origin is also sanctioned in regional human rights treaties. Yet across the globe, people of African descent still face the inter-generational burdens of discrimination and exclusion that slavery and colonialism generated. Has COVID-19 and the increased demands for dismantling of systemic racism opened the door for more innovative and effective ways to leverage these and other tools?

2.2 Revisiting UN standards on racial discrimination: is there space to sanction systemic racism?

Very few of the current legal instruments on racial discrimination mention racism, and none of the ones that do are treaties (Bradley 2019). Existing binding tools within the UN system do not necessarily support an approach that takes into account the practices, institutions, and systems that sustain or cause racial discrimination as itself a violation of state obligations. This is critical because by not embracing such an approach, they limit the possibilities of holding states responsible for the very existence of systemic racism.

Article 1 of the ICERD (1969) defines racial discrimination as 'any distinction, exclusion, restriction or preference' arising from 'race, color, descent or national ethnic origin', with the purpose or effect of 'nullifying or impairing' the enjoyment and exercise of human rights in all spheres of life. Racial discrimination can be found where there is a specific act (a distinction, exclusion, restriction, or preference), with either the purpose (intention) or effect (impact) of causing an objectively unjustified differentiated treatment, in this case, due to 'race'. There is consensus that for an act to amount to racial discrimination under the ICERD, it is not necessary to find both a discriminatory purpose and effect (Malaihollo 2017). Thus, if a state's actions or omissions cause racial discrimination towards an individual or group, as defined in Article 1, it may be found in breach of the ICERD, even in the absence of intention.

Indeed, the inclusion of 'effect' in the ICERD definition considers statutes, policies, or practices that are not be based on discriminatory grounds on their face, but which have consequences that significantly and unjustifiably impact a particular ethnic or racial group or individual negatively (Malaihollo 2017). Employing this lens, the Committee for the Elimination of Racial Discrimination (CERD) has used contextual information to call for the implementation of certain measures. The Committee has also recognized that 'racism and racial discrimination against people of African descent are expressed in many forms, notably structural and cultural' (CERD 2011, p. 2).

However, although the CERD has acknowledged the existence of systemic or structural racism against people of African, it has yet to build on whether that acknowledgment could, by itself, support finding a breach of obligations under ICERD in certain circumstances. From the current ICERD standards, it appears that there is a subtle but important difference: the beliefs, practices, policies, institutions and systems that may drive or give place to racial discrimination can and have been considered by the CERD. However, it appears that the existence of systemic racism (as a root cause of racial discrimination) has not yet been found as a breach of an international obligation, in this case, a duty to prevent discrimination based on race, derived from the prohibition of racial discrimination. Making this link can be crucial to find state responsibility for systemic racism and its impact on people of African descent.

Despite available data that could help to demonstrate its existence and impact on state actions and omissions, arguing the existence of 'systemic racism' as a violation of the ICERD is challenging. It also appears to be that this silence as to whether systemic racism can be a violation itself, has been, somehow, understood as lack of illegality, or in other words, as not necessarily opening space for potential state responsibility (Hill-Cawthorne 2020). The failure to acknowledge state responsibility for systemic racism is at the heart of the limited progress during the debate at the HRC.

Notwithstanding this current approach under ICERD standards, recent references to 'structural' or 'systemic' racism as drivers or roots of internationally wrongful acts can be found within the UN, in the latest publications of the Special Rapporteur on racism and of the Working Group of Experts of People of African descent. Both offices have pushed for the recognition by IHRL that discrimination against people of African descent and other racialized communities cannot be eradicated unless transformative measures that help change the structures that sustain racism are adopted. This requires recognizing the role that states play in maintaining the very existence of racism and racist structures, potentially considering their responsibility under international law beyond a clear definition of an 'act', as ICERD requires.

For example, the Special Rapporteur, in a 2019 report on reparations, argues that accounting for the historic wrongs of slavery and colonialism, particularly through guarantees of non-repetition and through building 'a just and equitable international order', is fundamental for 'the eradication of persisting structures of racial inequality, subordination and discrimination' (Achiume 2019, pp. 4, 6). By naming the 'racially discriminatory structures', the Special Rapporteur calls the international community to acknowledge that the contemporary manifestations of racial discrimination are not only connected to practices from the past, but are very much the result of systemic racism today, and that obligations to repair must be upheld in order to realize the promise of equality and non-discrimination for all (Achiume 2019, p. 8).

Strategic advocacy from grassroots organizations and civil society at the UN can continue to shape standards in this direction, building on the experiences that the George Floyd killing has generated and using other tools within IHRL in terms of state responsibility and reparations, as the current Special Rapporteur on racism has done. If racism is not named as the outrageous dehumanizing phenomenon that it is, bringing forward the prohibition of racial discrimination is harder, as the manifestations of systemic racism are by definition collective, structural, and patterned. George Floyd was one of too many, lost by policing practices rooted in racism. The thousands of people of African descent lost to COVID-19 are another example of how systemic racism jeopardizes human rights.

In reacting to the strong calls for reparations for systemic racism in the context of COVID-19, different UN mechanisms have put in evidence that one of the key barriers to achieve this goal is, first, recognizing the structural nature of racism that serves as a root cause of racial discrimination in all spheres of life, including in access to healthcare, in the criminal justice and policing systems, in the labor market, and in political participation.

Part of what makes such recognition difficult is the exclusion of the very existence of racism as a potential breach of obligations on behalf of states under IHRL. This may be possibly linked to how colonialist practices still shape international law today, or, as the Special Rapporteur stated, because 'international law has not fully been "decolonized"' (Achiume 2019, p. 19). Former colonial powers have shaped international law since its inception, as Third World approaches to international law (TWAIL) and critical legal theory scholarship have extensively discussed (Anghie 2005).

Using international law to frame racism as the result of unfulfilled obligations (in this case, eradicating the causes of racial discrimination) has proven to be particularly difficult, not just for apparent lack of political will, but also, because IHRL appears to somehow allow for this exclusion by omission. However, the Inter-American system may be paving the way.

2.3 Systemic racism as a potential violation of international obligations under the Inter-American system: the concept of structural discrimination

On April 2020, the Inter-American Commission on Human Rights (IACHR) gave a general overview on standards to follow while responding to the pandemic, stating that COVID-19 arrived in the Americas in a challenging context, including persisting 'structural discrimination' against particularly vulnerable people and communities, such as people of African descent (CIDH 2020a). The Organization of American States (OAS) and the Inter-American Court of Human Rights (IACtHR) followed similar terms, calling on states to adopt a differentiated and inclusive approach regarding people of African descent while implementing measures to respond to COVID-19 (Corte IDH 2020; OEA 2020).

In early June, the IACHR adopted a stronger tone regarding state obligations on discrimination and COVID-19 while condemning the 'murder' of George Floyd (CIDH 2020b). In a strong statement, the IACHR reiterated that the killings of people of African descent in the United States 'are not isolated acts of violence', but 'part of a historical and structural process of systematic discrimination' that is surrounded by 'historical impunity' (CIDH 2020b).

Subsequently, the IACHR reminded American states of their obligations to tackle racial discrimination in the region and to protect people of African descent, particularly women and girls, from structural, multiple, and intersectional discrimination (CIDH 2020c; 2020d). It also called for 'comprehensive reparations' that acknowledge the exclusion, discrimination, and stigmas faced by people of African descent, financially compensate for damages caused, and uplift the history and contributions of this community to our societies (CIDH 2020e).

These statements are based on standards on structural discrimination that have been developed by both the IACHR and the IACtHR in the last twenty years. At least since 2011, the IACHR has stated that people of African descent are 'deeply impacted by the persistence of racism' rooted in slavery and colonialism and that under the OAS Charter and the American Convention on Human Rights (ACHR), states must adopt measures specifically oriented to fulfill their rights without discrimination (CIDH 2011, p. 37).

In its jurisprudence, the IACtHR has used the concept of 'structural discrimination' for the analysis of complex, historical, and generalized situations linked to exclusion and marginalization, including gender-based violence, discrimination against LGBTQI people, and more recently poverty as a social condition under the ACHR (Ferrer Mac-Gregor 2017). For our purposes, structural discrimination may be characterized as discrimination that (a) is based on a historical, socioeconomical, and cultural context; (b) is manifested in systematic, massive, or collective patterns; and (c) occurs against a specific group considered as vulnerable or marginalized (Pelletier Quiñones 2014)

Structural discrimination includes practices, prejudices, and beliefs that sustain legal or de facto inequalities faced by a particular group of people due to a condition that is inherently theirs or that cannot be changed by pure will (Ferrer Mac-Gregor 2017). In contrast to the definition of racial discrimination derived from the ICERD, the concept of structural discrimination as defined by the Inter-American system may create space for acknowledging the very existence of systemic racism – manifested in practices, prejudices, and policies based on the color of our skin or our origins – as a potential breach of international obligations under the ACHR.

Unfortunately, the IACtHR missed an opportunity to apply this concept to racist practices in the cases of *Nadege Dorzema et al v. Dominican Republic* (2012) and *Expelled Dominicans and Haitians v. Dominican Republic* (2014), rejecting the requests of the representatives of the victims, the IACHR, and several amici curiae. However, in 2016 the concept of structural discrimination was applied in the complex context of poverty and discrimination: in the *Trabajadores de la Hacienda Brasil Verde* case, the IACtHR found that despite the abolition of slavery in 1888, the concentration of wealth followed colonial patterns, leading rural workers in Brazil, most of African descent, to submit to exploitative conditions of labor in order to survive, increasing their risk of enduring forced labor (2016, p. 27).

Due to the historical and sociocultural background of the phenomenon and the failure to adopt special measures to reverse it, the IACtHR declared Brazil in breach of its obligations under the ACHR to protect these workers from forced labor, because – among other reasons – they would not have been in that position but for the structural discrimination they had faced for generations due to their social condition (*Trabajadores de la Hacienda Brasil Verde* 2016, p. 28). It is worth noting that although the structural discrimination these workers likely faced due to race was not directly addressed in the ruling, this landmark case can give some insights on how to push for the application of structural discrimination to systemic racism, by building on the context and historical analysis.

The IACHR has used the concept of structural discrimination as a lens to develop standards on the rights of people of African descent, compensating for the lesser use of the term in the jurisprudence of the IACtHR related to racial discrimination. In doing so, it has stated that 'systemic racism' is a vehicle for human rights violations, such as racial profiling, extrajudicial killings, and non-realization of economic, social, and cultural rights (CIDH 2018). Thus, it has made extensive context analysis to understand how systemic racism enables structural discrimination against people of African descent.

Structural discrimination has already been embraced to develop or expand key obligations on equality and non-discrimination of other marginalized groups, such as the situation of women with disabilities (CRPD 2016). Perhaps one solution is to foster greater dialogue among key IHRL spaces: in 2018, UN experts and the IACHR Rapporteur on Racial Discrimination referred to structural drivers, manifestations, and solutions to tackle racial discrimination eight times (OHCHR 2020h). Borrowing developments from each other and incorporating them in their own work might be a path to follow in strengthening racial discrimination standards across the globe.

3 Conclusion: is there hope for transformation?

My goal in this chapter was not to perform a profound interpretation of jurisprudence, but rather, to try to find insights on how members of the IHRL community can push the boundaries of international law to continue to support the racial justice movement and do the anti-racist work our field requires. By analyzing developments at the intersection of COVID-19 and racial justice, it can be seen how black lives still do not matter enough for certain fora within IHRL.

Despite concerning data on the disproportionate impact of COVID-19 and the violent deprivation of a Black life on camera, in 2020, an urgent debate with the potential to contribute to reduce impunity was tergiversated into a sort of IHRL version of 'all lives matter'. Unfortunately, in many spaces, much lip service is paid to the fight for racial justice, but the implementation of effective guarantees of non-repetition stays short.

But that does not mean there is not a way. By aiming to understand how both the UN and the Inter-American system reacted to the pivotal moments related to racial justice, in an unprecedented context as COVID-19, it can only be hoped that these insights generate some important learnings. One learning appears to be that there is still work to do to strengthen IHRL standards in order to effectively tackle the root causes of racial discrimination, and one step is to build from the experiences of racialized communities and support the calls for transformative justice, for basic dignity through equality and non-discrimination.

Refinement of the legal concept of structural discrimination is still ongoing, but it can become an important tool in dismantling racism through legal standards, particularly where there is enough evidence to demonstrate that, in too many instances, racial discrimination cases are often not isolated, but rather a manifestation of something larger. The denouncing and documentation of the disproportionate impact that COVID-19 has had on people of African descent, including by increasing significant pre-existing inequalities, can be key for the continued push towards the recognition of state responsibility in sustaining (by action or omission) systemic racism, as a fundamental cause of racial discrimination.

Not embracing a structural approach to analyze racial discrimination is assuming that by targeting individual acts only, and not also the context that drives them, we will fix the problem. Understanding individual acts or specific country cases can surely help to strengthen the anti-racist work, but for it to be effective, our legalistic approach must be based in an understanding that such acts are a manifestation of systemic dynamics and therefore, the work must also target the causes and the responsibilities, not just the symptoms.

Besides strategic litigation and advocacy, there are other key actions that can be taken to help bring this into reality. One is to uplift the work of those expanding critical legal scholarship, for such an approach helps to understand not only how international law replicates systems of oppression, but also, how to begin to change them. Efforts must be made to support the development of knowledge by activists and communities through alternative channels and incorporate their reflections in our own processes. Academia must be a tool for social change.

Another action, already pushed for by Afro-human rights defenders and collectives across Latin America, is to challenge the invisibilization of Afro-voices. COVID-19 has shown how the lack of disaggregated data not only limits the effectiveness of measures, but also reinforces the exclusion of people of African descent. This is especially true in Latin America and the Caribbean, where systemic racism and colonization has left a legacy of adopting anti-Black identity rhetoric. Campaigns based on storytelling and visual data can help to tackle presumptions that blackness is not part of the Latin-American identity; or that killings of people of African descent in the Americas are a sad but isolated phenomenon.

One final action is to continue to develop networks that help accompany those impacted by the vices of systemic racism and bring their claims to key powerful spaces, such as the Palais des Nations. Being able to represent and tell reality in one's own words is a key step towards peace-building. For this, donors and INGOs must dedicate resources to strengthening the capacities of these Afro-movements and collectives, while not seeking to control their work, but rather aiming at making them stronger to persevere in the long fight ahead.

There is hope for change, but only if the IHRL system feeds from the energy and vision catalyzed by COVID-19 and takes action to fulfill the demands for truth, justice, accountability, and reparations. If, instead, the international human rights system opts to continue to treat cases such as George Floyd's as individual instances and address racial discrimination as if in a vacuum, then there is little hope. Which path are we going to take?

Note

1 Although the racial justice movement comprises all those being 'otherized' or racialized on the basis of White supremacy, this chapter will focus on racial justice for people of African descent. Throughout this chapter, I opt to capitalize Black and White, to reflect that although these are nouns created under the false premise that races exist at all, they have also become fundamental part of the identity of millions across the Americas, if not the world.

References

Achiume, ET 2019, *Report of the Special Rapporteur on Contemporary Forms of Racism, Racial Discrimination, Xenophobia and Racial Intolerance A/74/321*, Office for the High Commissioner on Human Rights (OHCHR), viewed 27 December 2020, https://undocs.org/A/74/321.

Amnesty International 2016, 'Waiting In Vain: Unlawful Police Killings in Jamaica and Relatives' Long Struggle For Justice', Amnesty International, viewed 26 December 2020, www.amnesty.org/en/documents/amr38/5092/2016/en/

Amnesty International 2019, '"If They Can Have Her, Why Can't We?": Gender-Based Torture And Other Ill-Treatment Of Women Engaged In Sex Work In The Dominican Republic', Amnesty International, viewed 26 December 2020, www.amnesty.org/en/documents/amr27/0030/2019/en/

Amnesty International 2020a, 'Human Rights in The Americas: Review of 2019', Amnesty International, viewed 25 October 2020, www.amnesty.org/en/documents/amr01/1353/2020/en/

Amnesty International 2020b, *America's at a Crossroads in Response to Covid-19*, viewed 25 October 2020, www.amnesty.org/en/latest/research/2020/03/americas-at-a-crossroads-in-response-to-covid19/

AMP Research Lab 2020, *The Color of Coronavirus: COVID-19 Deaths by Race and Ethnicity in the U.S.*, viewed 30 October 2020, www.apmresearchlab.org/covid/deaths-by-race#age

Anghie, A 2005, *Imperialism, Sovereignty and the Making of International Law*, Cambridge University Press, Cambridge.

Bambra, C, Riordan, R, Ford, J & Matthews F 2020, 'The COVID-19 Pandemic and Health Inequalities', *Journal of Epidemiology and Community Health*, vol. 74, no. 11, pp. 964–968.

Beckman, BL 2020, '#BlackLivesMatter Saw Tremendous Growth on Social Media. Now What?', *Mashable*, viewed 25 October 2020, https://mashable.com/article/black-lives-matter-george-floyd-social-media-data/

Bradley, AS 2019, 'Human Rights Racism', *Harvard Human Rights Journal*, vol. 32, pp. 1–58.

Caldwell, KL & Araújo, EM 2020, 'COVID-19 Is Deadlier for Black Brazilians, a Legacy of Structural Racism that Dates Back to Slavery', *The Conversation*, viewed 30 October 2020, https://theconversation.com/covid-19-is-deadlier-for-black-brazilians-a-legacy-of-structural-racism-that-dates-back-to-slavery-139430

Centers for Disease Control (CDC) 2020, *Demographic Trends of COVID-19 Cases and Deaths in the US Reported to CDC*, viewed 30 October 2020, https://covid.cdc.gov/covid-data-tracker/#demographics

Comisión Económica para América Latina y el Caribe (CEPAL) 2020a, *Afrodescendientes y la matriz de la desigualdad social en América Latina*, United Nations, Santiago.

Comisión Económica para América Latina y el Caribe (CEPAL) 2020b, 'Informe: el impacto del COVID-19 en América Latina y el Caribe', United Nations Sustainable Development Group, viewed 26 December 2020, https://unsdg.un.org/sites/default/files/2020-07/ES_SG-Policy-brief-COVID-LAC.pdf

Comisión Económica para América Latina y el Caribe (CEPAL) 2018, *Mujeres afrodescendientes en América Latina y el Caribe: deudas de igualdad*, United Nations, Santiago.

Comisión Interamericana de Derechos Humanos (CIDH) 2011, *La situación de las personas afrodescendientes en las Américas*, viewed 26 December 2020, www.acnur.org/fileadmin/Documentos/BDL/2012/8311.pdf

Comisión Interamericana de Derechos Humanos (CIDH) 2017, *Report on Poverty and Human Rights in the Americas*, viewed 26 December 2020, www.oas.org/en/iachr/reports/pdfs/Poverty-HumanRights2017.docx

Comisión Interamericana de Derechos Humanos (CIDH) 2018, *Afrodescendientes, violencia policial y derechos humanos en los Estados Unidos*, viewed 26 December 2020, www.oas.org/es/cidh/informes/pdfs/ViolenciaPolicialAfrosEEUU.docx

Comisión Interamericana de Derechos Humanos (CIDH) 2020a, *Pandemia y derechos humanos, Resolución 1/2020*, viewed 26 December 2020, www.oas.org/es/cidh/decisiones/pdf/Resolucion-1-20-es.pdf

Comisión Interamericana de Derechos Humanos (CIDH) 2020b, *The IACHR Expresses Strong Condemnation for George Floyd's Murder, Repudiates Structural Racism, Systemic Violence against Afro-Americans, Impunity and the Disproportionate use of Police Force, and Urges Measures to Guarantee Equality and Non-discrimination in the United States*, viewed 10 November 2020, www.oas.org/en/iachr/media_center/PReleases/2020/129.asp

Comisión Interamericana de Derechos Humanos (CIDH) 2020c, *CIDH condena acciones policiales violentas en Brasil e insta a adoptar medidas orientadas a combatir la discriminación social y racial*, viewed 10 November 2020, www.oas.org/es/cidh/prensa/comunicados/2020/187.asp

Comisión Interamericana de Derechos Humanos (CIDH) 2020d, *En anticipación al Día Internacional de la Mujer Afro-latinoamericana, Afrocaribeña y de la Diáspora, la CIDH llama a los Estados a adoptar medidas especiales para erradicar la discriminación múltiple que enfrentan las mujeres afrodescendientes en el contexto de la pandemia del COVID-19*, viewed 10 November 2020, www.oas.org/es/cidh/prensa/comunicados/2020/177.asp

Comisión Interamericana de Derechos Humanos (CIDH) 2020e, *IACHR Calls on the States of the Region to Eliminate all Forms of Racial Discrimination, Promote Cultural Change and Adopt Comprehensive Reparation Measures for People of Afro-descendance*, viewed 10 November 2020, www.oas.org/en/iachr/media_center/PReleases/2020/216.asp

Comisión Interamericana de Derechos Humanos (CIDH) 2020f, *IACHR Calls on the United States to Implement Structural Reforms in the Institutional Systems of Security and Justice to Counter Historical Racial Discrimination and Institutional Racism*, viewed 10 November 2020, www.oas.org/en/iachr/media_center/PReleases/2020/196.asp

Committee on the Elimination of All Forms of Racial Discrimination (CERD) 2020, *Prevention of Racial Discrimination, Including Early Warning and Urgent Action Procedures, Statement 1 (2020) United States of America*, viewed 10 November 2020, www.ohchr.org/Documents/HRBodies/CERD/earlywarning/statements/USA.PDF

Committee on the Elimination of All Forms of Racial Discrimination (CERD) 2011, *General Recommendation 34: Racial discrimination against people of African descent*, viewed 26 December 2020, https://digitallibrary.un.org/record/714927?ln=en

Committee on the Rights of Persons with Disabilities (CRPD) 2016, *General Comment No 3:Article 6:Women and Girls with Disabilities*, viewed 26 December 2020, www.ohchr.org/Documents/HRBodies/CRPD/GC/Women/CRPD-C-GC-3.doc

Corte Interamericana de Derechos Humanos (Corte IDH) 2020, *Declaración: Covid-19 y derechos humanos: los problemas y desafíos deben ser abordados con perspectiva de derechos humanos y respetando las obligaciones internacionales*, viewed 26 December 2020, www.corteidh.or.cr/tablas/alerta/comunicado/declaracion_1_20_ESP.pdf

The COVID-19 Tracking Project 2020, *The COVID Racial Data Tracker,* viewed 30 October 2020, https:// covidtracking.com/ race

Dickinson, E 2020, 'Police Killing Rouses Colombia's Lockdown Furies', *International Crisis Group*, viewed 29 October 2020, www.crisisgroup.org/latin-america-caribbean/andes/colombia/police-killing-rouses-colombias-lockdown-furies

Edwards, F, Lee, H, & Esposito M 2019, 'Risk of Being Killed by Police Use of Force in the United States by Age, Race–ethnicity, and Sex', *Proceedings of the National Academy of Sciences of the United States of America*, vol. 116, no. 34, pp. 16793–16798.

Expelled Dominicans and Haitians v Dominican Republic (2014) IACtHR.

Ferrer Mac-Gregor, E 2017, 'Acerca de la "discriminación estructural histórica" en razón de la posición económica (pobreza) de los trabajadores sometidos a trabajo esclavo', *Ius Constitutionale Commune en América Latina*, viewed 26 December 2020, https://archivos.juridicas.unam.mx/www/bjv/libros/10/4745/10.pdf

Google Trends 2020, *Protests for Racial Equality and Justice*, viewed 25 October 2020, https://trends.google.com/trends/story/US_cu_AsW8cXIBAADMNM_en

Gould, E & Wilson, V 2020, 'Black Workers Face Two of the Most Lethal Preexisting Conditions for Coronavirus – Racism and Economic Inequality', Economic Policy Institute, viewed 29 October 2020, www.epi.org/publication/black-workers-covid/

Hill-Cawthorne, L 2020, '"Racism Will Not Pass"…', *EJIL:Talk!*, viewed 10 November 2020, www.ejiltalk.org/racism-will-not-pass/

International Convention on the Elimination of All Forms of Racial Discrimination (1969) opened for signature 21 December 1965, 660 UNTS 195.

International Law Commission (ILC) 2002, *Draft Articles on the Responsibility of States for Wrongful Acts, with commentaries*, United Nations.

International Labour Organization (ILO) 2020, *Contagion or Starvation, the Dilemma Facing Informal Workers During the COVID-19 Pandemic*, viewed 30 October 2020, www.ilo.org/global/about-the-ilo/newsroom/news/WCMS_744005/lang--en/index.htm

Koeze, E & Popper, N 2020, 'The Virus Changed the Way We Internet', *The New York Times*, 7 April, viewed 25 October 2020, www.nytimes.com/interactive/2020/04/07/technology/coronavirus-internet-use.html

Latin America Risk Report 2020, *Colombia's Protests Signal a Region Primed for a New Protest Wave*, viewed 31 October 2020, https://bit.ly/2VZB8fl

Lima, MS, Sims, S, & Xavier, P 2020, 'For Black Brazilians, Covid-19 Is Deepening Painful Inequalities', *Bloomberg*, viewed 29 October 2020, www.bloomberg.com/news/articles/2020-06-26/for-black-brazilians-covid-19-is-deepening-painful-inequalities

Luhby, T 2020, 'US Black-white Inequality in 6 Stark Charts', *CNN*, viewed 29 October 2020, https://edition.cnn.com/2020/06/03/politics/black-white-us-financial-inequality/index.html

Malaihollo, M 2017, 'The International Convention on the Elimination of all Forms of Racial Discrimination – Reviewing Special Measures Under Contemporary International Law', *Groningen Journal of International Law*, vol. 5, no. 1, pp. 135–146.

Mapping Police Violence 2020, *Police Violence Map*, viewed 10 November 2020, https://mappingpoliceviolence.org/

McFadden, S 2020, 'Black Lives Matter Just Entered Its Next Phase', *The Atlantic*, viewed 25 October 2020, www.theatlantic.com/culture/archive/2020/09/black-lives-matter-just-entered-its-next-phase/615952/

McGonagle, D, Plein, S, O'Donnell, JS, Sharif, K, & Bridgewood, C 2020, 'Increased Cardiovascular Mortality in African Americans with COVID-19', *The Lancet Respiratory Medicine*, vol. 8, no. 7, pp. 649–651.

Muniz, B, Fonseca, B, & Pina, R 2020, 'Em duas semanas, número de negros mortos por coronavírus é cinco vezes maior no Brasil', *A Pública*, viewed 30 October 2020, https://apublica.org/2020/05/em-duas-semanas-numero-de-negros-mortos-por-coronavirus-e-cinco-vezes-maior-no-brasil/

Nadege Dorzema et al. v Dominican Republic (2012) IACtHR.

Noticias ONU 2018, *América Latina, no la más pobre pero sí la más desigual*, viewed 30 October 2020, https://news.un.org/es/story/2018/04/1431712

Organización de los Estados Americanos (OEA) 2020, *Guía práctica de respuestas inclusivas y con enfoque de derechos ante el COVID-19 en las Américas*, Secretaría General de la Organización de los Estados Americanos.

O Globo 2020, *Coronavírus é mais letal entre negros no Brasil, apontam dados do Ministério da Saúde*, viewed 30 October 2020, https://g1.globo.com/bemestar/coronavirus/noticia/2020/04/11/coronavirus-e-mais-letal-entre-negros-no-brasil-apontam-dados-do-ministerio-da-saude.ghtml

Office of the High Commissioner for Human Rights (OHCHR) 2020a, *Human Rights Council Holds an Urgent Debate on Current Racially Inspired Human Rights Violations, Systemic Racism, Police Brutality and Violence Against Peaceful Protests*, viewed 30 October 2020, www.ohchr.org/EN/NewsEvents/Pages/DisplayNews.aspx?NewsID=25971&LangID=E

Office of the High Commissioner for Human Rights (OHCHR) 2020b, *Disproportionate Impact of COVID-19 on Racial and Ethnic Minorities Needs to be Urgently Dddressed – Bachelet*, viewed 30 October 2020, www.ohchr.org/EN/NewsEvents/Pages/DisplayNews.aspx?NewsID=25916

Office of the High Commissioner for Human Rights (OHCHR) 2020c, *UN Experts Condemn Modern-day Racial Terror Lynchings in US and Call for Systemic Reform and Justice*, viewed 7 November 2020, www.ohchr.org/EN/NewsEvents/Pages/DisplayNews.aspx?NewsID=25933

Office of the High Commissioner for Human Rights (OHCHR) 2020d, *Statement from the UN Special Rapporteur on Contemporary Forms of Racism, Racial Discrimination, Xenophobia and Related Intolerance, and The Working Group of Experts on People of African Descent. Joined by The Special Rapporteur on the Rights of Freedom of Assembly and Association, and the Coordination Committee of the UN Human Rights Special Procedures*, viewed 7 November 2020, www.ohchr.org/en/NewsEvents/Pages/DisplayNews.aspx?NewsID=25969&LangID=E

Office of the High Commissioner for Human Rights (OHCHR) 2020e, *Statement by Michelle Bachelet, UN High Commissioner for Human Rights 17 June 2020*, viewed 7 November 2020, www.ohchr.org/EN/NewsEvents/Pages/DisplayNews.aspx?NewsID=25968&LangID=E

Office of the High Commissioner for Human Rights (OHCHR) 2020f, *Statement on the Human Rights Council Urgent Debate Resolution*, viewed 7 November 2020, www.ohchr.org/EN/NewsEvents/Pages/DisplayNews.aspx?NewsID=25977&LangID=E

Office of the High Commissioner for Human Rights (OHCHR) 2020g, *Statement on the Protests against Systemic Racism in the United States*, viewed 7 November 2020, www.ohchr.org/EN/NewsEvents/Pages/DisplayNews.aspx?NewsID=25927

Office of the High Commissioner for Human Rights (OHCHR) 2020h, *Joint Statement: "Confronting the Two Faces of Racism: Resurgent Hate and Structural Discrimination"*, viewed 7 November 2020, www.ohchr.org/EN/NewsEvents/Pages/DisplayNews.aspx?NewsID=22856&LangID=E

Parker, K, Menasce Horowitz, J, & Anderson, M 2020, 'Amid Protests, Majorities Across Racial and Ethnic Groups Express Support for the Black Lives Matter Movement', *Pew Research Center*, viewed 10 December 2020, www.pewsocialtrends.org/2020/06/12/amid-protests-majorities-across-racial-and-ethnic-groups-express-support-for-the-black-lives-matter-movement/

Parmar, S 2020, 'The Internationalisation of Black Lives Matter at the Human Rights Council', *EJIL:Talk!*, viewed 7 November 2020, www.ejiltalk.org/the-internationalisation-of-black-lives-matter-at-the-human-rights-council/

Pelletier Quiñones, P 2014, 'La discriminación estructural en la evolución jurisprudencial de la Corte Interamericana de Derechos Humanos', *Revista IIDH*, vol. 60, pp. 205–215.

Programa de las Naciones Unidas para el Desarrollo (UNDP) 2019, *Injusticia y desigualdad: nuevo informe del PNUD refleja el descontento en América Latina*, viewed 31 October 2020, www.latinamerica.undp.org/content/rblac/es/home/presscenter/pressreleases/2019/unfair-and-unequal--new-undp-report-sheds-light-on-discontent-in.html

Ramsden, P 2020, 'How the Pandemic Changed Social Media and George Floyd's Death Created a Collective Conscience', *LSE Blog*, viewed 25 October 2020, https://blogs.lse.ac.uk/medialse/2020/06/24/how-the-pandemic-changed-social-media-and-george-floyds-death-created-a-collective-conscience/

Schwab, K & Malleret, T 2020, *COVID-19: The Great Reset*, Forum Publishing, Geneva.

Semega, J, Kollar, M, Creamer, J, & Mohanty, A 2019, *Income and Poverty in the United States: 2018*, United States Census Bureau, viewed 27 December 2020, www.census.gov/library/publications/2019/demo/p60-266.html

Trabajadores de la Hacienda Brasil Verde v Brasil (2016) IACtHR.

United Nations Population Fund (UNFPA) 2020, 'Implicaciones del COVID-19 en la población afrodescendiente de América Latina y el Caribe', *Resumen Técnico*, UNFPA, viewed 27 December 2020, https://lac.unfpa.org/sites/default/files/pub-pdf/2-Covid-Afrodescendientes%20%281%29.pdf

UN News 2020a, *Citing 'Weight of History', Senior UN Officials of African Descent Issue Call to 'Go Beyond and Do More' to End Racism*, viewed 5 November 2020, https://news.un.org/en/story/2020/06/1066242

UN News 2020b, *Human Rights Council calls on top UN rights official to take action on racist violence*, viewed 5 November 2020, https://news.un.org/en/story/2020/06/1066722

UN Web TV 2020, *A/HRC/43/L.50 Vote Item: 1 – 44th Meeting, 43rd Regular Session Human Rights Council*, online video, viewed 5 November 2020, https://bit.ly/3oJUDEN

Washington Post 2020, *Fatal Force*, viewed 29 October 2020, www.washingtonpost.com/graphics/investigations/police-shootings-database/

7

COVID-19 AND VIOLENCE AGAINST WOMEN

Unprecedented impacts and suggestions for mitigation

Zarizana Abdul Aziz and Janine Moussa

The response to the COVID-19 pandemic has compelled a rethinking of ways of communicating, working, conducting business, and family life as well as accessing services, facilities, and justice. On the positive side, government restrictions have led to possibilities for flexible work hours, work from home opportunities, and the ability to spend more time with children, all of which have been part of women's rights demands. Face-to-face meetings have been replaced with online communications. The internet and other information communication technology (ICT) have become the primary means of maintaining social relationships, information sharing, working, learning and conducting business. While this shift facilitated a new reality of flexible working hours and work from home for some, it also brought heightened risks of online harassment, cyberattacks, hacking, and trolling. On the other hand, quarantine, movement restrictions, lockdowns, and social distancing mean heightened isolation and curtailed personal interaction with support networks as well as service providers. Empty streets, shuttered businesses, job losses, reduced transport options have all worked to deepen isolation and increase stress.

This chapter looks at the impact of the COVID-19 pandemic on violence against women, both offline and online and suggests ways to mitigate it. Part 1 looks at violence against women, its manifestations, and underlying causes. Part 2 examines how the COVID-19 pandemic has led to increased incidences of violence against women due to increased risk factors, increased social isolation, and increased internet presence and reliance.[1] Part 3 discusses the opportunities and challenges brought forth by the COVID-19 response with regard to the gender digital divide, access to services and justice, as well as workplace responsibility. Part 4 concludes with a set of targeted recommendations on the way forward.

1 Violence against women

The working definition of violence against women upon which this chapter relies is the 1993 UN Declaration on the Elimination ofViolence against Women which defines 'violence against women' as an act of gender-based violence (GBV) that results in, or is likely to result in, physical, sexual, psychological or economic harm or suffering to women, including threats of such acts, coercion or arbitrary deprivation of liberty, whether occurring in public or in private life. More particularly, gender-based violence is violence that is directed against a person because of her gender or that affects a person of that gender disproportionately and includes the following:

(a) acts that inflict physical, mental or sexual harm or suffering, threats of such acts, coercion, involuntary confinement, economic or financial deprivation and other deprivations of liberty;
(b) violence and abuse in the family including denial of support or access to adequate support or livelihood;
(c) sexual assault, harassment, sexual harassment and stalking;
(d) online violence; and
(e) trafficking and exploitation of women and girls (UN General Assembly 1993).

Violence against women is a form of gender-based violence. For the purposes of this chapter the two terms will be used interchangeably.

1.1 Domestic violence

World Health Organization data (WHO 2013) on prevalence of violence against women reveal that:

- One in three women experience physical or sexual violence, mostly by spouses and intimate partners;
- 30 percent of women who have been in a relationship report that they have experienced violence by their intimate partner;
- up to 38 percent of murders of women are committed by an intimate male partner.

Another United Nations study on killing of women found that 58 percent of all killings of women were committed by their intimate partners and family members, making the home the most dangerous place and family members the most dangerous people for women (UNODC 2018). This study included all gender-related killings of women and girls perpetrated globally, including forms that are prevalent across certain regions, such as dowry and killing under the pretext of honor.

The scope of violence against women has evolved over time to include structural violence and the recognition that it is rooted in gender inequality and discrimination manifested as societal power imbalances and social norms and culture (Abdul Aziz & Moussa 2016). Lack of strong societal condemnation as well as community and cultural attitudes towards domestic violence, including cultural views that support male authority over women, result in the acceptance and normalization of domestic violence (Abdul Aziz 2013). Lack of condemnation and prevalent cultural attitudes also trivialize or minimize the seriousness of domestic violence. Across the world even law enforcement personnel and judges are not immune from negative social perceptions. A South Australian Supreme Court judge, Justice Bollen, during a marital rape trial commented that 'rougher than usual handling' was acceptable when a husband was endeavoring to persuade his wife to engage in sexual intercourse (Lumley 2015). In 2016, a Spanish Court acquitted five men of sexual assault because the woman had kept her eyes closed and had a passive expression. Therefore, held the judge, she 'had not faced violence or intimidation, but had been abused' (Rosell 2018). The decision was overturned on appeal.

Domestic violence thrives in social isolation and seclusion, either by isolating or secluding the survivors or hiding the abuse from society. Female survivors of violence are often isolated from society by perpetrators. This occurs particularly in intimate partner violence or domestic violence, where the perpetrators live in the same household as the survivor. (While domestic violence overwhelmingly refers to intimate partner violence, it also includes violence committed by and against other members of the family, including in extended family settings where the wife often lives with her in-laws). This isolation was further enhanced during the COVID-19 pandemic with orders that kept families and individuals isolated by state order. These orders also removed women from their support and social networks (e.g., friends, relatives, hairdressers, family physicians).

1.2 Online VAW

As technology systems have developed, the online abuse of women has become a concerning and dangerous issue. ICT-related violence against women consists of acts of violence against women committed in part or fully through the use of ICT (Šimonović 2018). Common forms of ICT violence against women are cyber-stalking, cyber bullying, online harassment, and online sexual harassment. These forms of violence often involve repeated acts. While an individual incident may be a lawful expression of speech, repeated unwanted acts constitute unlawful harassment or stalking.

Enhancing the use of enabling technology to promote women's empowerment is one of the targets under the Sustainable Development Goals (UN General Assembly 2015). Yet, online violence against women is an obstacle to women accessing enabling technology. As women and girls spend more time online and increasingly live their lives through ICT, online or ICT-related gender-based violence is a major barrier influencing, curtailing, and preventing women's access and use of the internet and the digital space. Women have limited their online presence, closed their social media accounts and even stopped using mobile phones altogether after experiencing ICT violence, deepening their social isolation even as ICT assumes ever greater importance in social interaction, job and economic opportunities, and news and information delivery.

The ease with which data and images can be shared, liked, reposted, stored and downloaded means that there is more scope for repetition by the principal perpetrator (the person who first disseminates the image of data) and by others who are often recklessly indifferent as to whether the content constitutes violence against women and as to the harm that may ensue. For example, in *United States v. Sayer*, the perpetrator stalked his ex-wife online, created fictitious Facebook and Myspace pages in her name, disseminated non-consensual intimate media and made Yahoo messenger profiles to invite men to her home, thereby enlisting third parties to harass his ex-wife (*United States v. Sayer* 2014).

Yet, when ICT violence does not result in physical violence it tends to be trivialized and thus receive inadequate and inappropriate responses not only from law enforcement agencies and internet intermediaries, but also from women themselves who are more likely to block or ignore their assailants than report them (Pasricha 2016). One such instance is the non-consensual sharing of intimate images. Furthermore, victim-blaming under these circumstances is prevalent and survivors risk being prosecuted under obscenity/pornography laws for having created or participated in the creation of the intimate image which led to the image being in the possession of the principal perpetrator (Berkiempes 2019).

In other instances, freedom of speech has protected abusive men despite the woman's fear that results from social media posts (*Elonis v. United States* 2015). In *Elonis*, the accused argued that his threats against his wife and others were made for a 'therapeutic' purpose, 'to "deal with the pain" … of a wrenching event', or for 'cathartic' reasons and therefore he was protected under freedom of expression. The US Supreme Court partially upheld the defense and held that regardless of whether his wife felt threatened by the posts, the prosecution had to prove intention to threaten or at the very least recklessness – that is disregard of a risk of harm of which he was aware. The case was remanded for further proceedings.

Beyond social media, acts of digital voyeurism have evolved to encompass all forms of illicit filming. Women have been filmed in changing rooms and restrooms using hidden cameras by a growing army of voyeurs or by their former intimate partners (CNA Insider 2018; Paulo 2018).

Consent is pivotal in differentiating lawful from unlawful and harmful behavior. Defining consent is critical. Consent must relate to the exact act to which the consent, if any, is given – that is consent to share with the principal perpetrator cannot be extended to consent for the latter to disseminate the image/data. Consent may also be conditional or temporal, for example, for the duration of the relationship (BBC News 2015b). The harm, which the principal perpetrator initially commits by disseminating an image, is repeated each time the image is liked, downloaded, reposted and shared.

Another alarming twist is the trading of rape images or footage (BBC News 2015a; Ashraf 2016). These videos could initially have been used to blackmail survivors into not reporting to the police, and subsequently the footage would be 'stolen' and sold.

Though the resulting harm may not be physical, ICT violence against women is neither trivial nor temporary. In 2013, 17-year-old Nova Scotia (Canada) student Rehtaeh Parsons took her own life after being subjected to months of harassment and humiliation arising from the online dissemination of a photo of her alleged rape (Newton 2013). The principal perpetrators were handed probationary sentences (Barber 2015).

Perceived anonymity can encourage individuals – lulled by the reduction of non-verbal cues and the fact that they are communicating via a screen rather than with a live person – to become more uninhibited, both disclosing more and acting up more (Suler 2004). Geographical and temporal distance may also motivate people to become less sensitive to the consequences of their actions (Wong et al. 2018). Consequently, users act with less restraint, resulting in more frequent and intense ICT violence against women (Suler 2004). This aggravates the harm to survivors and violates a range of rights and freedoms including the right to privacy or respect for private life compared to other forms of more traditional media (*Editorial Board of Pravoye Delo and Shtekel v. Ukraine* 2011).

Gender hate speech includes hateful, demeaning, insulting, and vitriolic comments based on a person's gender (Abdul Aziz 2020). Other forms of ICT violence include, amongst others, dog piling (vicious mob attack of a person over a comment); disseminating altered photos or videos and uploading them to dating, pornography, or other kinds of websites (morphing/transmogrification); online grooming predation; doxing (searching and publicizing someone's personal data even if the data is publicly available e.g., in the public record – sometimes made more egregious when the disclosure is accompanied by images of the survivor); sextortion (e.g. extorting sex/sexual favors by threatening to disseminate intimate images including rape footage) (Kasulis 2020); cyber flashing (receiving unsolicited images of male genitalia); and sexual exploitation of women and girls driven by poverty. The live-streaming of child sexual abuse, sometimes facilitated by poverty-stricken family members, has boomed in countries with high levels of English, good internet access, and well-established money transfer systems (Holmes 2016).

2 Increased incidences of violence against women

In 2020 the world saw the unprecedented onset and subsequent rapid spread of COVID-19. The pandemic has compelled governments to issue social distancing guidelines, movement restrictions, and lockdowns. An estimated 2.73 billion women in 162 countries around the world live in countries where stay-at-home orders were in place (UN Women 2020a).

Responses to COVID-19, though necessary, have led to a spike in gender-based violence against women, which has been labeled as a 'pandemic within a pandemic'

(Mutongwiza 2020). The UN Population Fund (UNFPA) estimates that '6 months of lockdowns could result in an additional 31 million cases of gender-based violence' (UNFPA 2020).

In order to understand the impact of COVID-19 on violence against women, it is important to gauge how the response to COVID-19 amplifies or diminishes risk factors of violence against women, particularly domestic violence but other forms of violence as well. What is needed is critical mindfulness of the impact of pandemic responses on women. Once we better understand the impact of the COVID-19 response on violence against women, we can better tailor our responses and preventative measures to offset the foreseeable spike in violence against women.

2.1 *Increased risk factors*

The response to COVID-19 has resulted in the shuttering of retail establishments and businesses, with millions of men and women losing their jobs. It is estimated that about a quarter of all US jobs were disrupted by the pandemic (Morath 2020). To date, only an estimated 42 percent of those jobs have since been reinstated (US Bureau of Labor Statistics 2020). Similar patterns of job losses and accompanying economic impacts are repeated in countries globally triggering the worst recession since World War II with a projected 4.5 percent fall in global GDP (Gurría 2020).

These statistics however reflect only those jobs that governments count; the statistics do not take into account the informal work force. UN Women estimates that in South Asia, over 80 percent of women in non-agricultural jobs are in informal employment; in sub-Saharan Africa, the number is 74 percent, and in Latin America and the Caribbean, 54 percent (UN Women 2020c). Women in the informal sector are often left on the margins of labor law protection, paid sick leave, social benefits or insurance. They are vulnerable to abuse and exploitation – job losses are uncounted and uncompensated. Undocumented immigrants, already susceptible to abuse, are similarly situated. Neither category of women was extended COVID-19 financial relief packages, where available. Without sick leave, insurance or healthcare benefits, these women had no choice but to continue working amidst the pandemic and, if they were to contract COVID-19, they were unable to seek medical attention, stop working or quarantine. Because of this, some States have employed different strategies to extend access to health care to the most vulnerable as part of their overall response to COVID-19 (e.g., Portugal and Italy extended access to healthcare to migrants with pending applications and those whose permits were about to expire) (UN Women et al. 2020).

One sector that is almost wholly engaged by women, yet is one of the sectors with the fewest labor protections, is the domestic services sector. While most domestic workers lost their jobs (in the US, 93 percent of domestic workers lost their jobs by late March 2020), for those who have not lost their jobs, the pandemic has resulted in increased work, higher stress, and employer-imposed prohibitions against leaving the house/workplace (National Domestic Workers Alliance 2020). For millions of Asian and African migrant domestic workers, particularly in the

Middle East, these prohibitions have increased the risk of serious abuse (Human Rights Watch 2020).

Economic and financial insecurity together with poor coping strategies lead to conflict and violence in the family. Loss of income streams and fewer job prospects have also resulted in increased care responsibilities, a responsibility disproportionately placed on women that adds to increased tensions and conflict as well as risk of domestic violence. The increased daily contact brought about by quarantines and stay-at-home orders, confined living quarters, suspension of schools or its conversion to online education, can also be challenging for parenting and increase opportunities for violence and abuse.

2.2 Increased social isolation

Lockdowns and movement restriction orders exacerbate the risk of violence against women. At particular risk are female survivors of domestic violence who are often isolated from society by perpetrators, who are emboldened by the additional power and control presented by the pandemic responses (Šimonović 2020a). Loss of income also means more women are trapped in violent homes, limited by financial constraints.

Even under normal circumstances, the home can be the most dangerous place for women. A global study on gender-related killings of women and girls found that of a total of 87,000 women intentionally killed in 2017, 58 percent were killed by intimate partners or family members (UNODC 2018). This translates to 137 women across the world killed by a member of their own family every day. More than a third (30,000) of the women intentionally killed in 2017 were killed by their current or former intimate partner. During the pandemic, reports have emerged of an increase in domestic homicides in a number of affected countries (Bradbury-Jones 2020). The responses to COVID-19 such as lockdowns, quarantines and movement restrictions can intensify women's isolation and seclusion. Coupled with increased contact and presence with perpetrators, these factors heighten the risk of violence.

Despite this, the home is often seen as within the private sphere, a sanctuary for its members, away from the prying eyes of society and the law. In more conservative communities, survivors themselves frequently believe themselves to be transgressing social and cultural norms, while bringing shame and dishonor into the family, by seeking assistance.

2.3 Increased internet presence and reliance

With closure or restrictions on cinemas, dine-in restaurants, bars, theaters and concerts, the pandemic has compelled most people to live more of their lives online. We are now reliant on the internet to work, learn, and connect with family and friends. As of January 2020, there were an estimated 4.5 billion internet users globally – over half of the world's population (Internet World Stats 2020b). As of July

2020, that number has increased to 4.8 billion, equivalent to 62 percent of the world's population (Internet World Stats 2020a).

Online news, social media, live-streaming entertainment, online meetings, and online schooling have raised security and privacy concerns including ICT violence. In the United States, as early as April 2020, the Federal Bureau of Investigation (FBI) noted a 400 percent spike in cybercrimes reported to its Internet Crime Complaint Center (IC3), that is 3,000 to 4,000 complaints per day (Miller 2020).

Not surprisingly, users with limited digital skills, predominantly women and girls, are more at risk of information communication technology-related gender-based violence (UN Women 2020b). Schoolchildren who spend more time online may also be at risk, including the risk of online sexual exploitation. To date there have yet to be rigorous studies on increased incidences of ICT VAWG during the pandemic, apart from a few media reports, law enforcement statistics, and anecdotal evidence.

3 Challenges and opportunities

This section examines the challenges and opportunities the response to COVID-19 has brought to efforts to address and combat domestic violence and ICT violence against women.

3.1 Gender digital divide

The increased reliance on the internet brought on by the lockdowns has worsened the gender digital divide and exacerbated online ICT violence against women in particular. The gender digital divide refers to the measurable gap between women and men in their access to, use of, and ability to influence, contribute to, and benefit from ICTs (UN OHCHR 2017). The gender digital divide is both a consequence and cause of violations of women's human rights (Iglesias 2020).

Social distancing, job losses, and restricted mobility have resulted in women losing their internet access. Gender inequality at home may result in women having less access to limited computer and internet resources (Human Rights Watch 2020). Loss of internet access deepens the seclusion and isolation for survivors of domestic violence. Digital exclusion may likewise disproportionately affect women from marginalized communities, elderly women, women with disability, and displaced and refugee women. As resources go digital, the impact of gender digital divide is exacerbated.

Still, there has been greater awareness of development of safe technology that enhances service delivery to survivors. Even prior to the pandemic, there was a proliferation of ICT web-based and mobile phone applications with geolocation functions that provide free helplines and messaging services (some with safe code words) (Abdul Aziz 2018; UN Women et al. 2020). In India, the brutal rape and murder of a young woman in Delhi in 2013, provided the impetus for the development of many mobile phone apps in India (Dhar 2014). In the United States, the

Department of Health and Human Services weighed in through its *Apps Against Abuse* initiative which challenged developers 'to harness the power of mobile technology to help prevent dating violence and abuse' (Bivens & Hasinoff 2018).

Mobile apps are premised on women in the household being permitted to have phones by their abuser. Women, however, are less likely than men to own a mobile phone, a fact that is particularly apparent in low-medium income countries (e.g., in South Asia, women are 28 percent less likely than men to own a mobile phone and 58 percent less likely to use mobile internet) (GSMA 2019). As Human Rights Watch has observed, digital services 'assume a baseline of access', and many women do not even have a phone, much less a smartphone (Human Rights Watch 2020). Still, for women who do have mobile phones, mobile apps that have been deployed by both governments and private sector tech developers alike remain a viable safety tool during unprecedented lockdowns, quarantines, and social distancing to access services, particularly intervention services and facilities (UN Women 2020a).

3.2 Access to services and justice

The pandemic is negatively impacting and disrupting women's support networks and services. Stay at home and other orders restrict access by women to their support networks, including family and friends, health and medical personnel (many of whom are trained to identify domestic violence and serve as first responders), women's organizations and shelters, as well as access to law enforcement agencies and courts. The ability of, and opportunity for, survivors of domestic violence to seek help and intervention to escape or end the violence is severely restricted (WHO 2020). In Belarus, the pandemic response resulted in phone calls being substituted for regular assessment visits to families with domestic violence history (Human Rights Watch 2020). Protection orders, too, may be granted online. However, without ensuring privacy of the connection, survivors may not be able to communicate openly with police let alone attend court remotely to obtain protection orders.

Fear of COVID-19 spread amongst persons detained and in the prison population have also led to States drastically limiting arrests and detentions. These measures are likely to affect the intervention and detention rates of domestic violence cases (Johnson et al. 2020). This observation is borne out by reports from Argentina, Australia, Brazil, Canada, China, Cyprus, France, Germany, Singapore, Spain, the United Kingdom, and the United States that suggest an increase in violence against women and children (UN Women 2020a; Peterman et al. 2020). A non-profit organization working on intimate partner violence in China indicates that statistics of reported cases have increased three-fold with 90 percent of these cases related to the pandemic (Allen-Ebrahimian 2020). Another in Kyrgystan said that many women are too afraid to call police or crisis centers because 'their abusers are at home 24 hours a day, controlling their every step' (Kurmanbekova 2020). Survivor support services (crisis centers, social services, legal aid, even the criminal justice system) have had to scale back as resources are diverted toward the health response to the pandemic (WHO 2020; Šimonović 2020b). Some shelters have closed or been re-purposed as health centers. Those that remain have difficulty meeting with survivors (UN Women et al. 2020). Consequently, although domestic violence cases had increased, often requests for assistance to domestic violence helplines dropped as survivors faced difficulty asking for help during lockdowns (UN Women 2020a).

Furthermore, women's organizations offering crisis intervention services, including shelters, are negatively impacted by the economic crisis resulting from the pandemic. Not all service providers, particularly smaller providers, were able to invest in setting up remote service (Human Rights Watch 2020). This, apart from the lockdowns and movement restrictions, reduced their capacity to undertake advocacy and outreach programs as well as provide direct services to survivors of violence (UN Women 2020a).

3.3 Workplace responsibility

The convergence of home and work provides an opportunity for an additional level of scrutiny by the employer to prevent and respond to domestic violence. Employers are grappling with how to handle workplace safety in abusive homes and if there should be different approaches depending on whether the employee is the abuser or the survivor and in situations where both the survivor and abuser work for the same employer.

This convergence has provided employers the opportunity to take more active roles in preventing domestic violence and facilitating access to support services to ensure workplace safety and well-being of employees. The 2019 ILO Convention on Violence and Harassment applies to 'violence and harassment in the world of work occurring in the course of, linked with or arising out of work' amongst others 'in the workplace, including public and private spaces where they are a place of work' (International Labour Organization 2019a). Recommendation 206 on Violence and Harassment in article 8(c) provides that particular attention should be paid to the hazards and risks arising from discrimination, abuse of power relations, and gender, cultural and social norms that support violence and harassment (International Labour Organization 2019b). Recommendation 9 specifically mentions occupations where exposure to violence and harassment may be more likely, such as night work, work in isolation, health, hospitality, social services, emergency services, domestic work, transport, education or entertainment. Recommendation 18 sets out appropriate measures to mitigate the impacts of domestic violence in the world of work. These include leave for victims of domestic violence, temporary protection against dismissal for survivors of domestic violence, inclusion of domestic violence in workplace assessments, referral systems to public mitigation measures and awareness raising about the effects of domestic violence.

4 Conclusions and recommendations

Undoubtedly, the COVID-19 pandemic has disrupted every facet of life, from socializing and entertainment to learning and working. In many instances, it has intensified the risks of violence against women, both online and offline. Since the onset of the pandemic, sexual and other forms of violence against women have increased. Isolation and seclusion brought about by lockdowns, quarantines, stay-at-home orders and mobility restrictions have led to an escalation of domestic violence. Diminished social support for survivors has left many survivors trapped in situations of violence. Civil society organizations working on violence response including shelters (UN Women 2020a) face dwindling funds and lack the requisite capabilities to switch to rigorous online services.

ICT violence against women has intensified as women and children, as well as predators and trolls, spend increased hours online. The usual strategies on violence prevention have been derailed. Should the pandemic continue over the next six months or more, the long-term gains achieved in the struggle against violence against women and gender equality might be set back as well.

4.1 Recommendations

The unprecedented responses to COVID-19, while necessary, require States and society to be critically mindful of the impact of pandemic responses on women and girls. Some measures that States should consider including the following:

4.1.1 Domestic violence

- Allocate resources to address domestic violence in COVID-19 national response plans including effective police responses and safe medical protocols, exploring ways to provide survivors the ability to escape their seclusion and isolation and hence the violence if face-to-face interaction were to be reduced;
- Use of safe technology to provide online services with geolocation functions in reporting violence without alerting the perpetrators, including disguised applications and safe code words;
- Use of a forensic gathering app that assists survivors to record, encrypt, and store incidences of violence in a way that is safe, secure, and legally admissible (Johnson 2020);
- Implement coherent and holistic strategies on domestic violence during the pandemic including webinars with links to online resources and online services, emphasizing that law enforcement and justice processes are not suspended during the pandemic (e.g., China's hashtag #AntiDomesticViolenceDuringEpidemic) (UN Women 2020a);
- Designating safe spaces for survivors to report domestic violence such as pharmacies and grocery stores and safe (coded) ways to report domestic violence (UN Women 2020a);

- Declare prevention and response to violence against women programs and services including psychosocial support, crisis centers, shelters, and medico-legal interventions as part of essential services that remain fully operational during the pandemic and ensure these services are accessible during the COVID-19 pandemic;
- Recognize medical response to violence against women as critical in triaging to identify medical priorities during disruptions;
- Explore means to reach out to women with limited access to ICT including telephone and internet connectivity and devices;
- Create awareness and guidelines on safe bystander intervention in domestic violence and enlist the assistance of essential workers such as postal workers and delivery drivers to look out for signs of abuse and confidentially report them (UN Women 2020a);
- Develop and disseminate online safety advisories for women and children and bystander intervention strategies; and
- Work with employers to identify and intervene in domestic violence of and by employees working from home including convening domestic inquiries and taking disciplinary actions against perpetrators while facilitating assistance and support for survivors.

4.1.2 ICT violence against women

- Establish measures to address and prevent ICT violence that are informed by the experiences and perceptions of women and girls, including survivors of ICT violence;
- Develop and disseminate counternarratives to push back against ICT violence against women including gender hate speech;
- Implement dynamic behavior-shaping education programmes on ICT violence directed at specific groups, for example youth and students;
- Educate users on online safety and digital security;
- Legislate to prohibit all forms of ICT violence including sextortion, cyber flashing, morphing, trolling, doxing and live-streaming of sexual abuse content/material and non-consensual dissemination of intimate images, illicit digital voyeurism with a view to promoting women's equal access to ICT without fear of harassment and violence while ensuring that such legislation respects freedom of expression, and complies with human rights and constitutional norms;
- Establish a multi-stakeholder consultative body of government agencies, civil society, the tech community, and academics to develop good practices on preventing, responding to, and eliminating ICT VAWG;
- Collaborate with ICT intermediaries that provide access to, host, transmit and index content, products and ICT services to reduce the toxicity and violence associated with an internet/digital presence and use;

- Collaborate with ICT intermediaries to provide transparent accessible complaint and reporting mechanisms with a process for appeals; and
- Develop an alternative understanding of proprietary rights in images which are vested in the subject of the images/footage particularly if such image/footage constitute ICT violence against women.

Note

1 Both 'victim and 'survivor' are used to refer to the woman who has experienced violence, upon whom the violation/s has occurred. 'Victim' is used when referring to the crime associated with the violation/s. 'Survivor' speaks to the sense of empowerment our coordinated response strategies hope to instill. As the criminality of the violation is not the focus of this chapter, we use the term 'survivor' of violence throughout.

References

Abdul Aziz, Z 2013, 'Culture, Power and Violence in Domestic Violence Narrative', in M Mohamad & S Wieringa (eds.), *Family Ambiguity and Domestic Violence in Asia: Concept, Law and Process*, Sussex Academic Press, United Kingdom, pp. 53–77.

Abdul Aziz, Z 2017, 'Due Diligence and Accountability for Online Violence against Women', *Due Diligence Project*, viewed 28 November 2020, http://duediligenceproject.org/wp-content/uploads/2019/05/Paper-on-Due-Diligence-and-Accountability-for-Online-Violence-against-Women-make-this-active-link.pdf

Abdul Aziz, Z 2018, 'Expert Group Meeting of the UN Joint Global Programme on Essential Services for Women and Girls Subject to Violence "Optimal Entry Points for Safe Technology in the Provision of Essential Services"', unpublished.

Abdul Aziz, Z 2020, 'Online Violence against Women in Asia: A Multi-Country Study', *UN Women*, viewed 9 December 2020, https://asiapacific.unwomen.org/-/media/field%20office%20eseasia/docs/publications/2020/12/ap-ict-vawg-report-7dec20.pdf?la=en&vs=4251

Abdul Aziz, Z & Moussa, J 2016, *Due Diligence Framework: State Accountability Framework for Eliminating Violence against Women*, International Human Rights Initiative, Malaysia.

Allen-Ebrahimian, B 2020, 'China's Domestic Violence Epidemic', *Axios*, 7 March, viewed 10 December 2020, www.axios.com/china-domestic-violence-coronavirus-quarantine-7b00c3ba-35bc-4d16-afdd-b76ecfb28882.html

Ashraf, A 2016, 'A Dark Trade: Rape Videos for Sale in India', *Al Jazeera*, 31 October, viewed 10 December 2020, www.aljazeera.com/indepth/features/2016/10/dark-trade-rape-videos-sale-india-161023124250022.html

Barber, J 2015, 'Second Man Walks Free after Humiliation of Canadian Teen Rehtaeh Parsons', *The Guardian*, 15 January, viewed 10 December 2020, www.theguardian.com/world/2015/jan/15/rehtaeh-parsons-second-man-walks-free-humiliation-canadian-teen-killed-herself

BBC News 2015a, 'How a Rape was Filmed and Shared in Pakistan', 26 February, viewed 10 December 2020, www.bbc.com/news/world-asia-31313551

BBC News 2015b, 'Sex Tape Row: German Court Orders Man to Destroy Naked Images', 22 December, viewed 10 December 2020, www.bbc.com/news/world-europe-35159187

Berkiempes, V 2019, 'Maryland Court: Teen Girl who Sexted Friends Violated Child Pornography laws', *The Guardian*, 31 August 2019, viewed 10 December 2020, www.theguardian.com/us-news/2019/aug/31/maryland-court-teen-girl-video-law

Bivens, R & Hasinoff, A 2018, 'Rape: Is There an App for That? An Empirical Analysis of the Features of Anti-rape Apps', *Information, Communication and Society*, vol. 21, no. 8, p. 1050.

Bradbury-Jones, C 2020, 'The Pandemic Paradox: The Consequences of COVID-19 on Domestic Violence', *Journal of Clinical Nursing*, vol. 29, no. 13–14.

CNA Insider 2018, *South Korea's Digital Sex Crime Wave*, online video, viewed 10 December 2020, www.youtube.com/watch?v=n8EVv1FFl5I

Dhar, S, 2014, 'Women's Safety Schemes Go Mobile in India', *Inter Press Service*, 14 November, viewed 10 December 2020, www.ipsnews.net/2014/11/womens-safety-schemes-go-mobile-in-india/

Editorial Board of Pravoye Delo and Shtekel v. Ukraine, Eur. Ct. H.R., § 63, App. No. 33014/05, May 5, 2011.

Elonis v. United States, 575 U.S. (2015).

GSMA 2019, 'The Mobile Gender Gap Report 2019', viewed 10 December 2020, www.gsma.com/mobilefordevelopment/wp-content/uploads/2019/02/GSMA-The-Mobile-Gender-Gap-Report-2019.pdf

Holmes, O 2016, 'How Child Sexual Abuse Became a Family Business in the Philippines', *The Guardian*, 30 May, viewed 10 December 2020, www.theguardian.com/world/2016/may/31/live-streaming-child-sex-abuse-family-business-philippines

Human Rights Watch 2020, *Submission to the UN Special Rapporteur on Violence against Women, Its Causes and Consequences Regarding COVID-19 and the Increase of Domestic Violence against Women*, 3 July, viewed 10 December 2020, www.hrw.org/news/2020/07/03/submission-un-special-rapporteur-violence-against-women-its-causes-and-consequences

Iglesias, C 2020, 'The Gender Gap in Internet Access: Using a Women-Centred Method', *World Wide Web Foundation*, 10 March, viewed 10 December 2020, https://webfoundation.org/2020/03/the-gender-gap-in-internet-access-using-a-women-centred-method/

International Labour Organization 2019a, *C190-Violence and Harassment Convention (No. 190)*.

International Labour Organization 2019b, *R206-Violence and Harassment Recommendation (No. 206)*.

Internet World Stats 2020a, 'Usage and Population Statistics', viewed 28 November 2020, www.internetworldstats.com/stats3.htm

Internet World Stats 2020b, 'Internet Usage Statistics The Internet Big Picture', viewed 13 December 2020, www.internetworldstats.com/stats.htm

Johnson, K, Green, L, Volpellier, M, Kidenda, S, McHale, T, Naimer, K, & Mishori, R 2020, 'The Impact of COVID-19 on Services for People Affected by Sexual and gender-based Violence', *International Journal of Gynecology and Obstetrics*, vol. 150, no. 3, pp. 285–287.

Johnson, K 2020, 'This App Helps Domestic Violence Victims Collect the Evidence Needed to Charge Their Abusers', *A Mighty Girl*, 24 Oct., www.amightygirl.com/blog?p=26289

Kasulis, K 2020, 'New Arrest Amid Nationwide Anger over S Korea 'Sextortion' Case', *Al Jazeera*, 11 May, viewed 10 December 2020, www.aljazeera.com/news/2020/05/arrest-nationwide-anger-korea-sextortion-case-200511031427033.html

Kurmanbekova, A 2020, 'Women Risk Domestic Violence During Kyrgyzstan's Lockdown', *Human Rights Watch*, 8 April, viewed 13 December 2020, www.hrw.org/news/2020/04/08/women-risk-domestic-violence-during-kyrgyzstans-lockdown

Lumley, K 2015, *Without Fear or Favour, Affection or Ill Will: Addressing Gender Bias in NSW Judicial Education*, International Journal of the Legal Profession, vol. 22, no. 2, 212–225.

Miller, M 2020, 'FBI Sees Spike in Cyber Crime Reports during Coronavirus Pandemic', *The Hill*, 16 April, viewed 13 December 2020, https://thehill.com/policy/cybersecurity/493198-fbi-sees-spike-in-cyber-crime-reports-during-coronavirus-pandemic

Morath, E 2020, 'How Many U.S. Workers Have Lost Jobs During Coronavirus Pandemic? There Are Several Ways to Count', *Wall Street Journal*, 3 June, viewed 13 December 2020, www.wsj.com/articles/how-many-u-s-workers-have-lost-jobs-during-coronavirus-pandemic-there-are-several-ways-to-count-11591176601

Mutongwiza, L 2020, 'Gender Based Violence Is a Pandemic within a Pandemic', *London School of Economics Blog*, 23 April, viewed 13 December 2020, https://blogs.lse.ac.uk/africaatlse/2020/04/23/gender-based-violence-in-zimbabwe-a-pandemic-covid19-virus/

National Domestic Workers Alliance 2020, 'The Impact of COVID-19 on Domestic Workers', October 2020, viewed 13 December 2020, https://domesticworkers.org/sites/default/files/6_Months_Crisis_Impact_COVID_19_Domestic_Workers_NDWA_Labs_1030.pdf

Newton, P 2013, 'Canadian Teen Commits Suicide after Alleged Rape, Bullying', *CNN*, 10 April, viewed 28 November 2020, www.cnn.com/2013/04/10/justice/canada-teen-suicide/index.html

OECD Secretary-General Gurría, A 2020, '2020 Ministerial Council Meeting: The Path to Recovery: Strong, Resilient, Green and Inclusive', 28 October, viewed 28 November 2020, www.oecd.org/about/secretary-general/2020-ministerial-council-meeting-the-path-to-recovery-strong-resilient-green-and-inclusive.htm

Paulo, D 2018, 'In South Korea, A Society Faces up to an Epidemic of Sexual Harassment', *CNA Insider*, 24 February, viewed 28 November 2020, www.channelnewsasia.com/news/cnainsider/south-korea-sexual-harassment-revenge-porn-abuse-get-real-9987316

Pasricha, J 2016, 'Violence Online in India: Cyber Crimes against Women and Minorities on Social Media', *Feminism in India*, Freedom House Hyperlinkers Project, viewed 28 November 2020, https://feminisminindia.com/wp-content/uploads/2016/05/FII_cyberbullying_report_website.pdf

Peterman, A, Potts, A, O'Donnell, M, Thompson, K, Shah, N, Oertelt-Prigione, S & van Gelder, N 2020, 'Pandemics and Violence Against Women and Children', working Paper 528, *Center for Global Development*, viewed 28 November 2020, www.cgdev.org/sites/default/files/pandemics-and-vawg-april2.pdf

Rosell, V 2018, 'The "Wolf Pack" Case Showed the World How Spanish Law is Mired in Misogyny', *The Guardian*, 26 June, viewed 9 December 2020, www.theguardian.com/commentisfree/2018/jun/26/wolf-pack-case-spain-law-misogyny

Šimonović, D 2018, *Report of the Special Rapporteur on Violence against Women, Its Causes and Consequences on Online Violence against Women and Girls from a Human Rights Perspective,* U.N. Doc A/HRC/38/47.

Šimonović, D 2020a, 'States Must Combat Domestic Violence in the Context of COVID-19 Lockdowns', *United Nations Office of the Human Rights Commissioner*, 27 March, viewed 28 November 2020, www.ohchr.org/EN/NewsEvents/Pages/DisplayNews.aspx?NewsID=25749

Šimonović, D 2020b, *Report of the Special Rapporteur on Violence against Women, its Causes and Consequences on Intersection between the Coronavirus Disease (COVID-19) Pandemic and the Pandemic of Gender-based Violence against Women, with a Focus on Domestic Violence and the "Peace in the Home" Initiative,* U.N. Doc A/75/144.

Suler, J 2004, 'The Online Disinhibition Effect', *Cyber Psychology & Behavior*, vol. 7, no. 3, pp. 321–326.

UN General Assembly 1993, *Declaration on the Elimination of Violence against Women*, A/RES/48/104.

UN General Assembly 2015, *Transforming Our World: the 2030 Agenda for Sustainable Development*, U.N. A/RES/70/1.

UN OHCHR 2017, 'Promotion, Protection and Enjoyment of Human Rights on the Internet: Ways to Bridge the Gender Digital Divide from a Human Rights Perspective', A/HRC/35/9.

United Nations Office on Drugs and Crime (UNODC) 2018, 'Global Study on Homicide: Gender-related Killing of Women and Girls', *UNODC Research*.

United Nations Population Fund (UNFPA) 2020, 'Millions More Cases of Violence, Child Marriage, Female Genital Mutilation, Unintended Pregnancy Expected Due to the COVID-19 pandemic', 28 April, viewed 13 December 2020, www.unfpa.org/news/millions-more-cases-violence-child-marriage-female-genital-mutilation-unintended-pregnancies

UN Women 2020a, 'COVID-19 and Ending Violence Against Women and Girls', viewed 28 November 2020, www.unwomen.org/-/media/headquarters/attachments/sections/library/publications/2020/issue-brief-covid-19-and-ending-violence-against-women-and-girls-en.pdf?la=en&vs=5006

UN Women 2020b, 'Online and ICT Violence against Women and Girls During COVID-19', viewed 28 November 2020, www.unwomen.org/-/media/headquarters/attachments/sections/library/publications/2020/brief-online-and-ict-facilitated-violence-against-women-and-girls-during-covid-19-en.pdf?la=en&vs=2519

UN Women 2020c, 'Women in Informal Economy', viewed 28 November 2020, www.unwomen.org/en/news/in-focus/csw61/women-in-informal-economy#notes

UN Women, IDLO, UNDP, UNODC, World Bank and The Pathfinders 2020, 'Justice for Women Amidst COVID-19'.

US Bureau of Labor Statistics 2020, *Job Openings and Labor Turnover Summary*, viewed 6 October 2020, www.bls.gov/news.release/jolts.nr0.htm

United States v. Sayer, 748 F.3d 425 (1st Cir. 2014).

World Health Organization (WHO) 2013, 'Global and Regional Estimates of Violence against Women: Prevalence and Health Effects of Intimate Partner Violence and Non-partner Sexual Violence'.

World Health Organization (WHO) 2020, 'COVID-19 and Violence against Women: What the Health Sector/System Can Do', 7 April, viewed 28 November 2020, https://apps.who.int/iris/bitstream/handle/10665/331699/WHO-SRH-20.04-eng.pdf?ua=1

Wong, R et al., 2018, *Does Gender Matter in Cyberbullying Perpetration? An Empirical Investigation, Computers in Human Behaviour*, vol. 79, pp. 247–257.

8

COVID-19 AND DISABILITY

A war of two paradigms

Gerard Quinn

Moments of crises have a way of bringing deep truths to the surface. Instant reactions reveal a lot. In this instance, the immediate reactions to COVID-19 from policy makers have laid bare the degree to which changes that we thought were permanent in the context of disability were in fact temporary and fragile.

More than anything else, COVID-19 has revealed that the much-vaunted paradigm shift on disability – from the 'medical model' to the 'human rights model' – has yet to sink deep and permanent roots (MacKay 2006–7). Perhaps this was inevitable. Boundaries can shift within and between legal fields over time. But there is always an undertow of outdated ideas – a tug backward which acts as a brake on change. Normally this brake on change is useful in preventing wild policy swings with unpredictable results. It generally dissipates over time. But for a period at least, the two paradigms have seemed to uneasily co-exist and the earlier one sometimes comes to the fore, especially during periods of extreme crises as now.

So it is with COVID-19 and disability. COVID-19 has exposed the new 'rights-based' paradigm on disability as a framework that still exists on shaky stilts – too easily knocked to one side when competing exigencies take center stage. Many of the immediate policy and other responses can only be explained in terms of the resurgence and dominance of an old paradigm. Governments (and many people) did not experience any sense of contradiction at the time. Or, if there were any lingering doubts about the initial responses, they were put to one side almost as if the losses had to be allowed to lie where they fell until more considered responses could be made when under less pressure. In the heat of the moment, rights were a side-constraint to be avoided – not an automatic reflex to be built into the policy responses.

In the first part of this chapter, I shall draw out the contrast between the old paradigm based on the 'medical model' of disability and the newer 'human rights-based model', which pivots on dignity, autonomy, and inclusive equality. Here the literature is truly voluminous. I draw out the contrast only insofar as needed to demonstrate that the initial responses to COVID-19 in the context of disability owed much more to the old paradigm than to the new.

In the second part I shall explore how the older model helps explain the immediate response to COVID-19 in the context of disability. This can be seen in the lack of inclusive prevention, which had the perverse effect of stripping away fragile supports for persons with disabilities. It can be seen in egregious forms of unequal treatment when it came to the rationing of health care goods and services (e.g., ventilators). And it can be seen in the heightened degree of risk for persons with disabilities (and indeed many older persons) due to congregated settings/ institutionalization. Many other dimensions come to the fore, such as inadequate planning to ensure that inclusive education continues on new online and remote learning platforms. But for the sake of brevity in this chapter I will confine myself to the above three sets of impacts: lack of inclusive prevention, unequal treatment in healthcare rationing, and heightened risk from living circumstances.

The last section explores the lessons to be learned, especially as humankind will undoubtedly face new existential crises into the future. Perhaps the most telling feature of the initial responses was the conspicuous lack of consultation with civil society. This not only undermined the legitimacy of many of the responses but also detracted from their efficiency. Problems that were wholly predictable were missed. It is suggested that a key to the future success of a rights-based approach will be in-depth forward planning and adaptation alongside civil society – the *co-production* of legitimate and efficient responses to inevitable crises.

Reference will be made throughout to the highly impressive report of the Disability Rights Monitor (hereinafter, DRM) which was published on 23 October 2020. This project brought together some of the leading disability rights advocacy groups in the world, which together conducted a large-scale research study on all continents detailing the effects of COVID-19 and related policies on persons with disabilities. Its findings were based on a large survey that was circulated in several languages around the world. Both the analysis and the recommendations of the DRM report will be referenced where needed.

Reference will also be made throughout to the COVID-19 Guidance issued by the UN Office of the High Commissioner on Human Rights in May 2020 (hereinafter, OHCHR Guidance). At the outset, the Guidance observes that while international law does allow for emergency measures in response to significant threats, it also insists that such measures be 'proportionate to the evaluated risk, necessary and applied in a non-discriminatory way … and taking the least intrusive approach possible to protect public health' (UN OHCHR 2020a). It is highly questionable whether this was achieved in practice during the pandemic and especially in the context of disability.

An extremely useful resource to help policy makers think through the disability implications of the pandemic came in the shape of the COVID-19 Guidelines from the Australian Human Rights Commission (2020). These AHRC Guidelines will also be referred to where appropriate.

1 A war of two paradigms

Paradigms – or frameworks of reference – are important and operate at three different levels. First of all, they direct our attention toward certain realities or facts. Implicitly, they direct our gaze away from other realities that do not fit. In other words, they determine what is considered salient – or not, as the case may be. This means that some persons with disabilities were effectively treated as if invisible (e.g., blind persons living remotely or in rural areas) (Soldatic & Johnson 2019).

Second, paradigms provide or imply an implicit fund of normative departure points. We draw on these values to help us judge what we 'see'. Is the effective relegation in importance of blind persons living remotely an issue – or not? If the framework or paradigm already internalizes some sort of natural ordering of the human race, then probably not.

And finally, paradigms guide us in framing how we respond to what we 'see'. Our blueprints for change are both motivated and shaped by paradigms. Paradigms make some blueprints for change viable and relegate others in terms of importance. In short, paradigms exert a channeling effect on both perception and action.

Paradigm shifts can come about for many different reasons and can have dramatic effects. For example, in the past, to ignore a person with an intellectual disability in determining who gets medical treatment was not even 'seen' as an issue. It lacked salience. Invisibility operates at many levels to effectively exclude. Switching to the 'rights-based' paradigm sharply reverses this and gives equal visibility to persons with intellectual disabilities in any calculus about who gets treated and who does not.

Another way of bringing out the contrast between the old paradigm based on care or welfare and the newer one based on rights is to spotlight the difference between viewing persons with disabilities as 'objects' or as 'subjects'. Put simply, an object is an entity that one can manipulate or treat without considering its inherent agency or rights. A subject, by way of contrast, is not a thing and cannot be treated as a thing akin to property. It is an end in itself, possessing human agency, equal rights, and deserving respect. That is why the general struggle for equal personhood of persons with disabilities has been so central to the new paradigm. Of course, this places a premium on deep philosophical questions about who – or what – is a person (what are the essential ingredients of personhood). This is a rich and much neglected debate (Kittay & Carlson 2010).

In addition to this inbuilt bias against certain categories of persons with disability is the tendency in many societies (at least in market-driven societies) to judge or evaluate people according to the utility or 'use value'. Some persons are more useful than others. Some persons have skills that are in higher demand than others. It is but a short jump to the conclusion that some persons' lives are worth more than others and worth preserving before those others. We may have thought that hierarchies of this sort are a thing of the feudal past. However, hierarchical thinking often reasserts itself in the implicit ordering of society, whether based on judgments about use value or otherwise. Of course, these judgments are mostly counterfactual and based on stereotypes. But because they are buried so deep in culture, they hardly ever come to the surface, even though they explain much behavior (Kakoullis & Johnson 2020).

The rights-based framework inverts all the above. First of all, we start with the foundational premise of personhood – indeed *equal* personhood. This framing rejects the view that there is an implicit ordering of the human race in terms of relative 'use value' or otherwise. All persons regardless of the difference of disability (or age) are regarded as having equal worth and indeed an equal right to determine their own future and choose their own course of action.

Of some considerable relevance is the UN Committee on the Rights of Persons with Disabilities' view on what exactly equality means in the context of disability (UN CRPD 2018). The Committee's understanding is very far removed from traditional or juridical conceptions of equality that simply compared the treatment of one cohort (presumably disadvantaged) with another (the comparator). This approach has been disparaged as 'normatively empty' since it lets the analysis rest on the relativities of treatment. Instead, the Committee sees the equality ideal (which it calls 'inclusive equality') as resting on: (1) equal recognition as a person, (2) the positive accommodation of difference, (3) a participative dimension that emphasizes the equal right to belong, and (4) a (re)distribution dimension of resources to underpin the above. For our purposes what is important in this formulation is its explicit grounding in equal personhood and its emphasis that resources should be used to make this a reality and not to otherwise cushion persons with disabilities on the margins of society (Jacobs 2018).

Of course, the main legal expression of this new paradigm – the UN Convention on the rights of persons with disabilities (hereinafter, UN CRPD) – has been near-universally ratified. One would have thought that its values (and especially the extent to which it resets the framing on disability) would have had a dramatic impact in how policy makers react in crises, including COVID-19 – not so and quite the reverse. The Legal Realists have long admonished us to beware of the difference between the 'law in the books' and the 'law in action' (Pound 1910, p. 12). To formally adopt a legal instrument like the UN CRPD does not necessarily mean that the underlying shifts in values that the instrument represents have been internalized or accepted. The osmosis of international legal obligations into the DNA of domestic policymaking is a complex process and certainly not unilinear (Goodman & Jinks 2013). The natural reflex of most systems seems to be to genuflect before such instruments (especially when easy political capital can be obtained without too much cost) and then to keep them at arm's length when formulating domestic policy.

So, at one level, and looking on the subject from the perspective of legal sociology, it is not surprising to see the UN CRPD marginalized when it comes to the initial COVID-19 responses. The gap, however, between international normative commitments and domestic responses has been so egregious that governments themselves now openly concede that COVID-19 has revealed deep-seated and systemic inequalities (e.g., the European Union at 3rd Committee UN GA).

2 The triumph of an old paradigm in the immediate responses to COVID-19

Why the old paradigm came to the surface and drove many initial policy responses to COVID-19 in the context of disability remains a complex question. How it did so is more easily described. There was a myriad of ways in which this happened. Most of it has been graphically highlighted by the aforementioned DRM report of October 2020.

I will focus on three strands of actions which demonstrate the validity of my core thesis – that an old paradigm dominated and explains the initial policy responses as they touch on disability. These initial reactions span different economic and political systems. And they were as present in the developed North as they were in the developing South. This says a lot about the durable power of the old paradigm irrespective of political, economic, or legal systems or environments (Kakoullis & Johnson 2020).

2.1 Lack of inclusive preventive strategies

Preventive strategies have tended not to include any consideration of the situation of persons with disabilities. For example, curfew and lockdown measures were not adequately communicated to different groups of persons with disabilities. Sound medical advice did not get through to those who really needed it.

The DRM report highlights that this lack of accessible information was particularly true to those living in institutions: many respondents were worried that persons with disabilities [living] in institutions were cut off from society, without any knowledge of the state of emergency (DRM 2020, p. 25). This is why the UN OHCHR Guidelines specifically call for steps to be taken to 'support...the flow of accessible information to these groups' (listed under the heading 'Leaving No One Behind') (UN OHCHR 2020a, p. 2).

One result was that many persons with disabilities unwittingly flouted curfew and lockdown rules with the result that confrontation with the police was inevitable. As the DRM report states: 'Around the world persons with disabilities and their family members have had no choice but to break curfew rules to access food and essential medical supplies because no exceptions were made for them' (DRM 2020, p. 32). The DRM report continues: '[t]he testimonies [gathered by the DRM survey] reveal an alarming global phenomenon of police harassment, torture and murder of persons with disabilities and their family members' (DRM 2020, p. 33). Such a pattern of behavior is probably due less to malevolence than to a lack of sensitization on the part of police forces to the situation of persons with disabilities, as well as a lack of nuance in the governing regulations. One testimonial in the DRM report from Uganda stated: 'I know two PWDs who have been shot at because they were outside in curfew time. These were deaf people who didn't know what was happening' (DRM 2020, p. 33).

And this is why the European Disability Forum (EDF) has recommended that governments should put in 'place flexible mechanisms to authorize persons with disabilities (including support persons) to leave their homes during mandatory quarantines... when they experience difficulty with home confinement' (European Disability Forum 2020).

In addition, the support systems that enabled many persons with disabilities to live their own lives in the community and in their own homes (i.e. not their parents' homes) were uniquely vulnerable. It is important to realize that these support systems are specifically called for by the UN CRPD in order to enable the right to live independently and be included in the community. Article 19.2 affirms that states shall ensure that 'persons with disabilities have access to a range of in-home, residential and other community support services, including personal assistance necessary to support living and inclusion in the community, and to prevent isolation or segregation from the community' (UN CRPD 2006, art. 19(2)).

In the DRM survey 38 percent of respondents said that they lacked access to personal assistance (DRM 2020, p. 28). Since it was virtually impossible to guarantee the safety of care workers (personal assistants) because of (among other issues) the lack of personal protective equipment (PPE), they were generally withdrawn or opted to discontinue working.

Prevention strategies have had some peculiar and unintended results. Interestingly, support workers were mostly paid through emergency budget measures (which were wholly justified). However, these emergency budget measures tended to make no allowance for ways to ensure that other or alternative supports were available for the end-users – the primary reason why supports existed in the first place. Usefully, in their joint statement on 1 April 2020 the chair of the UN CRPD Committee and the UN Secretary General's Special Envoy on Accessibility stated: 'the range of support in the community, including rehabilitation services and home-care and personal assistance support, when necessary must be ensured and not discontinued as they are essential for the exercise of the rights of persons with disabilities' (UN CRPD 2020, para. 9). In as much as family or siblings took over responsibility, they too were generally left unsupported. In a major resolution on COVID-19 and disability, the European Disability Forum specifically pointed to the impoverishing impacts on caretakers who are usually women and mothers – the so-called 'feminization of poverty'.

Indeed, the DRM report asserts that as many as 33 percent of persons with disabilities were left with no family support (because family was unavailable) and no informal care at all *in lieu* of personal assistance (DRM 2020, p. 28). So persons with disabilities could not leave their homes, nor were services allowed/enabled to come to their homes.

The gender dimension here is quite significant. Women Enabled International (WEI) figured that this scenario entrapped many women and girls with disabilities living at home and further heightened their vulnerability to gender-based violence (WEI 2020, p. 1). In a significant report published in April 2020 and which was based on an extensive world-wide survey, WEI states:

> Home may be a safe place for most, but not for many women, girls, non-binary, trans, and gender non-conforming persons with disabilities, their homes are a place of fear. Women and girls with disabilities experience violence from partners and family members at least two to three times the rate of other women, and during lockdowns, shelter in place orders… these individuals will be even less able to escape violence, particularly if their usual supports are not available to them.
>
> *(WEI 2020, p. 16)*

This is much more than an inconvenience. This goes directly to the right to life of persons with disabilities. A particularly harrowing account of gender-based violence directed against women and girls with disabilities during the pandemic is provided in a report by the India-based NGO Rising Flame (Rising Flame 2020). The intersectional nature of the vulnerabilities exposed during the pandemic covering both persons with disabilities and the LGBTI community was brought to the fore by a report by Outright Action: 'Vulnerability Amplified: the Impact of COVID-19 Pandemic on LGBTIQ people' (2020).

The UN OHCHR Guidance specifically acknowledges that 'physical distancing, self-isolation and other emergency measures, need to take [into] account the needs of persons with disabilities who rely on support networks essential for their survival' (UN OHCHR 2020a, p. 2). Clearly, not enough attention was given to the inevitable consequences of withdrawing support for people already on the margin.

Unsurprisingly, there was a measurable uptick in homelessness of persons with disabilities. And those who were already homeless now went without even basic services on which they had hitherto relied. The DRM reports that 51 percent of respondents to their survey said that 'their government took no measures to protect the life, health and safety of persons with disabilities living on the streets or in homeless shelters' (DRM 2020, p. 37). That is why the UN OHCHR Guidelines specifically calls for the provision of emergency shelters with adequate services (under the subtitle Housing) (UN OHCHR 2020a, p. 2).

Many persons with disabilities who had been living in remote or rural areas were effectively abandoned. The European Disability Forum pointed to the danger of undetected violence and exploitation when persons with disabilities were effectively abandoned in their own homes. Living in such isolation, persons with disabilities tended to lack access to the basics including food, nutrition, and medical goods or services. It is estimated that some starved and many went without medicine. Reportedly, some persons with disabilities in Canada openly speculated about assisted suicide as a way out (Mulligan & Yawar 2020). On this point, the DRM report includes one Ugandan respondent's reflections on the psychological toll of isolation: 'due to isolation and social restrictions it has caused a lot of fear and psychological pain, anxiety, with uncertainty about what will happen next. This may culminate into an increase in mental health breakdowns and increase in suicide cases' (DRM 2020, p. 29).

Mandatory mask wearing has proven effective against the spread of the virus. Generally speaking, the regulations of guidelines governing such preventive measures usually contain exceptions. For example, children under two are generally exempted. If mask wearing is difficult, if not impossible, for some people with disabilities then they too are generally exempted. This would include those with muscular or skeletal disabilities or those who cannot breathe easily or normally or who might have trouble taking a mask on or off. Generally speaking, proof (i.e., medical proof) of a disability is not required to take advantage of these exemptions.

Some commentators have observed that the majority of businesses are unaware of these exemptions (Pendo et al. 2020, p. 11). Out of a fear of slippery slopes (persons without disabilities can too easily claim the disability exemption if no proof of a disability is required), businesses either demanded medical proof of disability or denied any accommodation. This has led some to call for mask wearing non-binding recommendations instead of mandatory legal requirements. The argument runs that store providers and others need more time to educate themselves about the disability exemptions.

So, the prevention strategies that should have reached many persons with disabilities and informed their behavior did not do so. To some extent this must have exacerbated their risk and inherent susceptibility to the virus as well as exposure to harsh law enforcement. Prevention strategies that removed services tended to have a decisively negative impact on persons with disabilities who disproportionately depended on them for their wellbeing. To a large extent, all of this was predictable but was ignored, likely due to the relative invisibility of the voices of persons with disabilities in crisis planning.

2.2 Unequal treatment in health care and medical responses

Most countries enact general legislation providing broad parameters for the operation of medical ethics. Ultimately, it is for the autonomous medical profession to decide for itself on the shape and content of their own ethical guidelines. Many medical schools in the world still lack modules on the sensitization of future professionals to patients with disabilities and their inherent rights. And most medical bodies have not in the past consulted widely with disability civil society groups in formulating their ethical guidelines.

The flashpoint had to do with the formulation of emergency ethical guidelines on how to prioritize cases when resources were severely constrained. At one point in the pandemic, it looked as if intensive care units would be overwhelmed and that scarce life-saving resources like ventilators would have to be rationed. Thankfully that did not happen everywhere. However, medical authorities had to prepare in case it might happen. That placed a premium on outlining priorities for care (and the rationing of care) and setting out a clear rationale for the same.

Typical of such medical guidelines (or 'triage' guidelines) were those of Pennsylvania. These guidelines provided that certain categories of persons with disabilities would be automatically relegated in importance or priority. This included primarily persons with intellectual disabilities. The operation of the exception worked automatically if one were simply part of the relevant group. That is, no individualized assessment needed to be made. Further, the guidelines allowed medical personnel to make judgments based on notions (implicit or otherwise) on the relative quality of life or the inherent worth of the lives of particular persons or groups with disabilities. It is plain that what is at play here is the old paradigm.

An interesting and entirely laudable pushback against these kinds of guidelines came in the form of a ruling by the Office of Civil Rights of the US Department of Health and Social Services (OCR-DHSS) in May 2020 (HHS 2020). The Pennsylvania guidelines would have allowed medical personnel to exclude (or relegate in importance) certain categories of persons with disabilities and, in addition, to make judgments based on imputed 'quality of life'. The State of Pennsylvania agreed with the OCR-DHSS to amend the guidelines along the following lines:

> removing criteria that automatically deprioritized persons on the basis of particular disabilities… requiring individualized assessments based on the best available, relevant, and objective medical evidence to support triaging decisions, and… ensuring that no one is denied care based on stereotypes, assessments of quality of life, or judgments about a person's 'worth' based on the presence or absence of disabilities.
>
> *(HHS 2020)*

The OCR noted at the outset that no federal civil rights law had been put into abeyance as a result of the onset of COVID-19. That meant that existing laws – including the Americans with Disabilities Act (ADA) and the corresponding non-discrimination provisions of the Rehabilitation Act continued in full force.

Parenthetically, it should be similarly noted that the UN CRPD does not contain a provision allowing for derogation during periods of emergency and no State Party has entered a reservation with respect to their obligations during or because of COVID-19. By definition, the UN CRPD continues to apply with full force even during the emergency (and perhaps especially during the emergency). This does not mean that retrenchment or retrogressive measures are totally prohibited provided they meet the requirements set up by the UN OHCHR Guidance outlined above (proportionality, necessity, non-discriminatory application, and opting for the least intrusive measures).

The first limb of the OCR settlement above states the obvious – that decisions based on status are utterly impermissible. To do so would explicitly problematize the person. Problematizing the person is the hallmark of the older disability paradigm.

The second limb in the OCR settlement still leaves space for assessments that deprioritize persons with disabilities – provided they are done so on an individualized basis. It should be noted that this has the effect of narrowing down room for status-based thinking – but does not preclude it altogether. To a certain extent, it reframes the question rather than conclusively resolving it.

The third limb is extremely welcome and clearly belongs to the newer paradigm on disability. The fact of the matter is that any consideration of the 'quality of life' of potential patients allows too much room for status-driven and stereotypical assumptions. Such considerations are highly – and perhaps inescapably – subjective. On a pretense of objectivity they seem to allow subjective judgments almost free rein. From a human rights perspective, this cannot be allowed.

Women Enabled International has drawn specific and detailed attention to the double discrimination experienced by women with disabilities in the context of triage guidelines as well as broader discrimination with respect to health services (WEI 2020, pp. 7–8). It recounts many harrowing testimonials about the fear of such discrimination by women and girls with disabilities.

The quest is to find a disability neutral (and indeed an age neutral) way of setting priorities. The OCR constrains this quest but does not preclude it. In a guidance note published by the Center for Dignity in Healthcare for People with Disabilities (Cincinnati), health care providers are admonished to 'ensure that the allocation of COVID-19 resources, supplies and care, are not based on inaccurate assumptions about life with a disability'. While useful, this does not deal with how to react when the assumptions are in fact accurate or rest on at least partially accurate surmisals (Alexander 1992).

Triage is of course at the sharper end of healthcare. The reality is that much healthcare provision falling short of triage was implicitly rationed in a way that disfavored persons with disabilities. Access to food and nutrition was also reportedly uneven (DRM 2020, p. 46). This is one reason why the World Bank COVID Crisis Response focused on food insecurity. The UN Food and Agriculture Organization (FAO) is also alert to food insecurity and gross inequalities as it affects persons with disabilities and others (FAO 2020).

Usefully, the UN OHCHR Guidance is to the effect that States should ensure that 'decisions on the allocation of scarce resources… are not based on pre-existing impairments, high support needs, quality of life assessments or medical bias against persons with disabilities' (UN OHCHR 2020a). This echoes strongly with the above OCR ruling.

At play here is not only Article 5 of the UN CRPD prohibiting unequal treatment, whether taken alone or in combination with Article 25 (right to health). It should be recalled that Article 25(f) of the UN CRPD specifically calls on States Parties to 'prevent discriminatory denial of health care of medical services or food and fluids on the basis of disability' (UN CRPD 2006).

2.3 Situations of heightened risk – congregated settings and institutions

A plurality of persons who died during COVID-19 died in congregated settings (Peisah et al. 2020). This mostly accounted for older persons with pre-existing conditions, co-morbidities, and disabilities. Institutions as such – and nursing homes are institutions – should not exist. Put another way, congregated settings certainly run counter to both the spirit and the letter of the UN CRPD. One might say this applies with equal force to those institutions that house older people and especially older persons with disabilities. A moot point is whether such settings should exist for older persons who do not have disabilities (or at least not obvious disabilities) (Capacity Australia 2020).

To the argument based on the UN CRPD that such places should not exist and should be transitioned out of existence is a newer argument based on the exigencies of public health. Put bluntly, such places are a petri dish allowing for the disease to spread easily and should be abolished or transitioned out of existence on the grounds of public health reasons alone. The COVID-19 crisis has made this clear.

First of all, the support workers in such institutions often work in more than one institution. Any infection they pick up travels with them from institution to institution. This is not their fault; they too should not be problematized. Instead, it speaks to the weakness of the general ecosystem put in place to ensure the continuity of service during periods of crisis.

Second, because their employment is usually low-paid and precarious, support workers often depend on public transport, which further heightens their risk as well as the risk of transmission to the residents. Employment tends to be either over-professionalized or over-precarious for those working in institutions. The 2017 McKinsey Report on the future of work envisions a qualitative transformation of these kinds of precarious caring roles – but this remains in the future (Manyika et al. 2020).

Third, even if the support workers could successfully protect themselves, there probably was not enough physical room in the relevant institutions for adequate 'social distancing'. Indeed, the job itself does not lend itself to distancing. This was especially so where residents were housed more than one to a room.

Fourth, PPE equipment was rationed out first to hospitals. Only later was consideration given to the distribution of PPE to congregated settings like institutions or nursing homes. One testimonial reported in the DRM recalled that 'the measures taken to protect persons [with disabilities and older persons] in institutions was a bit late coming, almost as an afterthought' (DRM 2020, p. 26). This was a direct result of relative invisibility: out of sight, out of mind.

Fifth, severe visitor restrictions were put in place – thus exacerbating the sense of isolation and loneliness in institutional settings. Of course, visitors did carry risks. But it is probably fair to say that those who were inclined to visit were also probably inclined to stay safe and to mitigate risks. They probably posed less risk than the formal care workers. And indeed, if the care workers were routinely tested then there was no reason not to test visitors to control risks. Cutting off this lifeline was cruel and arguably unnecessary and disproportionate.

It was not just visitors who were limited – bodies that might ordinarily be counted on to monitor conditions within such institutions were also limited (UN OHCHR 2020c). As the DRM report states:

> authorities have denied access to independent human rights authorities to monitor the health and safety of detainees. A Greek organisation of persons with disabilities described the psychiatric institutions [of Greece] as 'hermetically sealed with more absolute restrictions than before, with no possibility of visits, with no advocacy services and with no independent monitoring'.
>
> *(DRM 2020, p. 24)*

If there are no outside visitors or independent monitors allowed in then the risk is that untoward things happening in institutions will not be caught and remedied. In this regard, the UN Special Rapporteur on the rights of persons with disabilities noted in her appeal 'Who is Protecting the People with Disabilities' (17 March 2020), 'limiting their contact with loved ones leaves people with disabilities totally unprotected from any form of abuse or neglect in institutions'. And that is why the UN OHCHR Guidance states: 'limiting contact with families may be justified as part of emergency health measures but may result in people with disabilities and older persons being further exposed to neglect and abuse' (UN OHCHR 2020a).

All of the above accounts for one of the main recommendations of the DRM study: to accelerate an emergency de-institutionalization program throughout the world. The need for this was underscored by a joint statement of the chair of the UN CRPD Committee and the UN Special Envoy on Accessibility (UN OHCHR 2020b). The UN OHCHR Guidance also recommends that states 'should release persons with disabilities from institutions, nursing homes, psychiatric and other facilities whenever possible, and take measures to ensure the protection of those who are in such facilities' (UN OHCHR 2020a, p. 3).

At play here is Article 5 of the UN CRPD prohibiting unequal treatment. Segregation into congregated settings is an extreme form of unequal treatment which begs strong justification under Article 5. At play also is Article 19 which paints an entirely different picture of flourishing in the community in a home of one's own (the right to live independently and be including in the community). Taken together, these two provisions point strongly in the direction of de-institutionalization for persons with disabilities.

We have become used to the arguments for ending institutionalization under the UN CRPD. Now these arguments are powerfully reinforced by public health considerations. *A priori,* there is no reason to doubt the equal applicability of these norms to older persons – even those without disabilities (Steele et al. 2020; Steele et al. 2019). Logically, these arguments apply as much to older people, even those without disabilities, as it does to persons with disabilities (whether older or not).

3 Building back better – going beyond a slogan

What conclusions can be derived from the above? First, it is plain that the diverse responses to the pandemic – especially in the early days – owed almost nothing to a sense of the centrality of the rights of persons with disabilities. If anything, persons with disabilities were treated as if they were invisible. As suggested above, the early responses to the pandemic owe much to the dominance of an old paradigm which has not gone away and reasserts itself during moments of crisis.

Second, the dominance of the outdated paradigm has been reflected in how preventive measures unfolded without taking account of the diverse needs of persons with disabilities. It was reflected in the ease with which supports, which had been painstakingly built up over the years, were swept to aside, bringing a tide of misery in its wake. It was reflected in blatantly unequal triage and other healthcare rationing policies. Finally, it was reflected in the high proportion of 'excess' deaths due to institutionalization.

Third, the dominance of the old paradigm begs a profound question about how the centrality of the rights of persons with disabilities could have been embedded in policy responses from the outset. Clearly, the older paradigm still competes for attention. It should be obvious by now that the substantive provisions of the UN CRPD (e.g., equality, independent living) are not self-executing. Equal attention should be paid to the process-based rights of the treaty. More than likely, an appropriate as well as efficient response to the COVID-19 crisis could only have been done if persons with disabilities and their representative organizations had been involved in pandemic planning from the outset. After all, this is a (process-based) legal obligation incumbent on States Parties under the UN CRPD (UN CRPD 2006, art. 4(3)) and is strongly reinforced by the UN OHCHR Guidance. The process-based rights of the treaty are just as important as the substantive rights. If not adhered to then the Potemkin illusion of substantive rights literally dissolves before our eyes. This point was strongly emphasized by the previous UN Special Rapporteur on the rights of persons with disabilities in her Appeal of 17 March 2020 as well as by the European Disability Forum.

This option of policy co-production was probably resisted because of a perception that it would foreclose painful but needed options. However, the failure to include advocacy groups generated additional problems that could easily have been predicted and catered for at the outset. One latent fear of policymakers is that solutions on one 'ground' (e.g. disability) may complicate issues on other grounds. In her prodigious work, Linda Steele points out the many ways in which persons with disabilities have demonstrated real leadership during the pandemic and have been among the first to reach out intersectionally (Steele 2020; Spade 2020). By this she means that persons with disabilities have shown themselves adept at responsibly factoring in the policy implications for many groups beyond themselves.

Policy makers do not have to agree with every input from civil society. To govern is to choose. But to govern wisely without creating needless problems does require that those who are not at the table should have a voice. New accessibility laws in Canada stipulate how citizen participation is to work in the co-production of accessibility regulations and proves to be a model of sorts (Jacobs 2016).

Finally, many states engaged in bilateral assistance and many multilateral assistance programs are now reprioritizing their programs to take account of the COVID-19 emergency and the need to 'build back better'. The UN OHCHR Guidance specifically calls for this pivot (UN OHCHR 2020a).

In this regard, it should be understood that many, if not most, of the problems highlighted by the DRM report do not really go to resources (or to resource scarcity) as such. The problems came about because of the dominance of an old model in the immediate response and an unwillingness (or temporary inability) to center persons with disabilities (and other similarly situated groups) at the heart of the initial responses. Logically therefore, any redirection of development assistance to meet the exigencies of COVID-19 should aim to find ways of embedding a sense of the centrality of the rights of persons with disabilities in crisis planning and appropriate policy responses.

Given the proclivity of systems – all systems – to fall back on anachronistic frameworks of reference to guide action if left to their own devices, the single best investment of the international community would be to find ways of ensuring effective consultation and co-production of future policy. 'Build Back Better' will remain merely a nice slogan unless and until voices that were not at the table are given the prominence that they are due. This goes to both legitimacy as well as efficiency.

And given the fragility of support systems – systems that are vital not just for wellbeing but for life itself – investments should be made to assist states in developing their support ecosystem necessary to guarantee continuity of service (EASPD & EAN 2020). Most assuredly this should not include pouring money into existing service structures that have not served persons with disabilities well in the past and which have proven to be unreliable in an emergency.

Both Women Enabled International and Rising Flame have performed immense public service in detailing the disproportionate effects of COVID-19 policies on women and girls with disabilities. It is an imperative that future policy responses have to be much more attuned to the situations of heightened vulnerability in which women and girls with disabilities find themselves. Put more affirmatively, their agency and voice need to be at the fore in resetting how public policy adjusts in the future.

To be guarded against at all costs is reinvestment in institutions and other forms of congregated settings. Since the support ecosystem for persons with disabilities has shown itself to be exceptionally fragile, material investment – if forthcoming through international development assistance – should be used to spur innovation in service design and delivery. If a surge in development assistance is not tied to enhancing voices of persons with disabilities in the crisis planning process and is used instead to build back old sites of risk and susceptibility (like institutions) then nothing much will have changed.

The above rhymes closely with the tenor of the World Bank response to COVID-19 which deals with the responses in terms of (1) immediate relief, (2) restructuring efforts (especially in the economy), and (3) resilient recovery (World Bank 2020). A cross-cutting theme in the World Bank approach is the treatment of vulnerable groups including those with disabilities. Under the last heading, the World Bank specifically calls for improvements in the 'standards of services to ensure continuity of services' for persons with disabilities and others (World Bank Group 2020, p. 19).

At a regional level, it is to be noted that recent changes in the European Structural and Investment Funds (ESIF) (a sort of development assistance program internal to the EU and going to less developed regions and states) have created additional flexibility to allow EU Member States to respond to the COVID-19 crisis and to rebuild (European Commission 2020). De-institutionalization remains a priority even under the more flexible regime in the ESIF. These funds should be used to reconfigure the service ecosystem to be much more resilient and to ensure that relief efforts reach all including those with disabilities.

Humankind will undoubtedly face more pandemics as well as natural and humanitarian disasters in the future. The old paradigm on disability is both dangerous and ineffective. It is time to embed the new paradigm based on rights much more intentionally in how we position ourselves to face the future.

References

Alexander, L 1992, 'What Makes Wrongful Discrimination Wrong: Biases, Preferences, Stereotypes and Proxies', *University of Pennsylvania Law Review*, vol. 141.

Australian Human Rights Commission 2020, 'Guidelines on the Rights of People with Disabilities in Health and Disability Care during COVID-19', viewed 10 December 2020, https://humanrights.gov.au/our-work/disability-rights/publications/guidelines-rights-people-disability-health-and-disability

Capacity Australia 2020, 'Nursing Homes Should Be Abolished Global Debate', 2 September, viewed 10 December 2020, https://capacityaustralia.org.au/capacity-australia-international-debate-nursing-homes-should-be-abolished-september-2-2020/

Disability Rights Monitor (DRM) 2020, 'Disability Rights During the Pandemic: A Global Report on Findings of the COVID-19 Disability Rights Monitor', viewed 10 December 2020, https://covid-drm.org/assets/documents/Disability-Rights-During-the-Pandemic-report-web.pdf

European Association of Service Providers for Persons with Disabilities (EASPD) & European Aging Network (EAN) 2020, 'Ensuring EU Response to COVID-19 Tackles Threat of Social Care Emergency', 11 March, viewed 10 December 2020, www.easpd.eu/sites/default/files/sites/default/files/Publications/easpd-ean_letter_to_president_von_der_leyen_re._covid-19_0.pdf

European Commission 2020, 'Cohesion Policy Action against Coronavirus', viewed 10 December 2020, https://ec.europa.eu/regional_policy/en/newsroom/coronavirus-response/

European Disability Forum General Assembly 2020, *Resolution on Covid-19 and the Rights of Persons with Disabilities*.

Goodman, R & Jinks, D 2013, *Socializing States: Promoting Human Rights through International Law*, Oxford University Press, Oxford.

Health and Human Services (HHS) 2020, 'OCR Resolves Civil Rights Complaint Against Pennsylvania After it Revises its Pandemic Health Care Triaging Policies to Protect Against Disability Discrimination', 16 April, viewed 10 December 2020, www.hhs.gov/about/news/2020/04/16/ocr-resolves-civil-rights-complaint-against-pennsylvania-after-it-revises-its-pandemic-health-care.html

Jacobs, L 2016, '"Humanizing" Disability Law: Citizen Participation in the Development of Accessibility Regulations in Canada', *Revue Internationale des Gouvernements Ouverts*, vol. 3.

Jacobs, L 2018, 'The Universality of the Human Condition: Theorizing Transportation Inequality Claims by Persons with Disabilities in Canada, 1976–2016', *Canadian Journal of Human Rights*, vol. 7, no. 1.

Kakoullis, EJ & Johnson, K 2020, *Recognising Human Rights in Different Cultural Contexts: the United Nations Convention on the Rights of Persons with Disabilities*, Palgrave.

Kittay, EF & Carlson, L 2010, *Cognitive Disability and its Challenge to Moral Philosophy*, Wiley-Blackwell, Oxford.

MacKay, D 2006–7, 'The United Nations Convention on the Rights of Persons with Disabilities', *Syracuse Journal of International Law and Commerce*, vol 34, p. 323.

Manyika, J, Lund, S, Chui, M, Bughin, J, Woetzel, J, Batra, P, Ko, R, & Sanghvi, S 2017, 'The Future of Work: Jobs Lost, Jobs Gained, What the Future of Work Will Mean for Jobs, Skills and Wages', *McKinsey & Company*.

Mulligan, C & Yawar, M 2020, 'ODSP Recipients Calling for Help, Exploring Assisted Dying', 2 September, *CityNews*, 2 September.

OutRight Action International 2020, *Vulnerability Amplified: The Impact of the COVID-19 Pandemic on LGBTIQ People*, OutRight Action International, New York.

Peisah, C, Byrnes, A, Doron, I, Dark, M, & Quinn, G 2020, 'Advocacy for the Human Rights of Older People in the COVID Pandemic and Beyond: A Call to Mental Health Professionals', *International Psychogeriatrics*, vol. 32, no. 10.

Pendo, E, Gatter, R, & Mohapatra, S 2020, 'Resolving Tensions between Disability Rights Law and Covid-19 Mask Policies', *Maryland Law Review*, vol. 80, online 1.

Pound, R 1910, 'Law in Books and Law in Action', *American Law Review*, vol. 44.

Rising Flame 2020, 'Neglected and Forgotten: Women with Disabilities during the Covid Crisis in India', viewed 10 December 2020, https://risingflame.org/project/neglected-and-forgotten-women-with-disabilities-during-covid-crisis-in-india/

Soldatic, K & Johnson, K 2019, *Disability and Rurality: Identity, Gender and Belonging*, Routledge, Abingdon.

Spade, Dean 2020, *Mutual Aid: Building Solidarity During This Crisis (and the Next)*, VERSO, New York.

Steele, L 2020, *Disability, Criminal Justice and Law: Reconsidering Court Diversion*, Routledge, Abingdon.

Steele, L, Swaffer, K, Phillipson, L, & Fleming, R 2019, 'Questioning Segregation of People Living with Dementia in Australia: An International Human Rights Approach to Care Homes', *Laws*, vol. 8, no. 3, p. 18.

Steele, L, Carr, R, Swaffer, K, Phillipson, L, & Fleming, R 2020, 'Ending Confinement and Segregation: Barriers to Realising Human Rights in the Everyday Lives of People Living with Dementia in Residential Aged Care', *Australian Journal of Human Rights*. Published online (25 June 2020), viewed 16 March 2021, www.tandfonline.com/action/doSearch?AllField=linda+steele&SeriesKey=rjhu20

UN Committee on the Rights of Persons with Disabilities (CRPD) 2018, *General Comment 6 on Equality and Non-discrimination*, CRPD/C/GC/6.

UN CRPD 2006, *Convention on the Rights of Persons with Disabilities*, UN Doc. A/61/49.

UN CRPD Committee 2020, 'The Joint Statement of the Chair of the UN CRPD Committee and the UN Secretary General's Special Envoy on Accessibility', 9 June, viewed 10 December 2020, www.ohchr.org/EN/NewsEvents/Pages/DisplayNews.aspx?NewsID=25942&LangID=E

UN Food and Agriculture Organization (FAO), 'Addressing Inequality in Times of COVID-19', 18 June, viewed 10 December 2020, www.fao.org/3/ca8843en/CA8843EN.pdf

UN OHCHR 2020a, *Covid-19 Guidance*, viewed 10 December 2020, https://www.ohchr.org/Documents/Events/COVID-19_Guidance.pdf

UN OHCHR 2020b, 'Joint Statement: Persons with Disabilities and COVID-19 by the Chair of the United Nations Committee on the Rights of Persons with Disabilities, on behalf of the Committee on the Rights of Persons with Disabilities and the Special Envoy of the United Nations Secretary-General on Disability and Accessibility', United Nations Human Rights Office of the High Commissioner, viewed 13 December 2020, www.ohchr.org/EN/NewsEvents/Pages/DisplayNews.aspx?NewsID=25765&LangID=E

UN OHCHR 2020c, 'COVID-19: Who is Protecting the People with Disabilities? UN Rights Expert', *United Nations Human Rights Office of the High Commissioner*, 17 March, viewed 10 December 2020, www.ohchr.org/EN/NewsEvents/Pages/DisplayNews.aspx?NewsID=25725

Women Enabled International 2020, 'COVID-19 at the Intersection of Gender and Disability: Findings of a Global Human Rights Survey', viewed 10 December 2020, https://womenenabled.org/blog/covid-19-survey-findings/.

World Bank Group 2020, 'COVID-19 Response Approach Paper: Saving Lives, Scaling up Impact and Getting Back on Track', World Bank.

9

LIFE AND DEATH IN PRISONS

Hope Metcalf

When the coronavirus pandemic hit the small state of Connecticut, Carlos DeLeon knew he was in trouble. A city jail was no place for a sixty-three-year-old with chronic lung disease. Still, for a time, Carlos seemed to have a shot at avoiding COVID-19. The state had already determined that Carlos – who was halfway through a two-year sentence – posed little risk to the public and approved him for supervised release (Knowles 2020). There was one catch: the state had to approve his destination. No halfway house beds were available, so two of Carlos' sisters offered to house him, but the state determined their houses were 'unsuitable' (Krasselt 2020a). In March 2020, as the virus made its way through Connecticut's prisons and Carlos contracted the disease, his family became increasingly desperate. Activists picked up the demand for his release, gathering in front of the jail where he was held. Nothing happened. On April 13, 2020, Carlos became the first person in Connecticut to die from COVID-19 in state custody (Krasselt 2020b).

Carlos' death propelled a local movement to demand that the state take decisive action to rapidly decrease the state's prison population. They pointed to the fact that state could cut the prison population by nearly half simply by releasing people detained on technical parole violations and people who had less than ninety days left on their sentences; releasing most pretrial detainees would decrease the population by another 25 percent. Physical distancing would be much more feasible, protecting the lives of prisoners, staff, and the community at large.

Governor Ned Lamont refused to entertain these demands. Instead, the state announced it would quarantine individuals suspected of having the virus at Northern Correctional Institution, the state's supermax prison. Just one month earlier, the UN Special Rapporteur on Torture had denounced Northern where '[t]here seem[ed] to be a state-sanctioned policy aimed at purposefully inflicting severe pain or suffering, physical or mental, which may well amount to torture' (UN News 2020). Individuals were shipped from around the state and forced to wait out the virus in cold, concrete cells, getting aspirin and twice daily temperature checks. Prison officials, terrified of the virus and under pressure from the guards' union, implemented a twenty-four-hour lockdown, forbidding people from leaving their cells to eat, shower, or get fresh air. All outside communication – including calls to loved ones and lawyers – stopped.

Connecticut's punitive approach exacerbated the virus. Prisoners, fearful of being sent to Northern, downplayed their symptoms, fueling outbreaks across the system. By July, nearly 9 percent of the state's 11,000 prisoners had tested positive. The virus abated over the summer, but as community infection rates started to soar in the fall, prisons braced against a second surge. As of November 2020, the total infection rate among incarcerated people was more than five times that in the community (Marshall Project 2020).

For the eleven million people incarcerated across the globe, Carlos' personal tragedy and the state's foot-dragging would play out again and again over the coming months. Public health experts quickly named prisons 'a ticking time bomb' for their potential to spread the virus (UNAIDS 2020). In overcrowded and under-resourced criminal justice systems, the only viable prevention measures were broad and swift releases. Ultimately, however, the world's nations would release only 5 percent of prisoners, far too little to prevent the virus' spread (Human Rights Watch 2020a). Though making generalizations across borders is difficult, in a range of countries – Argentina, Brazil, Canada, France, Kenya, India, Indonesia, Iran, Russia, South Africa, the United Kingdom, and the United States – governments repeatedly chose to lock prisoners down rather than follow sound public health advice to decarcerate. Release proved to be politically unimaginable, even in the face of a deadly and highly communicable virus, even for people who had never been convicted or who posed little threat, and even though prison outbreaks would lead to community outbreaks.

Taking a further step back, COVID-19 shows the absurdity and cruelty of the prison writ large. Societies across the world rely on incarceration as a physical, social, political, and legal construct to separate people convicted of crimes from the general public. But we can no more keep the virus in or out than we can jail the problems – inequality, poverty, discrimination, mental illness, personal and intergenerational trauma – that send people to prison in the first place. Over-policed and under-resourced communities have long known that 'prisoner health is public health' (WHO Europe 2003).

The COVID-19 crisis should prompt human rights scholars and practitioners to reassess their relationship with punishment and prisons in particular. Human rights law is invaluable insofar as it affirms the essential dignity and humanity of incarcerated people. Yet, as the pandemic demonstrates, the rights afforded prisoners are no match for the system that detains them. Human rights law, which generally concerns itself with the *manner* rather than the *fact* of detention, grounds its tolerance of prisons in the concept of rehabilitation. That premise is misguided. In most parts of the world and for most of their 200-year history, prisons do exactly what they are designed to do: mete out punishment and maintain social order, typically along racial, ethnic and class lines. If the pandemic – which turned prisons deadly not just for the people caged there, but for society at large – failed to shift society's appetite for punishment, there is little reason to think moderate reforms will produce long-term change. The time to rehabilitate prison is over. So long as prisons are part and parcel of justice, cruelty will follow. Human rights must treat incarceration for what it is: a nineteenth-century technology that is incompatible with human dignity and equality.

1 A perfect storm

With the virus' global outbreak in early 2020, there was immediate and widespread recognition that prisons were a perfect vector: a captive population with high rates of underlying conditions, sleeping and eating in cramped and poorly ventilated spaces, and little access to basic hygiene and medical resources (Burki 2020). Global health experts have long recognized that infectious disease thrives behind bars (World Medical Association 2017). Communicable diseases such as tuberculosis pose a special risk, with transmission rates in prison being ten to 100 times higher than in the community (Penal Reform International 2019, p. 2). Prisons posed a threat not only to the people locked inside, but everyone who worked there, their families, and ultimately the broader community.

In the prison context, the principal measures to contain the virus – basic hygiene and physical distancing – were unattainable. Most systems – overcrowded or not – 'struggle to meet basic needs such as food, healthcare, clothing and even shelter in a safe, hygienic environment' (Penal Reform International 2020a, p. 15). Prisoners across the world commonly share a single toilet with dozens of others and are 'deprived of water for drinking and washing' (Jaiswal 2015). Overcrowding, found in 124 countries, made the spread of the disease inevitable (Penal Reform International 2020a, p. 17). In India, where the 2019 national occupancy rate was 118.5 percent, some jails topped 600 percent (Chakma 2020). In the United Kingdom, a majority of prisons are overcrowded, some by nearly 150 percent (HM Prison & Probation Service 2020a, p. 6). Official standards in the United States recommend only twenty-five square foot per person, but the actual figure is far lower, as many facilities cram dozens and sometimes hundreds of peoples on cots in a single dormitory. By comparison, passengers on cruise ships – which sustained the earliest COVID-19 outbreaks – have seventy-five square feet per person (Kajstura & Landon 2020).

Experts recognized that once the virus took hold in prison, the effects would be calamitous. Incarcerated people 'are distinguished by remarkably poor health profiles' (Kinner & Young 2018, p. 188), compounded by physical and mental stressors of prison life (Brinkley-Rubinstein 2013, p. 3). In Russia and the United States, people in prison have significantly higher rates of chronic illness and are more likely to die prematurely (Udo 2019, pp. 217–225; Massoglia & Remster 2019, p. 134; Pridemore 2014, pp. 215–233). By one measure, in the United States a person's life expectancy declines by two years for each year spent in prison (Patterson 2013, pp. 523–528).

The implications for COVID-19 were chilling. Most nations chronically underfund and understaff their prison health systems (Penal Reform International 2019, p. 29). In Brazil, notorious for its ill treatment of prisoners, one-third of prisons lack on-site healthcare facilities (Clarke 2020, p. 20), but long waits and staffing shortages are also common elsewhere. India and South Africa have acute and ongoing medical staffing shortages (Tata Trusts 2019, p. 46; Muntingh 2020). A 2018 report found that nearly half of English prisons provided inadequate medical care (Campbell 2018). In the United States, where most states charge copayments that exceed a prisoner's weekly pay, people routinely die of chronic but treatable conditions, such as hypertension and diabetes (Robbins 2019).

The best and only way to contain the virus was obvious: get as many people out of prison as quickly and as safely as possible. That strategy – termed de-densification – would permit prison officials to reduce the risk of contagion on the inside and to quarantine individuals if an outbreak occurred. Public health experts emphasized the importance of avoiding punitive approaches so that prisoners would not hide symptoms. By rapidly decreasing the population and limiting new admissions, experts counseled, prisons systems could focus resources and humanely implement physical distancing for the people who remained. With adequate spacing, testing, and controls on movement, an administrator could effectively create 'pods', so that people would retain some freedom and social connection within smaller groups (Williams et al. 2020). A consensus quickly emerged about categories appropriate for immediate release: pretrial detainees, people convicted of minor crimes, people almost at the end of their sentences, and people over sixty or with underlying conditions. By protecting the lives of those on the inside, governments could prevent future outbreaks and protect the greater good.

2 Two paths

As the world stood on the cusp of an unprecedented pandemic, two paths presented themselves: harden the walls or bring as many people home as possible to protect everyone's health. Some governments, such as Brazil and the United Kingdom, never attempted to de-densify, choosing to isolate prisons and the people inside. A few, such as the Philippines and Russia, crowded prisons even further, as they criminalized violations of public health guidelines (Rainsford 2020; Zeveleva 2020). Many others – Argentina, Canada, France, India, Indonesia, Iran, South Africa, and the United States – made early gestures towards de-densification but failed to take decisive action and, when the virus hit, doubled down on punishment. For millions of people incarcerated worldwide, the pandemic has meant being locked in a cell for twenty-three hours a day, shut away from family, lawyers, and any meaningful activity (Penal Reform International 2020b, p. 14).

Early on, a number of countries took swift action to drastically reduce the population. Iran grabbed headlines in early February by announcing the release of 54,000 prisoners (Zaghari-Ratcliffe 2020). Others – Nigeria, Myanmar, Indonesia, large jails in Canada and even the United States – followed in quick succession.

For a brief moment, it appeared that world leaders would embrace a public health approach to protecting their incarcerated citizens and the broader community from the pandemic.

Those hopes proved unfounded. Actions rarely matched rhetoric, and because most countries relied on discretionary mechanisms based on individual determinations – bail, compassionate release, parole, house arrest – systemic shortcomings were difficult to measure and even more difficult to implement. Thus, while Iran was being touted by prisoners' rights advocates globally as a model for decarceration, its security forces were killing prisoners who protested ongoing, severe overcrowding, and shortages of basic supplies, including soap and masks (Amnesty International 2020a). By late summer 2020, most of the thousands of prisoners who had been released during the temporary amnesty had returned to prison, where they lived as many as twelve people to a room (Amnesty International 2020c).

Iran may provide an extreme example of political doublespeak, but it stands in good company. A survey of countries hard-hit by the pandemic reveals a common pattern: initial steps towards discretionary releases, bureaucratic intransigence, prisoner unrest, and administrative crackdown. South Africa provides a good example. In early May 2020, in response to pressure from advocates, President Cyril Ramaphosa announced that the government would consider parole for approximately 19,000 'low-risk' prisoners (Reuters 2020). In theory, the releases would be the highest on the continent, amounting to 12 percent of the total prisoner population (Muntingh 2020, p. 5). In practice, however, that figure is likely far lower; experts and prisoners alike complained about the lack of transparency regarding the mechanisms and the actual numbers of prisoners released (Khoza 2020). For pretrial detainees, overcrowding in some places actually worsened due to the suspension of most criminal proceedings (Khoza 2020). Prisoners across the country – speaking in anonymity due to concerns about reprisals – began to complain about a decline in sanitation and a lack of basic essentials, such as soap and masks (Khoza 2020) and hunger strikes became commonplace (Koen, Nkosi, & Buso 2020). Meanwhile, independent monitors were not defined as essential services and thus denied access (Khoza 2020). As of 14 October 2020, 7,229 prisoners and prison officials had tested positive for COVID-19, more than three times the community rate (South Africa Department of Correctional Services 2020).

Other countries' emergency measures proved ephemeral. In Colombia, the government in March 2020 approved 4,000 prisoners for consideration for house arrest; as of 3 June, only 688 had met the requirements and been released (El Tiempo 2020). Canada's Safety Minister Bill Blair initially told the press that 600 of the country's 14,000 federal prisoners had been released for pandemic mitigation; in fact, they were routinely-scheduled releases (Ling 2020). Unlike provincial jails, which oversaw thousands of releases, the federal government relied on lockdowns and solitary confinement in lieu of de-densification. By July, infection rates reached as high as ninety per 100,000, ten times the community rate (Ouellet & Loiero 2020). Kenya's early release of 5,000 people barely made a dent in the country's overcrowding rate of over 200 percent; by October 2020, authorities were scrambling to build temporary shelters while rates began to skyrocket (Otieno 2020). Even in Indonesia, which initially approved, under pressure from activists, the release of 50,000 prisoners (one of the largest releases of any country), prisons remained at 176 percent capacity (Human Rights Watch 2020b).

Court-led reform also hit roadblocks. In March 2020, on its own initiative, the Supreme Court of India took up the question of preventing the spread of COVID-19 in India's overcrowded prisons. Effective physical distancing would require drastic and swift reductions; by one estimate, the state of Maharashtra alone would have to release 16,000 people, or two-thirds of the detained population (Dodhiya & Yadav 2020). But because India's system is overwhelmingly filled with low-level and pre-trial detainees, that outcome seemed feasible. The court ordered state governments to create a special process to consider granting bail to prisoners who were arrested or convicted of offenses with a maximum sentence of seven years (Supreme Court of India 2020).

The result was mixed. Some states – Maharashtra and Punjab – committed to releasing up to 50 percent of pretrial detainees (Raghavan & Tarique 2020). By late summer 2020, 68,264 prisoners had been released, a 17.2 percent decrease in the population (Lamba 2020), but new arrests nearly made up for the gap, as police in many places actually increased enforcement of petty offenses (Bokil, Sonavane, & Bej 2020). Judges across the country routinely rejected bail applications on technical grounds, such as the lack of documentation (Khandekar 2020). The process became politicized; protestors against India's discriminatory citizenship law found themselves excluded from bail (Amnesty International 2020b). By mid-October, as COVID-19 cases were climbing and Delhi's main jail was at 155 percent capacity, the state's High Court ordered those released on temporary bail to return to prison (Bokil, Sonavane, & Bej 2020).

France also fell short, even in the face of direct pressure from the European Court of Human Rights (ECHR). In January 2020, the ECHR held that that pre-pandemic crowding in France's prisons constituted an Article 3 violation (Boring 2020). Instead of decreasing the overcrowding, the government instead chose to contain the virus using a program of 'strict containment': prisons suspended all social visits, physical, and educational activities, while banning the use of masks or hand sanitizer for prisoners. Those measures were met with a wave of protests in forty prisons calling for de-densification, demands echoed on the outside by civil society groups, and the official state monitor (International Prison Observatory et al. 2020). The government responded aggressively to quell protests, but nonetheless took steps to de-densify; by 15 April, the prison population fell by nearly 10,000, lowering the overcrowding rate from 119 percent to 103 percent. Jails saw similar declines, from 138 percent to 116 percent capacity (Agence-France Presse 2020).

Even so, observers worried that measures were insufficient to protect either the dignity or the lives of those who remained (Prison Insider 2020a). Despite the ECHR's ruling, France took only hesitant steps towards further decarceration. Judges uniformly rejected applications by pretrial detainees, including those with underlying conditions. The Cour de Cassation observed that the pandemic 'cannot transform, in itself, a security measure and in particular pretrial detention … into inhuman and degrading treatment or a violation of the right to life…' (Avocats 2020). On 2 October, the Conseil Constitutionnel ordered the legislature to revise pretrial detention rules to bring France into compliance with the ECHR ruling; notably, the order was to take effect in March 2021 (Jacquin 2020).

Several countries – Brazil, the United Kingdom, and the United States – stand out for their especially punitive policies. Brazil's pandemic response in prison earned the moniker 'necropolitics': the ultimate exercise of state power to determine 'who lives and who dies' (Arantes 2020). In mid-March, the National Council of Justice issued modest guidelines to judges to control the spread of the virus through increasing alternatives to detention and early releases. Those guidelines met with outright hostility from President Jair Bolsonaro and his minister of justice, who accused advocates of using the pandemic as a pretext for mass releases (Dwamena 2020). Brazilian courts granted fewer than 15 percent of compassionate release requests; in Rio, that figure was close to zero. By late June 2020, the prison population had decreased by only 4 percent while the pandemic had increased by 800 percent (de Oliveira Andrade 2020).

Brazil's policies took a surreal and violent turn. To address overcrowding, the Bolsonaro administration proposed converting shipping containers into temporary isolation units (Sassine 2020). The government also banned all outside visits, prompting outrage among prisoners, who depended on family for food, medicine, and hygiene products (de Oliveira Andrade 2020). Meanwhile, the President vetoed legislation that would make masks mandatory in prisons. Government inaction prompted organizing by prisoners, who staged rebellions and breakouts (VOA News 2020). In response, the government subjected protest leaders to solitary confinement, beatings, and forced hunger and nudity (IACHR Complaint 2020b).

An urgent appeal to the Inter-American Commission for Human Rights, brought by more than 200 civil society groups, declaimed the 'genocidal character' of Brazil's pandemic prison policies, which threaten an incarcerated population that is overwhelmingly and disproportionately of African descent (IACHR Complaint 2020b). In response, the IACHR 'once again informed the Brazilian state that it must take measures to reduce overcrowding in penitentiaries, such as considering alternative measures, especially for those who are at particular risk' (IACHR Complaint 2020b). That possibility seems distant. Prisoners are five times more likely to die of the virus (Pauluze 2020), but Bolsonaro's popularity has surged (McCoy 2020).

When the pandemic hit the United Kingdom, life in prison came to a standstill. Prisoners could leave their cells for just thirty minutes per day to shower and exercise; all visits, education, and other programs ceased (HM Prison & Probation Service 2020, pp. 1–16). In early May, five prisoners committed suicide in just one week (Grierson 2020a). As lockdown stretched into its ninth month, the Chief Prison Inspector warned: '[t]he risk is you will end up doing irreparable damage to the mental health of a lot of prisoners' (Grierson 2020b).

The judiciary expressed discomfort with the harsh conditions but declined to intervene. In *R. v. Manning*, as UK prisoners entered the second month of lockdown, the Court of Appeal held that when setting sentences, judges 'could and in our view should keep in mind that the impact of a custodial sentence at the moment is likely to be greater during the current emergency than it would otherwise be'. Yet even for Manning himself, the Court of Appeals *increased* the defendant's sentence – from twelve to twenty-four months – at the request of the government. The Sentencing Council declined to adopt *Manning* more broadly on the grounds that the national sentencing guidelines, which encompass the proportionality doctrine, 'are sufficiently flexible to deal with all circumstances, including the consequences of the current emergency' (Sentencing Council 2020). Meanwhile, executive initiatives had negligible effect; of the 4,000 people eligible for early release, just 275 were able to meet requirements before the program ended in August 2020 (Grierson 2020c). Since the emergence of the pandemic, the United Kingdom's prison population fell less than 5 percent, and even that modest decrease is due primarily to a backlog of cases rather than changed policies or court orders (Ford 2020).

In the United States, despite widespread mobilization inside and outside prisons, progress stalled almost as quickly as it emerged. Many jails swiftly reduced populations, largely due to police departments becoming more selective about enforcing minor offenses such as property crimes (Widra & Wagner 2020). Releases from prisons were much harder to obtain and grossly inadequate to permit physical distancing. For example, as of August 2020, despite having released more than 14,000 people, California's state prisons still held 117 percent of their design capacity (Widra & Wagner 2020). By the end of the summer, releases across the country had slowed and, in many jails, the population had begun to increase (Widra & Wagner 2020). Ultimately, the United States would release 5.6 percent of its incarcerated population as a result of a patchwork of administrative actions and executive orders (Dolovich 2020, p. 6). Having failed to de-densify, most US prisoners were put on indefinite lockdown, three times more likely to die than their free counterparts (Saloner et al. 2020). The despair is overwhelming: '[w]e are helpless behind these locked doors' (Cromar 2020).

Prisoners found little sympathy from courts. In the federal system alone, an estimated 98 percent of habeas petitions on behalf of elderly and sick prisoners were denied (Blakinger & Neff 2020). Class actions, seeking release of individuals with underlying conditions as well as people pretrial or near the end of sentence, met with some initial success, only to stall or to be overturned on appeal (Dolovich 2020, pp. 16–18). Even the most basic remedies – the provision of cleaning supplies, for example – met with resistance among federal appeals courts. A case brought by two elderly prisoners in Texas, where 161 prisoners had died from COVID-19, illustrates the general trend. A federal district court agreed that Texas prisons had failed to give the plaintiffs routine access to soap and hand sanitizer and ordered relief. On appeal, the Fifth Circuit disqualified the suit because the plaintiffs had failed to fully exhaust internal administrative remedies. In the court's view – one seemingly shared globally: 'Special circumstances – even threats posed by global pandemics – do not matter' (*Valentine v. Collier*, p. 161).

3 The hard politics of prisons

Looking across these examples, before and after COVID-19, it is striking that virtually every nation has chronically failed to adequately care for the people whom it has decided to incarcerate. That fact is true regardless of whether the prison system is overcrowded, whether the detained population is increasing or decreasing, whether the nation is high or low-income, or whether it is in the North or South. A few notable – and frequently invoked – exceptions exist, but rather than providing any 'Nordic model' (Pratt 2020), they are best conceived as the exception that proves the general rule: suffering in prison is a feature, not an aberration.

The pandemic laid bare that truth. Decarceration was the best and only tool to protect the health of the people who lived and worked in prisons as well as the public health at large. Governments had ample tools to do so without significant risk to safety. For example, like Connecticut, France could have reduced its population by nearly two-thirds simply by releasing most pretrial detainees and people serving less than one year (Prison Insider 2020a, 2000b).

The calculus should have been straightforward, but governments largely ignored calls for release or did so halfheartedly and ineffectively. From a public health standpoint, that decision is irrational. But from a political standpoint, it is eminently reasonable, if not inevitable. For most segments of society, prisons are totemic of safety, and the people inside them are, by definition, to be feared and to be controlled. In Buenos Aires, thousands converted the nightly ritual of pot-banging – originally intended as a show of solidarity with healthcare workers – to protest *against* releases of pretrial detainees (Dube & Frydlewsky 2020). Release is unimaginable and intolerable, all the more so during a public health crisis.

Since the eighteenth century, prisons have been defended as an enlightened alternative to more overtly brutal forms of state sanction, such as capital punishment and public whippings. Prisons, the argument goes, channel the use of state force through democratic expressions of social norms and cement the rule of law. But, as decades of scholarship have demonstrated, that origin story stands at odds with history. The modern prison, which traces back to England and France, must be understood in the context of the rise of industrialism and efforts to control poor people (Rothman 1971; Foucault 1977; Roth 2014). If prison was 'classed' from the outset, it soon became 'raced', as European colonialist ideologies justified both the use of forced penal labor (even after declaiming slavery) and the expansion of colonial rule over local forms of customary justice (Bernault 2007, pp. 72–76). In post-slavery societies, such as the United States and Brazil, the social order preserved by prisons is distinctly racist. But the world over, '[p]ost-colonial regimes more often than not consolidated rather than dismantled the prison for their own purposes' (Aguirre 2007, p. 41). Penal severity derives from, thrives upon, and preserves inequality of all kinds. Thus, a visit to a jail virtually anywhere in the world reveals an array of people cast out from society: racial, ethnic, sexual, and religious minorities; sex workers; drug users and sellers; homeless people ; street vendors; migrants; and – overwhelmingly – poor people. In places like the banlieues of Paris, the favelas of Rio, the informal settlements of Mumbai and Cape Town, and post-industrial cities of the United States, incarceration's harms accrue and compound systemic inequalities and racist hierarchies. In that sense, prisons are profoundly anti-democratic (Thorpe 2015; Weaver & Lerman 2015).

It should come as no surprise, then, that during the pandemic democracies proved resistant to largescale releases. Action largely came through executive orders; courts generally proved reluctant to intervene. Rational and humane policies met outright popular resistance or the slow grind of political intransigence. In the United States and Brazil, where prisons show a through-line back to slavery, such institutional responses are unsurprising. But whether one is speaking of Muslims in France, *dalits* in India, West Papuans in Indonesia, drug users in the Philippines, these examples show how societies were willing to trade the greater public health for the preservation of social hierarchies. During the pandemic, public health measures were bound to falter at the prison gate. In the eyes of their own government, the people inside are already dead.

4 COVID-19 and prisons: an inflection point for human rights?

On 15 March 2020, as Carlos DeLeon lay dying in a Connecticut jail, Michelle Bachelet, UN High Commissioner for Human Rights, urged nations to act swiftly to forestall catastrophe for the 11 million people incarcerated worldwide. She expressed what advocates worldwide wanted to say: 'Imprisonment should be a measure of last resort, particularly during this crisis' (Bachelet 2020).

That proposition is wishful thinking under current human rights law, which provides that incarceration is a 'last resort' only for juveniles and people in administrative detention. Thus, initial statements by other human rights bodies were more measured, calling for governments to make 'concerted efforts' to decrease overcrowding or 'ensure consideration' of discretionary releases (CPT 2020; IACHR 2020a). But as the scale of the threat became clear, international bodies started to speak with a single voice. In early May, the WHO, UNAIDS, and UNDOC joined the High Commissioner in calling for 'a swift and firm response' to reduce overcrowding, urging governments 'to consider limiting the deprivation of liberty, including pretrial detention, to a measure of last resort' (WHO et al. 2020).

The legal bootstrapping by Bachelet and others underscores a fundamental tension within human rights. From its inception, the international human rights system recognized the uniquely vulnerable position of incarcerated people and advocates have often turned to its basic guarantees for procedural protections and minimum conditions as the few means to protect people outcast from their own societies. Yet human rights has little to say about the most fundamental question: what justifies taking someone's freedom? In contrast to pretrial detainees, who may only be held as a 'last resort' (Tokyo Rules 6.1), incarcerated people enjoy no such protections. The proportionality doctrine promises to take into account the harms inflicted by a criminal sentence but, as demonstrated by *R. v. Manning*, it has proven largely toothless (van Zyl Smit & Ashworth 2004). At base, human rights law has tolerated the inherent brutality of incarceration (Cover 1986) on the vague promise of 'reformation and social rehabilitation' (ICCPR art. 10.3). That bargain is the same one colonizers brought with them and, for more than two centuries, it has proven to be a bad deal.

The pandemic reinforces what penal abolitionists have been saying for decades: the time to rehabilitate the prison is over. It is 'inherently contradictory' to expect prisons, which 'involve[e] separation from family and community, hours of confinement in cells, forced cohabitation with other convicts, and exposure to harsh and sometimes violent conditions', to deliver anything that remotely resembles human betterment (Jacobson, Heard, & Fair 2017, p. 37). If states refused to protect prisoners to forestall a public health crisis, why should we expect them in normal times to provide adequate housing or medical care, let alone the mental health, vocational and educational supports necessary to surmount the socioeconomic factors that led people to prison in the first place?

There are no simple answers. Progress will not come through dogma or slogans. Nor will it come from begging small gains from corrupt systems or through the familiar lawyer's tools of procedural fairness or minimally humane conditions. Deep work must be done to envision and build support for new, rights-respecting ways that states can ensure the safety and dignity of all people. To do so, we will have to confront colonialism's long reach into contemporary forms of crime control and the complicity of human rights in those structures (Saito 2020, pp. 166–85).

The seeds for emancipation are there. In response to longstanding demands from civil society, human rights bodies are starting to acknowledge the inherent harms of incarceration and the urgent need for alternatives.[1] Meanwhile, an emerging transnational movement for racial justice is rekindling conversations about reparations and decolonization.[2] Zia Wasserman, a South African activist, urges us to think of the COVID-19 crisis as 'an opportunity' to show the closed hell of prison. The time to rehabilitate the prison is past: 'We must ask why they should be imprisoned in the first place' (Prison Insider 2020b).

Notes

1 For example, the Mandela Rules characterize incarceration as 'afflictive by the very fact of taking from these persons the right of self-determination by depriving them of their liberty' (Mandela Rules 3). The Tokyo Rules, while preserving the 'last resort' language for pre-trial detainees, acknowledge the harms from the carceral state and advise that non-custodial measures 'should be part of the movement towards depenalization and decriminalization instead of interfering with or delaying efforts in that direction' (Tokyo Rules 2.7). Recognizing both the individual harms and the system injustices of the carceral system in many parts of Africa, the African Commission on Human and Peoples' Rights has called for the decriminalization of petty offenses (ACHPR 2017).

2 In 2019, Tendayi Achiume, UN Special Rapporteur on racism, grounded calls for reparation in human rights principles and called for the 'decolonization' of international law, relied on by Member States to perpetuate economic and political inequalities (Achiume 2019, paras. 10–12).

References

African Commission on Human and Peoples' Rights (ACHPR) 2017, *Resolution on the Need to Develop Principles on the Declassification and Decriminalization of Petty Offences in Africa*, viewed 21 December 2020, www.achpr.org/sessions/resolutions?id=306

Agence-France Presse 2020, *10.000 détenus en moins dans les prisons françaises depuis le confinement*, viewed 21 December 2020, www.huffingtonpost.fr/entry/prison-confinement-coronavirus-surpopulation_fr_5e96d8cfc5b6ac7eb262fe0b

Aguirre, C 2007, *Prisons and Prisoners in Modernising Latin America*, in F Dikötter & I Brown, I (eds.), *Cultures of Confinement: A History of the Prison in Africa, Asia and Latin America*, Cornell University Press, Ithaca.

Amnesty International 2020a, *Iran: Prisoners Killed by Security Forces during COVID-19 Pandemic Protests*, viewed 21 December 2020, www.amnesty.org/en/latest/news/2020/04/iran-prisoners-killed-by-security-forces-during-covid19-pandemic-protests/

Amnesty International 2020b, *Human Rights Defenders Languish in COVID-19-hit Prisons as State Crackdowns Continue*, viewed 21 December 2020, www.amnesty.org/en/latest/news/2020/08/attacks-on-hrds-during-pandemic-report/

Amnesty International 2020c, *Iran: Leaked Official Letters Reveal State of Denial of COVID-19 Crisis in Prisons*, viewed 31 December 2020, www.amnesty.org/en/latest/news/2020/07/iran-leaked-letters-reveal-state-denial-of-covid19-crisis-in-prisons/

Arantes, M 2020, 'COVID-19 In Brazilian Prisons: Pandemic or a Necropolitical Project?', *Open Democracy*, 7 July, viewed 21 December 2020, www.opendemocracy.net/en/democraciaabierta/covid-19-brazilian-prison-pandemic-or-necropolitics/

Avocats, S 2020, 'Pre-Trial Detention: The Health Crisis Does Not in Itself Justify the Release from Prison', *Mondaq*, 30 September, viewed 21 December 2020, www.mondaq.com/france/operational-impacts-and-strategy/989684/pre-trial-detention-the-health-crisis-does-not-in-itself-justify-the-release-from-prison

Bernault, F 2007, *The Shadow of Rule: Colonial Power and Modern Punishment in Africa*, in F Dikötter F & I Brown (eds.), *Cultures of Confinement: A History of the Prison in Africa, Asia and Latin America*, Cornell University Press, Ithaca.

Bachelet, M 2020, 'Urgent Action Needed to Prevent COVID-19 "Rampaging through Places of Detention"', viewed 21 December 2020, www.ohchr.org/en/NewsEvents/Pages/DisplayNews.aspx?NewsID=25745&LangID=E

Blakinger, K & Neff, J 2020, 'Thousands of Sick Federal Prisoners Sought Compassionate Release. 98 Percent Were Denied', *The Marshall Project*, viewed 21 December 2020, www.themarshallproject.org/2020/10/07/thousands-of-sick-federal-prisoners-sought-compassionate-release-98-percent-were-denied

Bokil, A, Sonavane, N & Bej, S 2020, 'Push for Repopulation of Prisons during a Pandemic is Reckless', *Indian Express*, 2 November, viewed 21 December 2020, https://indianexpress.com/article/opinion/columns/coronavirus-jail-inmates-parole-6912890/

Boring, N 2020, 'France: European Court Of Human Rights finds France in Violation of European Human Rights Convention Due to Overcrowded Prisons', *Global Legal Monitor*, viewed at 21 December 2020, www.loc.gov/law/foreign-news/article/france-european-court-of-human-rights-finds-france-in-violation-of-european-human-rights-convention-due-to-overcrowded-prisons/

Brinkley-Rubinstein, L 2013, 'Incarceration as a Catalyst for Worsening Health', *Health & Justice*, vol. 1, no. 1, p. 3.

Burki, T 2020, 'Prisons Are "in No Way Equipped" To Deal with COVID-19', *The Lancet*, vol. 35 p. 1411.

Campbell, D 2018, 'Poor Healthcare in Jails is Killing Inmates, says NHS Watchdog', *The Guardian*, 27 October, viewed 21 December 2020, www.theguardian.com/society/2018/oct/27/prisoners-dying-poor-care-services-prisons-mental-health-care-quality-commission-report

Chakma, S 2020, 'The Status of COVID-19 in Indian Prisons', *National Campaign Against Torture*, viewed 21 December 2020, www.uncat.org/by-country/india/the-status-of-covid-19-in-indian-prisons/

Clarke, M 2020, 'COVID-19 Pandemic Leads to Unrest in Prisons around the Globe', *Prison Legal News*, viewed 21 December 2020, www.prisonlegalnews.org/news/2020/jul/1/covid-19-pandemic-leads-unrest-prisons-around-globe/

Cover, R 1986, 'Violence and the Word', *Yale Law Journal*, vol. 95, no. 1601.

Cromar, A 2020, 'Lockdown within a Lockdown', *Boston Globe*, 4 June, viewed 21 December 2020, www.boston.com/news/coronavirus/2020/06/02/mass-prison-coronavirus-pandemic

de Oliveira Andrade, R 2020 'Covid-19: Prisons Exposed in Brazil's Crisis', *The BMJ*, vol. 370.

Department of Correctional Services: Republic of South Africa 2020, viewed 21 December 2020, www.dcs.gov.za

Dodhiya, K & Yadav, VK 2020, 'As Covid-19 Cases Breach the 2,000-Mark in Prisons across Maharashtra, Lawyers to Press for Changes in High-Power Panel's Guidelines', *Hindustan Times*, 27 September, viewed 21 December 2020, www.hindustantimes.com/mumbai-news/as-covid-19-cases-breach-the-2-000-mark-in-prisons-across-maharashtra-lawyers-to-press-for-changes-in-high-power-panel-s-guidelines/story-d0pZBLWUuP1nlQB7lF80MK.html

Dolovich, S 2020, 'Mass Incarceration, Meet COVID-19', *University of Chicago Law Review Online*, viewed 21 December 2020, https://lawreviewblog.uchicago.edu/2020/11/16/covid-dolovich/

Dube, R & Frydlewsky, S 2020, 'Release of Prisoners in Bid to Contain Coronavirus Draws Fire in Argentina', *Wall Street Journal*, 16 May, viewed 21 December 2020, wsj.com/articles/release-of-prisoners-in-bid-to-contain-coronavirus-draws-fire-in-argentina-11589637601

Dwamena, A 2020, 'How Jair Bolsonaro and the Coronavirus put Brazil's Systemic Racism on Display', *The New Yorker*, 9 July, viewed 21 December 2020, www.newyorker.com/news/news-desk/how-jair-bolsonaro-and-the-coronavirus-put-brazils-systemic-racism-on-display

El Tiempo 2020, 'Decreto de excarcelación no ha dado resultado esperado': Minjusticia, El Tiempo, 4 June, viewed 21 December 2020, www.eltiempo.com/justicia/servicios/coronavirus-minjusticia-habla-de-poco-resultado-del-decreto-de-excarcelacion-502936

European Committee for the Prevention of Torture (CPT) 2020, *Statement of Principles Relating to the Treatment of Persons Deprived of Their Liberty in the Context of the Coronavirus Disease (COVID-19) pandemic*, viewed 21 December 2020, https://rm.coe.int/16809cfa4b.

Ford, M 2020, 'What's Happened to the Prison Population during COVID-19?', *Centre for Crime and Justice Studies*, 9 July, viewed 21 December 2020, www.crimeandjustice.org.uk/resources/whats-happened-prison-population-during-covid-19

Foucault, M 1977, *Discipline and Punish*, Pantheon Books, New York.

Grierson, J 2020a, 'Alarm over Five Suicides in Six Days at Prisons in England and Wales', *The Guardian*, 28 May, viewed 21 December 2020, www.theguardian.com/society/2020/may/28/alarm-over-five-suicides-in-six-days-at-prisons-in-england-and-wales

Grierson, J 2020b, 'Covid: Prisoner Mental Health at Risk of "Irreparable Damage"', *The Guardian*, 19 August, viewed 21 December 2020, www.theguardian.com/society/2020/oct/20/covid-prisoner-mental-health-at-risk-of-irreparable-damage

Grierson, J 2020c, 'Early-release Scheme for Prisoners in England and Wales to End', *The Guardian*, 20 October, viewed 21 December 2020, www.theguardian.com/society/2020/aug/19/prisons-inspector-england-wales-warns-of-mental-health-problems-from-severe-coronavirus-restrictions

HM Prison and Probation Service 2020, 'COVID-19: National Framework for Prison Regimes and Services', viewed 21 December 2020, https://assets.publishing.service.gov.uk/government/uploads/system/uploads/attachment_data/file/889689/prisons-national-framework.pdf

Human Rights Watch (HRW) 2020a, 'Covid-19 Prisoner Releases Too Few, Too Slow', viewed 21 December 2020, www.hrw.org/news/2020/05/27/covid-19-prisoner-releases-too-few-too-slow

Human Rights Watch (HRW) 2020b, 'Covid-19 Spreads in Indonesia's Crowded Prisons', Viewed 21 December 2020, www.hrw.org/news/2020/08/26/covid-19-spreads-indonesias-overcrowded-prisons

Inter-American Commission on Human Rights (IACHR) 2020a, *Resolución No. 1/2020, pandemia y derechos humanos en las Americas*, viewed 21 December 2020, www.oas.org/es/cidh/decisiones/pdf/Resolucion-1-20-es.pdf

Inter-American Commission on Human Rights (IACHR) 2020b, *IACHR Expresses Concern over the Situation of People Deprived of their Freedom in Brazil during the COVID-19 Pandemic*, viewed 21 December 2020, www.oas.org/en/iachr/media_center/PReleases/2020/195.asp

International Covenant on Civil and Political Rights (ICCPR) 1967, *Art. 10.3*, viewed 26 December 2020, https://treaties.un.org/doc/Treaties/1976/03/19760323%2006-17%20AM/Ch_IV_04.pdf

International Prison Observatory: French Section 2020, *Health Crisis in Prison: The Council of State is Locked in Inaction'*, viewed 21 December 2020, https://oip.org/communique/crise-sanitaire-en-prison-le-conseil-detat-senferme-dans-linaction/

Jacobson, J, Heard, C, & Fair, H 2017, 'Prison: Evidence of Its Use and Overuse', *Institute for Crime & Justice Policy Research*, viewed 21 December 2020, www.prisonstudies.org/sites/default/files/resources/downloads/global_imprisonment_web2c.pdf

Jacquin, J 2020, 'Conditions de détention: Le Conseil constitutionnel éxige une loi pour faire respecter la dignité humaine en prison', *Le Monde*, viewed 21 December 2020, www.lemonde.fr/societe/article/2020/10/02/conditions-de-detention-le-conseil-constitutionnel-exige-une-loi-pour-faire-respecter-la-dignite-humaine-en-prison_6054482_3224.html

Jaiswal, A 2015, '1 Toilet for 12 Prisoners: CAG Pulls up State for Poor Sanitation in Jails', *Times of India*, viewed 21 December 2020, https://timesofindia.indiatimes.com/city/raipur/1-toilet-for-12-prisoners-CAG-pulls-up-state-for-poor-sanitation-in-jails/articleshow/48288672.cms

Kajstura, A & Landon, J 2020, 'Since You Asked: Is Social Distancing Possible behind Bars?', *Prison Policy Initiative*, viewed 21 December 2020, www.prisonpolicy.org/blog/2020/04/03/density/

Khandekar, O 2020, 'Covid-19 in Prison: Is India Doing Enough?', *Mint*, viewed 21 December 2020, www.livemint.com/mint-lounge/features/covid-19-in-prison-is-india-doing-enough-11594096672458.html

Khoza, A 2020, 'How South African Prisons Are Managing Covid-19', *New Frame*, viewed 21 December 2020, www.newframe.com/how-south-african-prisons-are-managing-covid-19/

Kinner, S & Young, J 2018, 'Understanding and Improving the Health of People Who Experience Incarceration: An Overview and Synthesis', *Epidemiologic Reviews*, vol. 40, no. 1, pp. 4–11.

Knowles, H 2020, 'Carlos DeLeon was Cleared for Early release. He Died of Covid-19 before It Could Happen', *Washington Post*, 1 May, viewed 21 December 2020, www.washingtonpost.com/nation/2020/05/01/carlos-deleon-connecticut-inmate-coronavoris/

Koen, D, Nkosi, N & Buso, N 2020, 'St Albans Inmates on Prolonged Hunger Strike over Alleged Beatings and Growing Covid-19 Concerns', *Sowetan Live*, 14 July, viewed 26 December 2020, www.sowetanlive.co.za/news/south-africa/2020-07-14-st-albans-inmates-on-prolonged-hunger-strike-over-alleged-beatings-and-growing-covid-19-concerns/

Krasselt, K 2020a, 'Inmate Dead of Coronavirus Was Scrambling to Return to Bridgeport', *CT Post*, 14 April, viewed 21 December 2020, www.ctinsider.com/news/coronavirus/ctpost/article/Family-Inmate-dead-of-coronavirus-had-a-place-to-15199820.php

Krasselt, K 2020b, 'A Sad, Angry Farewell to CT's First Inmate Coronavirus Victim', *The Middletown Press*, 28 May, viewed 21 December 2020, www.middletownpress.com/news/coronavirus/article/A-sad-angry-farewell-to-CT-s-first-inmate-15302007.php

Lamba, S 2020, 'Covid-19 Spread in Jails Lays Bare Systemic Flaws', *Tribune india News Service*, viewed 21 December 2020, www.tribuneindia.com/news/comment/covid-19-spread-in-jails-lays-bare-systemic-flaws-102458

Ling, J 2020, 'The Government Said It's Releasing Many Inmates to Combat COVID-19. It's not', *VICE News*, viewed 21 December 2020, www.vice.com/en/article/jgey9p/the-government-said-its-releasing-many-inmates-to-combat-covid-19-its-not

Marshall Project 2020, *A State-by-state Look at Coronavirus in Prisons*, viewed 21 December 2020www.themarshallproject.org/2020/05/01/a-state-by-state-look-at-coronavirus-in-prisons#prisoner-state

Massoglia, M & Remster, B 2019, 'Linkages between Incarceration and Health' *Public Health Reports*, vol. 134(1_suppl), pp. 8S–14S.

McCoy, T 2020, 'The Coronavirus Has Hammered Brazil. But Somehow, Bolsonaro is Getting More Popular', *Washington Post*, 24 August, viewed 21 December 2020, www.washingtonpost.com/world/the_americas/brazil-bolsonaro-coronavirus/2020/08/24/47a22cf6-e17a-11ea-8dd2-d07812bf00f7_story.html

Muntingh, L 2020, 'Africa, Prisons and COVID-19', *Journal of Human Rights Practice*, viewed 21 December 2020, www.ncbi.nlm.nih.gov/pmc/articles/PMC7499662/

Otieno, J 2020, 'Three Prisoners Dead, 1700 Infected with Covid-19' *The Star*, viewed 21 December 2020, www.the-star.co.ke/news/2020-10-24-three-prisoners-dead-1700-infected-with-covid-19/

Ouellet, V & Loiero, J 2020, 'COVID-19 Taking a Toll in Prisons', *CBC News*, viewed 21 December 2020, www.cbc.ca/news/canada/prisons-jails-inmates-covid-19-1.5652470

Patterson, E 2013, 'The Dose–response of Time Served in Prison on Mortality: New York State, 1989–2003', *American Journal of Public Health*, vol. 103 no. 3, pp. 523–528.

Pauluze, T 2020, 'Coronavirus Lethality among Brazilian Prisoners Is Five Times that of the General Population', *Folha De Sao Paulo*, 5 May, viewed 21 December 2020, www1.folha.uol.com.br/cotidiano/2020/05/letalidade-do-coronavirus-entre-presos-brasileiros-e-o-quintuplo-da-registrada-na-populacao-geral.shtml

Penal Reform International 2019, 'Global Prison Trends Special Focus 2019: Healthcare in Prisons', viewed 21 December 2020, https://cdn.penalreform.org/wp-content/uploads/2019/05/PRI-Global-prison-trends-report-2019_WEB.pdf.

Penal Reform International 2020a, *Global Prison Trends 2020*, viewed 21 December 2020, https://cdn.penalreform.org/wp-content/uploads/2020/05/Global-Prison-Trends-2020-Penal-Reform-International-Second-Edition.pdf.

Penal Reform International 2020b, *Coronavirus: Healthcare and Human Rights of People in Prison*, viewed 21 December 2020, https://cdn.penalreform.org/wp-content/uploads/2020/03/FINAL-Briefing-Coronavirus.pdf.

Pratt, J 2008, 'Scandinavian Exceptionalism in an Era of Penal Excess', *The British Journal of Criminology*, vol. 48, no.2, pp. 119–137.

Pridemore, W 2014, 'The Mortality Penalty of Incarceration', *Journal of Health and Social Behavior*, vol. 55, no. 2, pp. 215–233.

Prison Insider 2020a, 'France: Inequality of Life During an Epidemic', viewed 21 December 2020, www.prison-insider.com/en/articles/france-l-inegalite-des-vies-en-temps-d-epidemie

Prison Insider 2020b, 'South Africa: Sounding the Alarm', viewed 21 December 2020, www.prison-insider.com/en/articles/south-africa-sounding-the-alarm

Raghavan, V & Tarique, M 2020, 'India's Jails Are Vastly Overcrowded. Here Are Some Ways to Protect inmates from Covid-19', *Scroll.in*, 8 April, viewed 21 December 2020, https://scroll.in/article/958334/indias-jails-are-vastly-overcrowded-here-are-some-ways-to-protect-inmates-from-covid-19

Rainsford, S 2020, 'Coronavirus: Russia Includes Jail Terms to Enforce Crackdown', *BBC News*, 31 March, viewed 21 December 2020, www.bbc.com/news/world-europe-52109892

Reuters 2020, 'South Africa to Parole 19,000 Prisoners to Curb Coronavirus', 8 May, viewed 21 December 2020, www.reuters.com/article/us-health-coronavirus-safrica/south-africa-to-parole-19000-prisoners-to-curb-coronavirus-idUSKBN22K1I8?il=0

Robbins, D 2019, 'For Some in Ga. Prisons and Jails, Diabetes has Meant a Death Sentence', *The Atlanta Journal – Constitution*, 12 April, viewed 21 December 2020, www.ajc.com/news/state--regional-govt--politics/for-some-prisons-and-jails-diabetes-has-meant-death-sentence/wVz7xy1g4ujG3ClhH1visJ/

Roth, M 2014, *An Eye for an Eye: A Global History of Crime and Punishment*, Reaktion Books, London.

Rothman, D 1971, *Discovery of the Asylum*, Routledge, New York.

Saito, N 2020, *Settler Colonialism, Race, and the Law*, New York University Press, New York.

Saloner, B et al. 2020, 'COVID-19 Cases and Deaths in Federal and State Prisons', *JAMA*, vol. 324 no. 6, pp. 602–603.

Sassine, V 2020, 'Contêineres para isolar presos podem gerar "contaminação em massa" por Covid nos presídios, alerta MPF', *O Globo*, viewed 23 December 2020, https://oglobo.globo.com/sociedade/conteineres-para-isolar-presos-podem-gerar-contaminacao-em-massa-por-covid-nos-presidios-alerta-mpf-24421485

Sentencing Council 2020, *The Application of Sentencing Principles during the Covid-19 Emergency*, viewed 21 December 2020, www.sentencingcouncil.org.uk/news/item/the-application-of-sentencing-principles-during-the-covid-19-emergency/

Supreme Court of India, 2020, *In re: Contagion of COVID-19 in Prisons*, viewed 30 December 2020, https://images.assettype.com/barandbench/2020-03/1d900e00-41c0-4a6a-a348-78bdcf26f0f7/In_re_Contagion_of_COVIC_19_Virus_in_Prisons.pdf

Tata Trusts 2019, *India Justice Report*, viewed 21 December 2020, www.tatatrusts.org/upload/pdf/overall-report-single.pdf

Thorpe, R 2015, 'Democratic Politics in an Age of Mass incarceration', in A Dzur, I Loader & R Sparks (eds.), *Democratic Theory and Mass Incarceration*, Oxford University Press, Oxford.

Tokyo Rules, 'Alternatives to Imprisonment and Restorative Justice (the Tokyo Rules)', *Wits Justice Project*, viewed 26 December 2020, www.witsjusticeproject.co.za/uploads/Tokyo-Rules.pdf

Udo, T 2019, 'Chronic Medical Conditions in U.S. Adults with Incarceration History', *Health Psychology*, vol. 38, no. 3, pp. 217–225.

UNAIDS 2020, 'COVID-19 in Prisons – A Ticking Time Bomb', viewed 23 December 2020, www.unaids.org/en/resources/presscentre/featurestories/2020/may/20200513_prisons

UN News 2020, 'Connecticut Prison Warning: Prolonged Solitary Confinement May "Amount to Torture" Expert Warns', viewed 26 December 2020, https://news.un.org/en/story/2020/02/1058311.

Valentine v. Collier, 978 F.3d 154 (5th Cir. 2020).

van Zyl Smit, D & Ashworth, A 2004, 'Disproportionate Sentences as Human Rights Violations', *The Modern Law Review*, vol. 67, pp. 541.

VOA News 2020, 'Inmates in Brazil Prison Protest Suspension of Visits', viewed 30 December 2020, www.voanews.com/covid-19-pandemic/inmates-brazil-prison-protest-suspension-visits

Weaver, V & Lerman, A 2015, *Arresting Citizenship: The Democratic Consequences of American Crime Control*, University of Chicago Press, Chicago.

WHO Europe 2003, *Declaration on Prison Health as Part of Public Health,* viewed 23 December 2020, www.euro.who.int/__data/assets/pdf_file/0007/98971/E94242.pdf

WHO, UNAIDS, UNDOC & OHCHR 2020, 'Joint Statement on COVID-19 in Prisons and Other Closed Settings', viewed 23 December 2020, www.who.int/news/item/13-05-2020-unodc-who-unaids-and-ohchr-joint-statement-on-covid-19-in-prisons-and-other-closed-settings.

Widra, E & Wagner, P 2020, 'Jails and Prisons Have Reduced Their Populations in the Face of the Pandemic, but not Enough to Save Lives', *Prison Policy Initiative*, viewed 23 December 2020, www.prisonpolicy.org/blog/2020/08/05/jails-vs-prisons-update-2/

Williams, B, Ahalt, C, Cloud, D, Augustine, D, Rorvig, L & Sears, D 2020, 'Correctional Facilities in the Shadow of COVID-19: Unique Challenges and Proposed Solutions', *Health Affairs*, viewed 23 December 2020, www.healthaffairs.org/do/10.1377/hblog20200324.784502/full/

World Medical Association (WMA) 2017, 'Declaration of Edinburgh on Prison Conditions and the Spread of Tuberculosis and Other Communicable Diseases', viewed 23 December 2020, www.wma.net/policies-post/wma-declaration-of-edinburgh-on-prison-conditions-and-the-spread-of-tuberculosis-and-other-communicable-diseases/

Zaghari-Ratcliffe, N 2020, 'Coronavirus: Iran Temporarily Frees 54,000 Prisoners To Combat Spread', *BBC News*, 3 March 2020, https://www.bbc.com/news/world-middle-east-51723398

Zeveleva, O 2020, 'COVID-19 Has Been Devastating for Russia's Prisoners', *RIDDLE Russia*, viewed 23 December 2020, www.ridl.io/en/covid-19-has-been-devastating-for-russia-s-prisoners/

10

SEIZING OPPORTUNITIES TO PROMOTE THE PROTECTION OF THE RIGHTS OF ALL MIGRANTS

Ian M. Kysel

The COVID-19 pandemic has simultaneously challenged the notion that human mobility is an inevitable constant of life in the twenty-first century, while also revealing that migrants are essential members of our communities, such that the health and wellbeing of migrants is as vital to the safety of our communities as anyone else's. No one is safe, as the saying goes, unless everyone is safe (United Nations 2020a).

But everyone is not safe.

Indeed, States have failed to adequately respect, protect, and fulfill the human rights of migrants, including refugees. Since the declaration of a pandemic by the World Health Organization (WHO) in March 2020, and in the absence of evidence-based or lawful justification, States around the globe have sealed borders, even to asylum-seekers; failed to protect migrants from – and even promoted – racism and xenophobia, including as a result of barriers to access to information; returned or encouraged the return of migrant laborers without payment of compensation or wages and allowed exploitation of 'essential' migrant workers; failed to guarantee migrants access to COVID-19 testing or to health systems; and neglected to ensure continuity of education to migrant children – among many other abuses. All of these trends uniquely harmed people on the move.

Fortunately, not all States have solely implemented retrograde measures that harm migrants. Progressive steps include ensuring that border closures remained porous to certain categories of migrants; releasing some migrants from detention; and regularizing or extending status to migrants during the pandemic. While this crisis continues to unfold, international human rights law is a vital tool for evaluating shortcomings in the pandemic response. Multilateral cooperation to recognize and protect the human rights of *all* migrants, including refugees, will likewise be a critical prerequisite to paving a path to the post-pandemic.

This chapter argues that State responses to the pandemic have uniquely harmed migrants, including refugees. Part 1 will survey some of these harms and then apply international human rights law to show that these harms violated State obligations to people on the move. Part 2 will then survey the latest law and governance developments, arguing that human rights law will be a key tool in structuring multilateral cooperation to facilitate human migration and develop policy that is resilient to future crises. It remains uncertain whether States will seize the opportunity to do so, or (re)assert sovereign control over human mobility in a manner that is shortsighted and brittle in the face of future shocks. What is clear, however, is that civil society could play a key role in advancing rights-based migration law and governance for the post-pandemic.

1 The COVID-19 pandemic and international migration

The COVID-19 pandemic has at best hardened existing fault lines when it comes to international migration. It has provided 'an object lesson in the nature of international migration law', a system 'marked by failed multilateralism and legal fragmentation', with no global treaty organizing migration flows or restating the rights of *all* migrants (Kysel & Thomas 2020). Indeed, globally, the rights of all migrants,[1] regardless of the cause of their migration, 'receive comprehensive elaboration and thus protection only indirectly', through general human rights law (Kysel 2016). Whether because of or despite this *status quo*, the pandemic brought a cascade of abuses against migrants, including refugees, which violated State human rights obligations.

1.1 The impact of State responses to the pandemic on people on the move

The full extent of abuses against migrants, including refugees, is both beyond the scope of this chapter and yet to be revealed. Five areas of State practice during this pandemic illustrate the challenges that have been and continue to be faced by people in the context of human mobility: (1) the closures of borders, including to those fleeing persecution and torture, and the problems faced by stranded migrants; (2) mistreatment based in racism and xenophobia, including that fueled by barriers to access to information; (3) the mass repatriation of migrant workers, without regard for lost wages or benefits, and the exploitation of migrant 'essential' workers; (4) the widespread barriers to migrants' access to health treatment; and (5) the failure to ensure the education of migrant children.

Certainly, States have not *only failed* migrants. As discussed below, a few governments took actions that benefited migrants, such as by ensuring family unity in the context of border closures and allowing even temporary migrants to return to host States; releasing migrants from detention; and extending or granting status as a response to the pandemic. Overall, and while the contours of State responses to the pandemic are still evolving, the trend has been regressive.

One of the defining early features of the pandemic was the closure of borders – even to those fleeing persecution. The United States, for example, invoked public health authority, trumpeting its subsequent expulsion of tens of thousands, including unaccompanied children seeking refuge (Dickerson 2020). Malta procured the assistance of merchant ships in the Mediterranean in order to intercept asylum-seekers and return them to Libya (Kingsley & Willis 2020). Researchers documented Greek authorities dragging asylum-seekers arriving on Greek islands and to territorial waters back out to sea and leaving them adrift in inflatable, motor-less rafts (Mann & Keady-Tabbal 2020). States on the Bay of Bengal and the Andaman Sea refused disembarkation to Rohingya refugees fleeing by boat (Beech 2020).

The United Nations High Commissioner for Refugees (UNHCR) reported that, at the height of the pandemic, 168 countries fully or partially closed their borders, with ninety of them – just under *half* of United Nations Member States – making no exception for people seeking asylum (UNHCR 2020a). Around the world, closed borders left thousands of migrants, including refugees, stranded, queued, or pushed back to or away from their countries of origin or host countries (UN News 2020). Some border controls arguably followed a discriminatory logic, as Matiangai Sirleaf (2020) suggests was evident in early US travel restrictions, reflecting a 'racialized' view of the disease and echoing a deeper and longstanding intersection between race, migration, and global health. Observers pointed to additional restrictions on migrants' departure – not just entry – as evidence of the proverbial 'shifting border', extending the 'reach of sovereign authority to regulate movement far beyond [any] country's actual territorial edges' (Shachar 2020). Others argued the pandemic brought deterrence measures against refugees in particular 'to their logical conclusion … largely suspend[ing] … asylum' in many places (Ghezelbash & Tan 2020).

Migrants, including refugees, around the globe also faced spikes in racism and xenophobia linked to the pandemic. In many countries, government leaders brazenly fanned the flames of discrimination. The United Nations Special Rapporteur on contemporary forms of racism, racial discrimination, xenophobia and related intolerance, E. Tendayi Achiume, pointed early in the pandemic to 'brutal acts of violence' and other attacks against people known or perceived to be of Chinese or other East Asian descent, including migrants (OHCHR 2020a). The United Nations Secretary-General spoke of a worldwide 'tsunami of hate and xenophobia' and a rise in anti-foreigner sentiment used to justify the targeting of migrants or those perceived to be migrants, including online (United Nations 2020b; IOM 2020d).

The United Nations Special Rapporteur on the promotion and protection freedom of opinion and expression reported on instances of States engaged in direct interference with the ability of independent media to question governments about pandemic response and that internet shutdowns rendered even basic health information difficult to obtain (OHCHR 2020f). Political leaders, including the then President of the United States, fueled this, amplifying slurs proliferating on the internet (Timberg & Chui 2020). One study found that top-down misinformation from public figures accounted for almost three-quarters of online social media engagement (Brennan et al. 2020). In response to what has been called a parallel 'infodemic', the United Nations launched a campaign to deliver trusted information and counter disinformation contributing to such harms (The Lancet 2020; United Nations 2020e). Special Rapporteur Achiume (2020) concluded that the pandemic 'lay[] bare just how dangerous climates of intolerance, and of racialized and religious suspicion and fear, can be to the social fabric required to sustain prosperous and safe communities'.

A third area of harm has been the impact of the pandemic on migrant workers. Lockdowns of migrant worker camps garnered widespread attention from the start of the pandemic (Pattisson & Sedhai 2020). Singapore notoriously all but completely failed to ensure adequate health measures in sprawling dorms housing migrant workers, leading to exploding rates of transmission despite an otherwise assertive broader response (Tan 2020). In the face of abuses, hundreds of thousands of migrant workers, if not many more, returned from overseas (Slater et al. 2020). Such has been the speed and scale of these repatriations that civil society activists have called for a transitional justice mechanism to facilitate resolution of claims of wage theft and wrongful termination (Justice for Wage Theft 2020).

Working conditions for many migrant workers who have not returned have been dire, with private employers imposing significant restrictions (Jordan 2020; Human Rights Watch 2020a). Barriers to the regular labor market for refugees have long been well-documented, suggesting workplace abuses may have particularly harmed refugees during the pandemic (Zetter & Ruaudel 2016). Perhaps the most dramatic of harms was the inadequate supply of personal protective equipment to migrants (including those in the care work sector, in which migrant health workers and particularly migrant women, comprised a significant proportion of 'essential' workers) and those disproportionately harmed by contracting the disease as a result (Eckenwiler 2020; Michaels & Wagner 2020). In short, the already endemic exploitation of migrant workers created the conditions for abuse of migrant workers during the crisis to be ubiquitous.

Barriers to access healthcare were also widespread for migrants during the pandemic, and in particular for refugees. The International Organization for Migration (IOM) estimates that, before the pandemic, fewer than one in two States provided access to health services to migrants, regardless of legal status (UNHCR 2020e). Among other things, systematic barriers to accessing health care and the determinants of health, further compounded by restrictions implemented by States and employers, put migrants at a substantial additional risk of negative health outcomes (Pernitez-Agan et al. 2020; OECD 2020). The United Nations Committee on the Protection of the Rights of All Migrant Workers and Members of their Families and the United Nations Special Rapporteur on the human rights of migrants jointly reported that, in some countries, migrants experienced the highest levels of contagion and death of any group (OHCHR 2020b). Returning migrants were frequently stranded in shelters or concentrated in rural border areas 'ill-equipped to monitor, test or treat COVID-19 cases' (Kapilashrami et al. 2020). In this way, return migration brought on by the pandemic itself created conditions accentuating disproportionate harms to migrant health.

Such challenges were further exacerbated for migrants held in detention facilities, compounding the risks of contagion because of poor conditions and physical proximity, inviting comparisons to being like burning buildings (Hsu 2020). In the United States, for example, which has the largest immigration detention capacity of any State, the system quickly became a vector for the spread of COVID-19, with the government fighting to prevent any release (Kerwin 2020). While migrants and advocates were able to use the courts to obtain release in some cases, US government officials argued that migrants were safer in detention (O'Toole & Carcamo 2020). Public health experts countered that the release of immigration detainees was a public health imperative (Lopez et al. 2020).

Health experts also expressed alarm about the safety of those in refugee camps, warning that 'concern about an outbreak of COVID-19 in … camps cannot be overstated' (Kluge et al. 2020). Among other things, pre-pandemic conditions – overcrowding, absence of basic determinants of health, including clean water and soap, sufficiency of medical capacity and limited access to health information – made camp settings a place of acute risk (Kluge et al. 2020). Limited testing and the rising second wave of the pandemic showed growing spread of the virus in camp settings throughout the fall of 2020 (UNHCR 2020b; Godin 2020).

It seems unlikely that United Nations entities will secure vaccine capacity for those on the move other than by relying on States to allocate doses. IOM has recently concluded a memorandum of understanding with the Global Alliance for Vaccines and Immunizations in part to ensure 'the distribution of any potential COVID-19 vaccine [is] as fair and equitable as possible' and the 'inclusion of migrants, internally displaced persons (IDPs) and refugees in governments' COVID-19 responses, in particular vaccination efforts' (IOM 2020a). United Nations agencies have thus called from the earliest days for migrants, including refugees, to receive equal access to health services and be incorporated in State responses to the pandemic (OHCHR, IOM, UNHCR, & WHO 2020; OHCHR 2020b).

Finally, States have failed to ensure access to education for migrant children during the pandemic. Before the pandemic, many of the more than 30 million migrant children, including refugee children, worldwide faced significant impediments to accessing education (in some cases because of the migration status of their parents) (You et al. 2020; Human Rights Watch 2020b). Less than half of all school-age refugee children were enrolled in school, dropping to one in four for secondary school; UNHCR and UNICEF have warned that some students might never return to schooling after prolonged disruptions during the pandemic (UNHCR & UNICEF 2020).

Denial of access to education brought even more devastating consequences for the many millions of migrants, including refugees, who are among the nearly half of children who depend on school for meals and to gain access to health services and – vitally important during the pandemic – health information (United

Nations 2020c). In places where schooling went virtual, migrant children living without household computers or access to reliable internet or electricity faced often insurmountable barriers to education (You et al. 2020). The United Nations Special Rapporteur on the right to education reported that some governments affirmatively 'deprioritised education for refugee communities' during the pandemic (OHCHR 2020e). The true extent of State failures and their human cost in this as in other areas may not be clear for some time.

Fortunately, some States have taken positive actions that benefited those on the move. Three illustrative progressive steps taken by a few States are representative of the positive developments.

Border closures in a few States contained notable exceptions. Most significantly, this included the ability of family members of migrants with regular status to enter. For example, both immediate and extended family members of permanent residents of Canada; immediate family members of permanent residents of Australia; and non-married partners of residents of Finland all benefited from exceptions to restricted borders (IATA 2020). Other States' border closures permitted migrants – both those in a settled status and temporary migrants – to return to their host countries. Among those permitted to cross otherwise impermeable borders were international students in Canada (Macklin 2020).

Another area where a few States diverged substantially from the trend was in relation to migrant detention. Many countries detain a substantial proportion of migrants in connection with their arrival and processing at the border, proceedings to determine their status as a migrant and/or removal and repatriation; this trend has only grown in recent decades (Sampson & Mitchell 2013). As the pandemic spread, some States released migrants from detention – though sometimes only in response to court orders or other advocacy by or on behalf of migrants. The United Nations has pointed to Spain for having emptied most immigration detention facilities in light of the pandemic, as well as to Zambia for having announced the release of all migrants from immigration detention and to the United Kingdom and Mexico for releasing large numbers from detention in response to court challenges (United Nations Migration Network 2020).

Finally, a few States took steps to regularize or defer enforcement measures against migrants during the pandemic. Arguably the most significant of these was Portugal's decision to grant those with a pending application a temporary residence permit. This move was significant, as it enabled tens of thousands to access health care, social protection, and employment on an equal basis with citizens (PICUM 2020). Italy's regularization, also important, focused on the agricultural sector as well as the domestic and care work sector and on those already in Italy at the start of the pandemic. It provided two tracks for migrants in an irregular situation to secure temporary residence permits – first, if their employer applied on their behalf in order to formalize an existing or new employment relationship and, second, to permit those holding an expired residence permit to apply for a new six-month permit to look for work (Palumbo 2020). Benefits for migrants were clearly the exception, but nonetheless remarkable.

Positive treatment of migrants occurred alongside cascading affirmations that migrants were already essential members of our communities. Certainly, the rhetorical commitment to migrants as 'essential' is not without complexity. As noted above, a number of States failed to ensure effective protection of migrant workers in positions deemed 'essential'. In some States, this recognition focused on those in an irregular situation: as many as 5 million undocumented migrants in the United States filled jobs deemed 'essential' to the nation's critical infrastructure, including in health care (Jawetz 2020). Given that immigrants made vital contributions to the COVID-19 response (constituting about a third of 'key labor' in Europe), commentators called for removing barriers to migration (Fasani & Mazza 2020; Dempster & Smith 2020). A network of municipal leaders, led by the Mayors Migration Council, launched a campaign to build a COVID-19 recovery inclusive of migrants, urging that '[i]n times of crisis, it's up to mayors to ensure no one is left behind' (Mayors Migration Council 2020). It remains to be seen how much the rhetoric will support the proliferation of new or expanded pathways to regular migration or regularization. But these are still welcome affirmations against the backdrop of harms surveyed above.

1.2 Applying the human rights framework to treatment of people on the move during the pandemic

The application of human rights law to evaluate State treatment of migrants, including refugees, has long presented significant challenges. A substantial one is that the scope of the law's inclusion of people on the move is contested. Although States have, in fact, developed a baseline of rights applicable to all migrants, including refugees, they have often been reluctant to apply it (Chetail 2013; Kysel 2016). Indeed, at the national level, new data suggest that States do not consistently recognize even the most basic international norms protecting all migrants in national law (Gest, Kysel, & Wong 2019).

In part to create a tool that might obviate barriers to compliance during the pandemic, a group of experts gathered in the spring of 2020 to develop guidance for States on applying international human rights law to human mobility. The resulting document, *Principles of Protection for Migrants, Refugees, and Other Displaced Persons* (*14 Principles*), applied law found in widely ratified treaties and relevant jurisprudence to key challenges during the pandemic (Aleinikoff et al. 2020). The *14 Principles* address the following:

> (1) Equal Treatment and Non-Discrimination; (2) Right to Health; (3) State Obligations to Combat Stigma, Racism and Xenophobia; (4) Restrictions on Movement Between States; (5) Restrictions on Movements Within States; (6) Non-Return and Access to Territory; (7) Enforcement of Immigration Law, Including Detention; (8) Right to Protection of Life and Health of Persons in Camps, Collective Shelters and Settlements; (9) Right to Information; (10) Protection of Privacy; (11) Gender Considerations;

(12) Marginalized Groups; (13) Labor Rights of Workers; (14) Rights and their Limitations.

The *14 Principles* were endorsed as an authoritative restatement of international law by more than 1,000 scholars worldwide and cited by the United Nations Secretary-General for the proposition that rights have not been 'sufficiently taken into account' during the pandemic (United Nations 2020b). Indeed, the *14 Principles* provide a tool for evaluating how the abuses of migrants, including refugees, described in the preceding subsection, violate the law. States also took positive measures – among them those that reflected the rights of migrants to family unity; rights of liberty and security of person; and a range of other rights implicated by regularizations.

For migrants, and in particular refugees, who have faced hardened borders during the pandemic, international law is clear. Foremost, the law requires that restrictions on the right to leave as well as on the right to re-enter one's home State be imposed only in exceptional circumstances and be limited to those necessary and proportionate to legitimate aims; most importantly here, protecting public health (Aleinikoff et al. 2020). Border restrictions must also recognize and protect the rights of refugees and others entitled to humanitarian protection, including ensuring protection against *refoulement*, or return to a risk of persecution, to arbitrary deprivation of life, or to torture or other cruel, inhuman, or degrading treatment or punishment (Aleinikoff et al. 2020); UNHCR 2020c; OHCHR 2020b; OHCHR 2020c).

For refugees or those otherwise protected against return by international law, the denial of access to territory both prevented evaluation of humanitarian claims (and access to accompanying rights to affirmative protection) and risked return to harm, whether to persecution or merely to an elevated risk of contracting the novel coronavirus. The widespread, blanket closures of borders were disproportionate, particularly in light of guidance by WHO early in the pandemic that such restrictions on the movement of people are generally 'ineffective' during public health emergencies (except perhaps for very short periods at the beginning of an outbreak in order to gain time to implement effective measures) and amassing evidence that migration restrictions are of decreasing significance as a tool of pandemic control as this pandemic has unfolded (World Health Organization 2020; Russell et al. 2020). Such disproportionality was all the more acute in situations where closures left migrants stranded, including in great numbers, at international borders. The use of borders to restrict mobility without tailoring for public health guidance or legal obligations violated State duties to protect the international human rights of migrants.

States are prohibited from discriminating against migrants based on their status, including actual or perceived health status, race, or other protected ground (Aleinikoff et al. 2020). The law requires States to consider migrants, including refugees, in their public health response and take proactive steps to combat stigma and discrimination, even that on behalf of third parties (Aleinikoff et al. 2020; OHCHR 2020b; OHCHR 2020c). Human rights law also underscores the importance of accurate and timely information about disease and how it can be transmitted as well as the obligation to clearly communicate, for example, that viruses are not synonymous with nationality, in order to proactively protect migrants from discrimination. That some State officials either took disproportionate action against people on account of their status as a migrant or even intentionally fanned the flames of racism and xenophobia in the midst of the pandemic violated these State duties.

International human rights law requires that States safeguard the labor rights of migrants, including refugees, to workplace safety, to remuneration, to freedom of association, and to protective equipment and basic sanitation (at least on an equal basis with nationals) (Aleinikoff et al. 2020). States also have a duty to incorporate migrant workers in economic recovery policies (OHCHR 2020b). Finally, States must ensure access to cross-border justice, such as when repatriated migrant workers have wage or other legal claims in their former host States (ILO 2020; IACHR 2019). The pandemic brought widespread rights violations to migrant workers' rights.

International human rights law requires that, just as with nationals, migrants, including refugees, be given access to essential medicines, prevention, and treatment in a non-discriminatory manner (Aleinikoff et al. 2020). Relatedly, the right to health includes the right to access food, water and sanitation, safe shelter, and education – key determinants of health (Aleinikoff et al. 2020; OHCHR 2020c). For those in camp settings, international human rights law requires States to take steps necessary for prevention, treatment, and control of pandemic disease (Aleinikoff et al. 2020). This includes access to health services in a language migrants understand and to sanitary and health measures ranging from soap to testing and contact tracing (Aleinikoff et al. 2020; OHCHR 2020c). When States failed to incorporate migrants into their emergency responses or excluded migrants, including refugees, from the ability to access healthcare and the determinants of health during the pandemic, they failed to protect migrants' right to health.

International human rights law requires that States provide children with special measures of protection and ensure that the best interests of the child is a primary consideration (Aleinikoff et al. 2020). States also have duties to make primary education compulsory and free to all migrant children, including refugee children (Aleinikoff et al. 2020; Bench et al. 2013). The failure of States to ensure access to or continuity of education to migrant children, including refugees, on the basis of equality with nationals violated these duties. As the UN Secretary-General has noted, the crisis 'exacerbat[ed] pre-existing educational disparities' for the most vulnerable, including the displaced, accentuating the 'formidable challenges' the world faces in fulfilling the 'promise of education as a basic human right' (United Nations 2020b).

Finally, international human rights law protecting migrants applies during crises – indeed, it was designed by States to do so. Thus, any restrictions on rights must be provided by law and reasonable, necessary, and proportionate (Aleinikoff et al. 2020; OHCHR 2020d). Suspension of certain rights is permissible during an emergency but only if strictly required and consistent with international obligations (Aleinikoff et al. 2020; International Commission of Jurists 1985). Notably, when it comes to provisions of key human rights treaties which do permit formal suspension in time of emergency by 'derogation' communicated to other treaty partners, certain rights are non-derogable (International Commission of Jurists 1985). Among these are protections against *refoulement*. While dozens of States have derogated from a limited number of provisions of the International Convenant on Civil and Political Rights, questions remain about whether States have adequately ensured protection of vulnerable populations from disproportionate harm even in the application of what might otherwise be a permissible derogation; no derogation is permissible from the International Convenant on Economic, Social and Cultural Rights nor does the Refugee Convention include a blanket derogation clause applicable to crises (Lebret 2020; OHCHR 2020d; Edwards 2012).

2 Meeting the challenges and seizing the opportunities to come

The future of human migration, its extent, and how States will endeavor to manage it, particularly in the name of public health, remains uncertain. Indeed, there have already been efforts by scholars to think through the consequence of this pandemic on migration (Frontiersin.org 2020; Achiume et al. 2020). In both the immediate and long term, there are a number of significant challenges – in addition to the abuses outlined above – that raise complex rights and governance challenges. Fortunately, there are promising developments at the international and regional level which may give States the tools (if the political will develops) to better coordinate and thereby ensure more consistent recognition and protection of migrant and refugee rights. At the very least, global civil society will remain at the vanguard in driving a migrants' rights agenda.

2.1 Challenges on the horizon

It is unclear how migration will resume as States call for more 'management' of migration in the name of 'health-proofing' mobility (IOM 2020b). This may well lead to more surveillance of migrants and invasion of privacy, even as migrants often lack either the legal standing or opportunity to push back against such encroachments (OHCHR 2020e). Of course, before the pandemic, governments were expanding reliance on the use of digital surveillance tools to regulate migration. Migrants, including refugees, and especially those who are also stateless, have often borne the brunt of innovation and use of technology (Institute on Statelessness and Inclusion 2020). Further, use of technology has often discriminated against migrants, whether by intent or impact, on account of race and/or status as a migrant (OHCHR 2020e). This raises significant questions about how efforts to 'health-proof' mobility systems might actually expand the reliance on technology to subject migrants to real-time digital surveillance and enforcement systems, with concomitant negative consequences for the rights of migrants, or, to the contrary, whether they might 'integrate health and protection imperatives' (Chetail 2020).

Perhaps the most significant uncertainty in evaluating the long-term horizon of international migration law and governance comes from global climate change. Certainly, much of the forecasting of the likely effect on migration of global climate change has suggested increased internal migration will be the greatest mobility impact (World Bank 2018). Yet some modeling suggests that certain migration corridors will experience substantial transnational migration as a consequence (Lustgarten 2020). The COVID-19 pandemic may not have substantially affected the pace of change, but discussions have already turned to looking at the pandemic as a 'test case' for evaluating the world's preparedness to respond to the disparate effects of climate crises on migrants, including refugees (UNHCR 2020d). Seen through this light, the future does not look bright.

2.2 Legal and governance developments

Fortunately, despite tremendous uncertainty about the future, new avenues for multilateral cooperation create new opportunities for States to collaborate on migration governance – and on the protection of the rights of migrants. In the past few years, States have negotiated two new non-binding agreements: a Global Compact for Safe, Orderly and Regular Migration and a Global Compact on Refugees. While distinct, both agreements focus on encouraging cooperation on implementing new and detailed policy commitments. The United Nations has also elevated IOM to be a formal part of the United Nations system and created the new Network on Migration, composed of United Nations entities with mandates that touch on migration.

The Network has been active during the pandemic, creating a space for dialogue among States and collaboration with civil society. The Network issued important pieces of policy guidance for States, allowing key humanitarian actors to speak with one voice. For example, the Network issued a call for a suspension of forced returns (IOM 2020c). The Network, through one of its working groups that included members of civil society, also issued detailed guidance on immigration detention, calling for a moratorium (UN Migration Network 2020). Both of these documents reflected human rights principles and the potential of the Network to mainstream human rights in global migration policy. While UNHCR is a member of the Network, it also separately oversees implementation of the Global Compact on Refugees, and reported that, despite the pandemic, the agreement has led to greater inclusion of refugees in national systems and development plans (UNHCR 2020f).

The United Nations Secretary-General has also actively contributed to debates about COVID-19 and migration, arguing that responding to the pandemic and protecting the human rights of migrants are not mutually exclusive (United Nations 2020b). The Secretary-General has thus called for further strengthening migration governance through implementing both Global Compacts and compliance with human rights law as a key pillar of State responses (United Nations 2020b). Most recently, the Secretary-General has argued that, when it comes to migration, the pandemic has been a 'disrupter, but also a leveller [*sic*]' and has shown the potential for the Compact for Migration in particular to help States navigate new challenges in the post-pandemic (United Nations 2020d).

While it remains uncertain how States will leverage the new Compacts and United Nations infrastructure after the pandemic – and whether they will use the crisis as an opportunity to affirm the rights of all migrants as part of a more robust governance of migration – there are also important parallel opportunities for regional leadership.

Not long before the WHO declared the COVID-19 pandemic, the Inter-American Commission on Human Rights adopted what may be the most comprehensive and progressive restatement of the human rights of all migrants ever issued by an international body. This document, the Inter-American Principles on the Human Rights of Migrants, Refugees, Stateless Persons and Victims of Trafficking (*Inter-American Principles*), was the result of a multi-year partnership between the Commission's Rapporteurship on the rights of migrants and the International Migrants' Bill of Rights (IMBR) Initiative (IACHR 2019). The *Inter-American Principles* contain a number of provisions relevant to the challenges of human migration in the current pandemic and beyond. For example, several of the eighty provisions recognize migrants' rights to health and to labor rights, rights to liberty, and security of person, against discrimination, to cross-border justice, and the rights of child migrants. This effort is just one example of how regional leadership could help put migrants' rights at the center of migration policy.

These new legal and governance configurations create new platforms for information- and data-sharing and expand opportunities to shape discussions with and among States. Taking migration governance out of the shadows could lead to new points of departure for the promotion of progressive reforms anchored in a rights-based approach. Despite these new avenues for coordination at the global and regional levels, State responses to the pandemic eschewed multilateralism.

2.3 The potential for civil society leadership

In addition to the promise of new legal and governance structures, new configurations among global civil society also present an avenue of opportunity when it comes to reshaping global migration law and policy and protecting migrants' rights.

The process of the negotiation of the Global Compacts brought together networks of civil society activists engaged on migration issues in new ways. Indicative of this, several groups launched the Civil Society Action Committee, a platform that helps coordinate engagement on migration policy and governance (Civil Society Action Committee 2020). Many members are representative of or networked with regional and national social movements led by or supporting migrants. Relatedly, a number of civil society groups have united around a pledge to include refugees in decisions that affect them (Global Refugee Led Network 2018). These new configurations have taken as an opening the commitment by the United

Nations to incorporating civil society voices in a whole-of-society approach to implementing the Global Compacts. The pandemic has also created new avenues for participation by civil society in virtual migration governance discussions. Civil society engagement with international migration governance and refugee protection is arguably at an all-time high.

Civil society leadership can result in alliances within and across regions and conduits for sharing lessons learned about retrograde or best practices. Civil society can exert coordinated pressure on States domestically and in global fora and hold States and governance networks accountable. Civil society activists could be the key actors to pressure both international organizations like the United Nations Network as well as States to implement modalities of cooperation on the governance of migration that recognize and protect a baseline of rights for all migrants. The development and use of soft law – like *14 Principles of Protection* and the *Inter-American Principles* – to restate this existing baseline 'can be a powerful catalyst in the development of legal norms that constrain states as a matter of formal obligation' (Kysel & Thomas 2020).

Even though the COVID-19 pandemic has brought a raft of rights abuses against migrants, and very little use of multilateral institutions to coordinate State response, the tools necessary to build a new era of migration lay ready. Indeed, because migration control and the treatment of migrants have been such prominent dimensions of the pandemic response around the world, COVID-19 may well create a unique opportunity for civil society to force States to build back better on migration and truly safeguard the rights of all people on the move.

3 Conclusion

States have responded to the COVID-19 pandemic in ways that have uniquely harmed migrants, including refugees – leaving them stranded at borders or pushed back to persecutors; subjected to violent racist or xenophobic attacks; fired from jobs or forced to work without personal protective equipment; denied access to healthcare; or, in the case of migrant children, unable to go to school. Though States have already agreed to a common baseline of rights protecting all migrants, including refugees, they have not complied with it. The pandemic revealed an erosion of the protection of rights, even those seen to be subject to broad consensus. There were exceptions: A few States have taken progressive actions consistent with migrants' rights: releasing migrants from detention and extending status; allowing border-crossing. Multilateral cooperation to address the movement of people across international borders is also at a low point. And major new challenges loom on the horizon, beginning with restarting mobility in the post-pandemic and running through to climate change. Fortunately, there are new tools in the governance toolbelt, including non-binding Global Compacts for Migration and on Refugees and a new United Nations Network as well as progressive developments at the regional level. States may yet take these up to craft a new, rights-respecting architecture to facilitate migration. If they do, it will likely be civil society leading the way, compelling States to recognize and protect the rights of all migrants, regardless of the reason for their movement across international borders.

Note

1 There is no widely adopted international law definition of migrant. I use 'migrant' to include refugees, in the sense of 'any person outside of a State in which [they are] a citizen or national or, in the case of a stateless [person, their] State of birth or habitual residence' (Bench et al. 2013). This definition was developed by the International Migrants Bill of Rights (IMBR) Initiative, and has since been adopted by international authorities (OHCHR 2014; IAHCR 2019). The rights of migrants who are also refugees are defined under specific legal instruments. This definition of migrants therefore excludes internally displaced persons; this chapter excludes internal mobility (as well as the forms of *immobility* that accompanied the COVID-19 pandemic (Martin & Bergmann 2020)). In focusing on international mobility and the human rights obligations of host States, this chapter likewise does not consider the treatment of migrants by their States of nationality, which has been a shifting phenomenon during the COVID-19 pandemic (Mégret 2020).

References

Achiume, ET, 2020, 'A Conversation with U.N. Special Rapporteur E. Tendayi Achiume: COVID-19, Racism, and Xenophobia', viewed 30 December 2020, www.justsecurity.org/70410/a-conversation-with-u-n-special-rapporteur-e-tendayi-achiume-covid-19-racism-and-xenophobia/

Achiume, ET, Gammeltoft-Hansen, T, & Spijkerboer, T 2020, 'Introduction to the Symposium on COVID-19, Global Mobility and International Law', *American Journal of International Law*, vol. 114, pp. 312–316.

Aleinikoff, TA et al. 2020, 'Human Mobility and Human Rights in the COVID-19 Pandemic: Principles of Protection for Migrants, Refugees and Other Displaced Persons', *International Journal of Refugee Law*.

Beech, H 2020, 'Hundreds of Rohingya Refugees Stuck at Sea With "Zero Hope"', *New York Times*, 1 May, viewed 30 December 2020, www.nytimes.com/2020/05/01/world/asia/rohingya-muslim-refugee-crisis.html

Bench, Z et al. 2013, 'International Migrants Bill of Rights', *Georgetown Immigration Law Journal*, vol. 28, no. 9.

Brennan, JS, Simon, F, Howard, PN, & Nielsen, RK 2020, 'Types, Sources, and Claims of COVID-19 Misinformation', *Reuters Institute*, 7 April, viewed 30 December 2020, https://reutersinstitute.politics.ox.ac.uk/types-sources-and-claims-covid-19-misinformation

Chetail, V 2020, 'COVID-19 and Human Rights of Migrants: More Protection for the Benefit of All', *IOM UN Migration*, viewed 30 December 2020, https://publications.iom.int/system/files/pdf/covid19-human-rights.pdf

Chetail, V 2013, 'The Human Rights of Migrants in General International Law: From Minimum Standards to Fundamental Rights', *Georgetown Immigration Law Journal*, vol. 28, no. 1, pp. 225–255.

Civil Society Action Committee 2020, 'Which Way Forward on the Implementation of the Global Compact For Migration in the Era of COVID-19?', viewed 30 December 2020, https://csactioncommittee.org/wp-content/uploads/2020/12/Which-way-forward-on-GCM-Implementation-final-layout.pdf

Dempster, H & Smith, R 2020, 'Migrant Health Workers Are on the COVID-19 Front Line. We Need More of Them', *Center for Global Development*, 2 April, viewed 30 December 2020, www.cgdev.org/blog/migrant-health-workers-are-covid-19-frontline-we-need-more-them

Dickerson, C 2020, '10 Years Old, Tearful and Confused After a Sudden Deportation', New York Times, 20 May, viewed 30 December 2020, www.nytimes.com/2020/05/20/us/coronavirus-migrant-children-unaccompanied-minors.html

Eckenwiler, L 2020, 'Health Workers Born outside of the US Are Essential in Our Fight against the Coronavirus. Sadly, America is Failing them', *Business Insider*, 15 November, viewed 30 December 2020, www.businessinsider.com/migrant-foreign-born-healthcare-workers-america-covid-19-coronavirus-pandemic-2020-11

Edwards, A 2012, 'Temporary Protection, Derogation and the *1951 Refugee Convention*', *Melbourne Journal of International Law*, vol. 13, pp. 1–41.

Fasani, F & Mazza, J 2020, 'Immigrant Key Workers: Their Contributions to Europe's COVID-19 Response', *IZA Institute of Labor Economics*, viewed 30 December 2020, http://ftp.iza.org/pp155.pdf

Fronteirsin.org 2020, 'Research Topic: Migration in the Time of COVID-19: Comparative Law and Policy Responses', www.frontiersin.org/research-topics/13787/migration-in-the-time-of-covid-19-comparative-law-and-policy-responses#overview

Gest, J, Kysel, I, & Wong TK 2019, 'Protecting and Benchmarking Migrants' Rights: An Analysis of the Global Compact for Safe, Orderly and Regular Migration', *International Migration*, vol. 57, no. 6.

Ghezelbash, D & Feith Tan, N 2020, 'The End of the Right to Seek Asylum? COVID-19 and the Future of Refugee Protection', European University Institute, viewed 30 December 2020, https://papers.ssrn.com/sol3/papers.cfm?abstract_id=3689093

Global Refugee Led Network 2018, 'Who We Are', viewed 30 December 2020, www.globalrefugeelednetwork.org/who-we-are/

Godin, M 2020, 'COVID-19 Outbreaks Are Now Emerging in Refugee Camps. Why Did it Take so Long For the Virus to Reach Them?', *TIME*, 9 October, viewed 30 December 2020, https://time.com/5893135/covid-19-refugee-camps/

Hsu, S 2020, 'U.S. Might Separate Families after Federal Judge Orders ICE to Free Migrant Children', *Washington Post*, 7 July, viewed 30 December 2020, www.washingtonpost.com/local/legal-issues/us-may-separate-families-after-federal-judge-orders-ice-to-free-migrant-children/2020/07/07/a1758ad6-c067-11ea-b178-bb7b05b94af1_story.html

Human Rights Watch 2020a, 'Maldives: COVID-19 Exposes Abuse of Migrants', viewed 30 December 2020, www.hrw.org/news/2020/08/25/maldives-covid-19-exposes-abuse-migrants#

Human Rights Watch 2020b, 'COVID-19 and Children's Rights', viewed 30 December 2020, www.hrw.org/news/2020/04/09/covid-19-and-childrens-rights#_Toc37256528

IACHR 2019, *Principles on the Human Rights of Migrants, Refugees, Stateless Persons and Victims of Human Trafficking*, viewed 30 December 2020, www.oas.org/en/iachr/decisions/pdf/Resolution-4-19-en.pdf

IATA 2020, 'COVID-19 Travel Regulations Map', viewed 30 December 2020, www.iatatravelcentre.com/international-travel-document-news/1580226297.htm

ILO 2020, 'Protecting Migrant Workers during the COVID-19 Pandemic', viewed 30 December 2020, www.ilo.org/wcmsp5/groups/public/---ed_protect/---protrav/---migrant/documents/publication/wcms_743268.pdf

IOM 2020a, 'Gavi and IOM Join Forces to Improve Immunization Coverage for Migrants', viewed 30 December 2020, www.iom.int/news/gavi-and-iom-join-forces-improve-immunization-coverage-migrants

IOM 2020b, 'Remarks Made by the Director General at the Briefing for Member States held on 15 April 2020', viewed 30 December 2020, http://governingbodies.iom.int/system/files/en/briefings/Remarks%20made%20by%20the%20Director%20General%20at%20the%20briefing%20for%20Member%20States%20held%20on%2015%20April%202020.pdf

IOM 2020c, 'Forced Returns of Migrants Must be Suspended in Times of COVID-19', viewed 20 December 2020, www.iom.int/news/forced-returns-migrants-must-be-suspended-times-covid-19

IOM 2020d, 'Countering Xenophobia and Stigma to Foster Social Cohesion in the COVID-19 Response and Recovery', viewed 30 December 2020, www.iom.int/sites/default/files/documents/countering_xenophobia_and_stigma_130720.pdf

IOM 2020f, 'Cross-Border Human Mobility Amid and After COVID-19', viewed 30 December 2020, www.iom.int/sites/default/files/defaul/pp_cross-border_human_mobility_amid_and_after_covid-19_policy.pdf

Institute on Statelessness and Inclusion 2020, *Locked in and Locked Out; The Impact of Digital Identity Systems on Rohingya Populations*, viewed 30 December 2020, https://files.institutesi.org/Locked_In_Locked_Out_The_Rohingya_Briefing_Paper.pdf

International Commission of Jurists 1985, *Siracusa Principles: on the Limitation and Derogation Provisions in the ICCPR*, viewed 30 December 2020, www.icj.org/wp-content/uploads/1984/07/Siracusa-principles-ICCPR-legal-submission-1985-eng.pdf

Jawetz T 2020, 'Immigrants as Essential Workers During COVID-19', *Center for American Progress*, 28 September, viewed 30 December 2020, https://cdn.americanprogress.org/content/uploads/2020/09/28102223/JawetzImmigrantsCOVID-testimony1.pdf?_ga=2.155661874.827889528.1608065444-1607758317.1607101569

Jordan, M 2020, 'Migrant Workers Restricted to Farms Under One Grower's Virus Lockdown', *New York Times*, 19 October, viewed 30 December 2020, www.nytimes.com/2020/10/19/us/coronavirus-tomato-migrant-farm-workers.html

Justice for Wage Theft 2020, 'Call for an Urgent Justice Mechanism for Repatriated Migrant Workers', viewed 30 December 2020, https://justiceforwagetheft.org/en/page/c1cu5etiltr

Kapilashrami, A et al. 2020, 'Neglect of Low-income Migrants in Covid-19 Response: A South Asian Perspective on the Failures of Global and National Public Health Policies', *BMJ*, 29 May, viewed 30 December 2020, https://blogs.bmj.com/bmj/2020/05/29/neglect-of-low-income-migrants-in-covid-19-response/

Kerwin, D 2020, 'Immigration Detention and COVID-19: How a Pandemic Exploited and Spread through the US Immigrant Detention System', *Center for Migration Studies*, viewed 30 December 2020, https://cmsny.org/wp-content/uploads/2020/08/CMS-Detention-COVID-Report-08-12-2020.pdf

Kingsley, P & Willis, H 2020, 'Latest Tactic to Push Migrants From Europe? A Private, Clandestine Fleet', *New York Times*, 30 April, viewed 30 December 2020, www.nytimes.com/2020/04/30/world/europe/migrants-malta.html

Kluge, H, Jakab, Z, Bartovic, J, D'anna, V, & Severoni, S, 2020, 'Refugee and Migrant Health in the COVID-19 Response', *The Lancet*, vol. 395, pp. 1237–1239.

Kysel, I 2016, 'Promoting the Recognition and Protection of the Rights of All Migrants Using a Soft-Law International Migrants Bill of Rights', *Journal on Migration and Human Security*, vol. 4, no. 2, pp. 29–44.

Kysel, I & Thomas, C 2020, 'The Contested Boundaries of Emerging International Migration Law in the Post-Pandemic', *AJIL* Unbound, vol. 114.

The Lancet 2020, 'The COVID-19 Infodemic', vol. 20, no. 8, viewed 30 December 2020, www.thelancet.com/journals/laninf/article/PIIS1473-3099(20)30565-X/fulltext

Lebret, A 2020, 'COVID-19 Pandemic and Derogation to Human Rights', *Journal of Law and the Biosciences*, vol. 7, no. 1.

Lopez, W, Kline, N, LeBrón, A, Novak, N, De Trinidad Young, ME, Gonsalves, G, Mishori, R, Safi, B, & Kysel, I 2020, 'Preventing the Spread of Covid-19 in Immigration Detention Centers Requires the Release of Detainees', *American Journal of Public Health*, vol. 111, no. 1, pp. 110–115.

Lustgarten, A 2020, 'The Great Climate Migration', *New York Times Magazine*, 23 July, viewed 30 December 2020, www.nytimes.com/interactive/2020/07/23/magazine/climate-migration.html

Macklin, A 2020, '(In)Essential Bordering: Canada, COVID and Mobility', *Frontiers in Human Dynamics*, viewed 30 December 2020, www.frontiersin.org/articles/10.3389/fhumd.2020.609694/abstract

Mann, I & Keady-Tabbal, N 2020, 'Torture by Rescue: Asylum-Seeker Pushbacks in the Agean', *Just Security*, 26 October, viewed 30 December 2020, www.justsecurity.org/72955/torture-by-rescue-asylum-seeker-pushbacks-in-the-aegean/

Martin, S & and Bergmann, J 2020, 'Shifting Forms of Mobility Related to COVID-19', *IOM UN Migration*, viewed 30 December 2020, https://publications.iom.int/system/files/pdf/shifting-forms.pdf

Mayor's Migration Council 2020, 'Joint Statement: Inclusive COVID-19 Response and Recovery', viewed 30 December 2020, www.mayorsmigrationcouncil.org/mmc-covid19

Mégret, F 2020, 'Homeward Bound? Global Mobility and the Role of the State of Nationality During the Pandemic', *AJIL Unbound*, vol. 114.

Michaels, D & Wagner, G 2020, 'Occupational Safety and Health Administration and Worker Safety During the COVID-19 Pandemic', *JAMA*, vol. 324, no. 14, pp. 1389–1390.

OECD 2020, 'What is the Impact of the COVID-19 Pandemic on Immigrants and their Children?', 19 October, viewed 30 December 2020, https://read.oecd-ilibrary.org/view/?ref=137_137245-8saheqv0k3&title=What-is-the-impact-of-the-COVID-19-pandemic-on-immigrants-and-their-children%3F

OHCHR, IOM, UNHCR, & WHO 2020, 'The Rights and Health of Refugees, Migrants and Stateless Must be Protected in COVID-19 Response', viewed 30 December 2020, www.unhcr.org/neu/36015-the-rights-and-health-of-refugees-migrants-and-stateless-must-be-protected-in-covid-19-response.html

OHCHR 2014, 'Recommended Principles and Guidelines on Human Rights at International Borders', viewed 30 December 2020, www.ohchr.org/Documents/Issues/Migration/OHCHR_Recommended_Principles_Guidelines.pdf

OHCHR 2020a, 'States Should Take Action against COVID-19-Related Expressions of Xenophobia, Says UN Expert', viewed 30 December 2020, www.ohchr.org/en/NewsEvents/Pages/DisplayNews.aspx?NewsID=25739&LangID=E

OHCHR 2020b, 'UN Committee on Migrant Workers & UN Special Rapporteur on the Human Rights of Migrants, Joint Guidance Note on the Impacts of the COVID-19 Pandemic on the Human Rights of Migrants', viewed 30 December 2020, https://reliefweb.int/sites/reliefweb.int/files/resources/CMWSPMJointGuidanceNoteCOVID-19Migrants.pdf

OHCHR 2020c, 'COVID-19 and the Human Rights of Migrants: Guidance', viewed 30 December 2020, www.ohchr.org/Documents/Issues/Migration/OHCHRGuidance_COVID19_Migrants.pdf

OHCHR 2020d, 'Emergency Measures and COVID-19: Guidance', viewed 30 December 2020, www.ohchr.org/Documents/Events/EmergencyMeasures_COVID19.pdf

OHCHR 2020e, 'Report of the Special Rapporteur on Contemporary Forms of Racism, Racial Discrimination, Xenophobia and Related Intolerance', viewed 30 December 2020, www.ohchr.org/EN/newyork/Documents/A-75-590-AUV.docx

OHCHR 2020f, 'Report of the Special Rapporteur on the Promotion and Protection of the Right to Freedom of Opinion and Expression', UN Doc. A/HRC/44/49, viewed 30 December 2020, https://undocs.org/A/HRC/44/49

O'Toole, M & Carcamo, C 2020, 'Citing Coronavirus, Trump Officials Refuse to Release Migrant Kids to Sponsors – and Deport Them Instead', *Los Angeles Times*, 12 May, viewed 30 December 2020, www.latimes.com/politics/story/2020-05-12/trump-officials-coronavirus-refuse-releasing-migrant-kids

Palumbo, L 2020, 'The Italian Plan for Regularisation: Real Progress for Migrants' Rights?', *Migration Policy Centre*, 8 June, viewed 30 December 2020, https://blogs.eui.eu/migrationpolicycentre/italian-plan-regularisation-real-progress-migrants-rights/

Pattison, P & Sedhai, R 2020, 'Covid-19 Lockdown Turns Qatar's Largest Migrant Camp into "Virtual Prison"', *The Guardian*, 20 March, viewed 30 December 2020, www.theguardian.com/global-development/2020/mar/20/covid-19-lockdown-turns-qatars-largest-migrant-camp-into-virtual-prison

Pernitez-Agan, S, Bautista, M, Lopez, J, Sampson, M, & Wickramage, K 2020, 'Bibliometric Analysis on COVID-19 in the Context of Migration Health', *Migration Health Research*, 22 June, viewed 30 December 2020, https://migrationhealthresearch.iom.int/sites/healthresearch/files/migration-health/bibliometric_analysis_on_covid-19_in_the_context_of_migration_health_version2.0_1.pdf

PICUM 2020, 'Regularising Undocumented People in Response to the COVID-19 Pandemic', viewed 30 December 2020, https://picum.org/regularising-undocumented-people-in-response-to-the-covid-19-pandemic/

Russell, T, Wu, J, Clifford, S, Edmunds, W, Kucharski, A & Jit, M, 'Effect of Internationally Imported Cases on Internal Spread of COVID-19: A Mathematical Modelling Study', *The Lancet*, v. 6, E.12–20, viewed 16 March 2020, www.thelancet.com/journals/lanpub/article/PIIS2468-2667(20)30263-2/fulltext

Sampson, R & Mitchell, G 2013, 'Global Trends in Immigration Detention and Alternatives to Detention: Practical, Political and Symbolic Rationales', *Journal on Migration and Human Security*, vol. 1, no. 3, pp. 97–121.

Shachar, A 2020, 'Borders in the Time of COVID-19', *Ethics & International Affairs*, viewed 30 December 2020, www.ethicsandinternationalaffairs.org/2020/borders-in-the-time-of-covid-19/

Sirleaf, M 2020, 'Entry Denied: COVID-19, Race, Migration, and Global Health', *Frontiers in Human Dynamics*, viewed 30 December 2020, www.frontiersin.org/articles/10.3389/fhumd.2020.599157/full

Slater, J, Fahim, K, & McQue, K 2020, 'Migration, in Reverse', *Washington Post*, 1 October, viewed 30 December 2020, www.washingtonpost.com/graphics/2020/world/coronavirus-migration-trends-gulf-states-india/

Tan, Y 2020, 'Covid-19 Singapore: A "Pandemic of Inequality" Exposed', *BBC News*, 17 September, viewed 30 December 2020, www.bbc.com/news/world-asia-54082861

Timberg, C & Chiu, A 2020, 'As the Coronavirus Spreads, So Does Online Racism Targeting Asians, New Research Shows', *Washington Post*, 8 April, viewed 30 December 2020, www.washingtonpost.com/technology/2020/04/08/coronavirus-spreads-so-does-online-racism-targeting-asians-new-research-shows/

United Nations 2020a, 'None Safe until All Are, Secretary General Stresses', viewed 30 December 2020, www.un.org/press/en/2020/sgsm20059.doc.htm

United Nations 2020b, 'Policy Brief on People on the Move', viewed 30 December 2020, www.un.org/sites/un2.un.org/files/sg_policy_brief_on_people_on_the_move.pdf

United Nations 2020c, 'Policy Brief: Education during COVID-19 and Beyond', viewed 30 December 2020, www.un.org/development/desa/dspd/wp-content/uploads/sites/22/2020/08/sg_policy_brief_covid-19_and_education_august_2020.pdf

United Nations 2020d, 'Global Compact for Safe, Orderly and Regular Migration: Report of the Secretary General', viewed 30 December 2020, https://migrationnetwork.un.org/sites/default/files/docs/english.pdf

United Nations 2020e, '"Verified" Initiative aims to Flood Digital Space with Facts amid COVID-19 Crisis', viewed 30 December 2020, www.un.org/en/coronavirus/%E2%80%98verified%E2%80%99-initiative-aims-flood-digital-space-facts-amid-covid-19-crisis

UN News 2020, 'Migrants Stranded "All over the World" and at Risk from Coronavirus', viewed 30 December 2020, https://news.un.org/en/story/2020/05/1063482

UNHCR 2020a, 'UNHCR's Gillian Triggs Warns COVID-19 Severely Testing Refugee Protection', viewed 30 December 2020, www.unhcr.org/en-us/news/press/2020/10/5f7de2724/unhcrs-gillian-triggs-warns-covid-19-severely-testing-refugee-protection.html

UNHCR 2020b, 'UNHCR Global COVID-19 Emergency Response', viewed 30 December 2020, https://reporting.unhcr.org/sites/default/files/13112020_UNHCR%20Global%20COVID-19%20Emergency%20Response.pdf

UNHCR 2020c, 'Key Legal Considerations on Access to Territory for Persons in Need of International Protection', viewed 30 December 2020, https://www.refworld.org/docid/5e7132834.html

UNHCR 2020d, 'COVID-19 Crisis Offers Lesson on Climate Response for Refugees', viewed 30 December 2020, www.unhcr.org/news/stories/2020/12/5fc7e3444/covid-19-crisis-offers-lesson-climate-response-refugees.html

UNHCR 2020e, 'UNHCR, IOM and UNHCR Chiefs Stress that COVID-19 Underlines the Urgent Need for Universal Health Coverage', viewed 30 December 2020, www.unhcr.org/en-us/news/press/2020/12/5fd35fc94/iom-unhcr-chiefs-stress-covid-19-underlines-urgent-need-universal-health.html

UNHCR 2020f, 'Report of the United Nations High Commissioner for Refugees', viewed 30 December 2020, www.unhcr.org/en-us/excom/bgares/5f69c6ca4/report-united-nations-high-commissioner-refugees-covering-period-1-july.html

UNHCR & UNICEF 2020, 'As COVID-19 pandemic continues, forcibly displaced children need more support than ever,' viewed December 30, 2020, https://www.unhcr.org/en-us/news/press/2020/4/5e9d4c044/covid-19-pandemic-continues-forcibly-displaced-children-need-support.html

UN Migration Network, 'COVID-19 and Immigration Detention: What can Governments and Other Stakeholders Do?', viewed 30 December 2020, https://migrationnetwork.un.org/sites/default/files/docs/un_network_on_migration_wg_atd_policy_brief_covid-19_and_immigration_detention.pdf

The World Bank 2018, 'Groundswell: Preparing for Internal Climate Migration', viewed 30 December 2020, https://openknowledge.worldbank.org/handle/10986/29461

World Health Organization 2020, 'Updated WHO Recommendations for International Traffic in Relation to COVID-19 Outbreak', 29 February, viewed 30 December 2020, www.who.int/news-room/articles-detail/updated-who-recommendations-for-international-traffic-in-relation-to-covid-19-outbreak

You, D, Lindt, N, Allen, R, Hansen, C, Beise, J & Blume, S 2020, Migrant and Displaced Children in the Age of COVID-19: How the Pandemic is Impacting Them and What We Can Do to Help, *Migration Policy Practice*, vol.V, no. X, pp. 32–39, viewed 16 March 2021, https://www.unicef.org/media/68761/file

Zetter, R & Ruaudel, H 2016, 'Refugees' Right to Work and Access to Labor Markets – An Assessment', *KNOMAD*, viewed 30 December 2020, www.knomad.org/sites/default/files/2017-03/KNOMAD%20Study%201%20Part%20I-%20Assessing%20Refugees%27%20Rights%20to%20Work_final.pdf

PART 3

Cornerstones for social cohesion

11

A PARADIGM SHIFT FOR THE SUSTAINABLE DEVELOPMENT GOALS?

Human rights and the private sector in the new social contract

Amanda Lyons

Virtually no conversation about COVID-19 recovery is focused on returning us to the status quo. Most commentators see the massive and multidimensional disruptions as an opportunity for actors to advance their agendas in transformational ways – for better or for worse. COVID-19 has been described as: a 'fork in the road', a 'crossroads', the 'opportunity to course-correct', a 'global wake-up call', 'a defining moment for modern society', a 'once-in-a-generation opportunity', the 'rebirthing of society', the New Social Contract, and the chance for 'the Great Reset'. There is a resounding consensus around the general aspiration to #Build Back Better.

This chapter will explore the possibility of the COVID-19 pandemic and related crises leading to one of two paradigm shifts – either a consolidation of stakeholder capitalism with the private sector in the driver's seat or a more rights-favorable course correction that alters the power dynamics between the public and the private sector, with the focus on people as rights-holders. In particular, the chapter will consider the fate of the United Nations' (UN) 2030 Agenda for Sustainable Development and its potential to serve as a vehicle for advancing just, sustainable, and rights-affirming recovery policies. Could the crisis create the conditions for the 2030 Agenda and its 17 Sustainable Development Goals (SDGs) to deliver on the promised transformations of economic, social, and environmental policies?

Many have reflected on the role of crises in creating the conditions for otherwise unimaginable advances, when 'seemingly impossible ideas suddenly become possible' (Klein 2020). Crisis as a catalyst is familiar in the field of transitional justice, for example, and it is embedded in the origins of the global human rights project itself, born out of the ashes of the Great Depression and World War II (Young 2020). Considering the deep economic, social, and environmental crises that are the backdrop to COVID-19, we should be aiming for nothing less.

At the global level, a prevalent thread in the calls for a transformative recovery is to scrap the outdated, ineffective, or unjust models of the past in favor of 'new' ones.

There are important calls for a new social contract to not only guide us out of the devastation caused during the pandemic, but also to save us from the pre-existing crises of inequality, poverty, hunger, closing of democratic and civic spaces, environmental degradation, and climate change (Guterres 2020).

As Klaus Schwab, founder and executive chairman of the World Economic Forum, describes:

> Seeing the failures and fault lines in the cruel light of day cast by the corona crisis may compel us to act faster by replacing failed ideas, institutions, processes and rules with new ones better suited to current and future needs. This is the Great Reset.
>
> *(Schwab & Malleret 2020)*

Yet, for this new social contract, there are drastically divergent proposals in terms of what exactly we need to abandon and what new structures we need to build, which ideas are the 'old ideas', and which are transformative. There are a wide range of possible paradigm shifts, each producing different groups as winners and losers (Bergman 2020).

This chapter considers possible paradigm shifts relating to human rights and the private sector. In the efforts to promote a transformative recovery and in the calls to scrap the old in favor of the new (or supposedly new), where does the 2030 Agenda for Sustainable Development fit? And what about the far less glamorous international human rights framework?

To explore these questions, section 1 offers first a human rights-based assessment of the Agenda's design and implementation to date to highlight the strengths and weaknesses in terms of its potential for guiding an integrated, transformative recovery from COVID-19. Section 2 then highlights particular dimensions of the COVID-19 crisis and responses that would suggest an opening for finally advancing a more rights-favorable paradigm with the chance to deliver on the transformations called for by the SDGs. Section 3, on the other hand, sets out two prominent trends – pressure for austerity and the consolidation of stakeholder capitalism – which are likely to intensify in the crisis and which undermine efforts to course correct on the SDGs in favor of rights-affirming transformations. The chapter concludes that a human rights-based approach to the SDGs is critical to maximize the transformative potential of putting the 2030 Agenda at the heart of the global and national COVID-19 recovery efforts. That rights-based approach must pragmatically engage in the 'nitty gritty' of policymaking and explicitly interact with the formal human rights framework (Sharp 2018).

1 Assessing the 2030 Agenda for Sustainable Development as a vehicle for transformation

Many expert observers have alerted that the COVID-19 crisis poses a serious challenge to the implementation of the 2030 Agenda (Santos-Carrillo,

Fernández-Portillo, & Sianes 2020). Already in May 2020 the UN's stock-taking report on the SDGs declared that the pandemic had 'abruptly disrupted implementation towards many of the SDGs and, in some cases, turned back decades of progress' (Jensen ed. 2020, p. 3).

At the same time, UN agencies and experts, states, and the private sector are centering the 2030 Agenda in their public calls for and commitments to a transformative, just, and sustainable recovery from the pandemic (United Nations 2020a; WEF 2020c). The Agenda is invoked as an alternative to short-termism and a framework to advance an integrated approach to economic, social, and environmental challenges (Hawkes 2020). UN Secretary-General António Guterres has urged states to link public spending to achieving the Sustainable Development Goals citing the 'moral obligation to ensure that the trillions of dollars for COVID-19 recovery – money that we are borrowing from future generations – does not leave them burdened by a mountain of debt on a broken planet' (Guterres 2020).

These are also strained efforts to assert the continued relevance of this centerpiece global development agenda, which was adopted in a very different context and for which progress has been at best 'uneven' (Jensen 2020, p. 3). Five years into the fifteen-year agenda, it is widely acknowledged that even pre-COVID-19 we were not on track to achieve the SDGs (United Nations 2020b).

Nonetheless, as Kate Donald (2020, p. 366) noted before the pandemic, the 2030 Agenda has become an 'unavoidable reference point' with which human rights advocates must contend. Judging from UN and member state pronouncements, the Agenda is poised to retain its place as the preferred framework for signaling longer-term economic, social, and environmental aims in national and international recovery plans.

1.1 Strengths in the 2030 Agenda that support rights-favorable transformations

The critical contribution of the 2030 Agenda is the overarching integrated aim to 'end the tyranny of poverty' while remaining within ecological boundaries. Considerations of jobs, gender equality, oceans, economic growth, rule of law, and partnerships appear in the integrated agenda specifically because of their relation to this overarching aim.

The Agenda recognizes that achieving this aim is not a challenge only for developing countries, which were the focus of the 2000 Millennium Development Goals, but in fact is necessarily a shared urgency and responsibility of all countries (Winkler & Williams 2017). There is a recognition embedded in the Agenda that global crises require cooperation and solidarity. The Agenda is therefore important as a shared platform for concerted language and consensus to facilitate global cooperation.

The 2030 Agenda also acknowledges the link to the other set of globally shared (universal) standards and expectations – the international human rights framework.

The 2030 Agenda preamble asserts that it is 'grounded in the Universal Declaration of Human Rights'. While there are important limitations imposed by not building the Agenda around existing rights and the corresponding State obligations, as discussed further below, many observers acknowledge that the momentum and political reach of this kind of goal-setting and aspirational language can breathe life into human rights language (MacNaughton 2017; Donald 2020). Arguably, the SDGs could then be a valuable vehicle for advancing and operationalizing emergent or longstanding human rights demands.

Despite the SDGs' purposively loose ties to the human rights framework, advocates have strategically emphasized the links and consistencies between the SDGs and human rights to try to anchor the Agenda in the human rights framework after the fact. The UN Committee on Economic, Social, and Cultural Rights (2019, p. 1) has declared that the 2030 Agenda 'powerfully expresses the essence' of the codified human rights.

Advocates have latched onto several dimension of this human rights 'essence' in the SDGs that are especially relevant for considering the relevance of the Agenda in the context of COVID-19 recovery. The adoption of a multidimensional definition of poverty creates space to advance rights-based approaches that expose systemic inequalities in terms of resources, capabilities, power, and security (Sepúlveda Carmona 2021; de Schutter 2020a). The emphasis on leaving no one behind and interrogating development outcomes to make visible the most marginalized and vulnerable is consistent with a human rights-based approach. Other important features include the emphasis on participation, the inclusion of a stand-alone goal on justice, and the inclusion of several 'zero targets' as compared to others that stop short of full realization (such as target 1.2 to reduce poverty by half by 2030) (Donald 2020, p. 369). Finally, the SDGs have been important for building momentum and pressure to raise marginalized issues where there is no other feasible entry point – for example, the rights of LGBTI persons.

The importance of these virtues of the 2030 Agenda and the paradigm shift they represent in terms of global development debates should not be underestimated. However, the overarching aim of eradicating the multidimensional phenomenon of poverty while protecting the planet has been undermined by critical weaknesses in the orientation and implementation of the Agenda.

1.2 Vices in the 2030 Agenda that undermine rights-based agendas

Alongside the positive momentum on which to hitch human rights-based efforts, there are important points of weakness in the 2030 Agenda that undermine efforts to advance human rights. These are key to assessing the Agenda's value as a vehicle for transformation and systems change in favor of human rights in the context of pandemic recovery.

1.2.1 The Agenda is untethered from, and supplants, the human rights framework

The human rights community has made important efforts to inform the development, interpretation, and review of the SDGs in alignment with human rights standards, but this is a tenuous tie. Despite concerted advocacy for rights-based framing, the language of human rights was explicitly rejected in the drafting of the 2030 Agenda as states called for 'fresh language'. The text adopted in the 2030 Agenda has been further slogan-ized for the purpose of the massive marketing effort around the goals. This makes the SDGs appear more accessible, concrete, and engaging than the seemingly convoluted human rights framework – not just for the public but for diplomats and national policy makers as well (Donald 2020).

This untethering from the human rights framework obscures the importance of a rights-based approach in fully achieving the Goals. The slogan of 'leave no one behind' does capture the essence of the rights-based approach, but without rights built into the design and monitoring of the agenda, this call is not operationalized (CESCR 2019; Saiz & Donald 2017). As the former Special Rapporteur on extreme poverty and human rights Philip Alston (2020, p. 11) summarized: '[t]he SDGs are replete with references to transformation, empowerment, collaboration, and inclusion. But these concepts are illusory if people are unable to exercise their human rights'. The aversion to rights-based approaches in SDG discussions is cause for doubting the real interest and political will to ensure development policies actually leave no one behind.

The concern is not only that human rights are overlooked in implementation, but that demands for rights-based approaches are deflated and explicitly rejected by the dominance of the SDGs, completely untethered from the intimately related human rights framework. The consequences are described further below.

In the battle for resources, the SDGs may dominate at the cost of human rights – in multilateral engagement, programmatic priorities, and political weight. Rights-based approaches may find acceptance and resonance in areas that do not rock the boat too much. But on the most important questions for addressing root causes of poverty and environmental destruction, it is clear that rights-based claims are sidelined: examples include extreme inequality, corruption, illicit funds, tax evasion, corporate accountability, communities' veto power, and gender justice, including the care economy and reproductive rights.

For the 2030 Agenda to reach its Goals and guide transformative and just COVID-19 recovery efforts, this tenuous and contentious relation to human rights-based claims must be intentionally counteracted.

1.2.2 The cafeteria approach to the SDGs

Although one of the most heralded features of the 2030 Agenda is its integrated approach, the first five years have shown that the Agenda is easily, and frequently, severable. This allows for a cafeteria-style approach of take what you wish and walk past the rest. The 'cherry-picking' and 'something for everyone' nature of the SDGs has been widely denounced. The parts of the Agenda getting the 'short shrift' are precisely those elements that 'would require most profound structural change or changes in power distribution. These are the elements that are, arguably, most important for human rights realization' (Donald 2020, p. 382).

The most significant consequence of this vice is that it allows states and private actors to pick up and showcase their engagement with a particular goal, target, or indicator that will cast them in a favorable light. Actors can gain the reputational benefit of aligning behavior with a part of the Agenda without inviting any corresponding evaluation of practices that undermine other components of the Agenda or even contradict the overarching goals of eradicating poverty and protecting the planet. This is increasingly recognized as the practice of 'SDG-washing' (Niewenkamp 2017). An especially familiar example is a multinational company's focus on women's empowerment under SDG 5 while the same company continues business models and practices that systematically undermine human rights and the environment, including with specific gendered harms. On a policy level, the focus is on indicators related to economic growth as independent and automatically positive, without an integrated assessment of negative impacts on other targets and the overall agenda from efforts to generate that growth.

The High Level Political Forum on Sustainable Development is the UN platform responsible for the 'follow-up and review' of the SDGs at the global level. Each year has prioritized the review of a few goals, but for the 2021 session the priority is to address this lack of a holistic and integrated approach to the Agenda.

In the context of COVID-19, the SDGs are being heralded as the guide to ensure that in economic recovery efforts we take an integrated approach sensitive to the short and long-term issues related to poverty, inequality, and the environment. However, the implementation of the Agenda has not yet lived up to this promise. Whether COVID-19 presents the opportunity to start to deliver on the SDGs' transformative vision is precisely the question.

1.2.3 First, do no harm

Lost in the framing of leaving no one behind is the need to first transform the policies and practices that drive inequality and hold people back. From a human rights perspective, a critical bias in the overall design of the SDGs is the lack of a 'first, do no harm' baseline (Mining Working Group 2015). In human rights terms, there is a focus on the obligation to fulfill, but not to respect and protect. This is facilitated by the cafeteria-style approach of selective engagement and showcasing.

Therefore, the challenge is not only to maximize contributions from development but also to curb those economic policies and practices that cause harms and undermine the aims of the 2030 Agenda. In addition to maximizing efforts to deliver on key development aims, priority must be given (first) to transforming the dynamics known to create vulnerability and inequality in the enjoyment of economic, social, and culture rights, including food, water, education, health, and social security. The priorities in this sense would be staples of the predominant pro-growth development framework: the extractive development model, whether minerals, fossil fuels, industrial agriculture, or biofuels; globalization and concentration of supply chains; foreign direct investment; tax privatization; and intellectual property regimes (Young 2020). These have particular impacts on the lives and rights of people living in poverty and erode the state's capacity to advance on the 2030 Agenda as a whole.

We should be cautious when the SDGs are brought into the COVID-19 recovery orientation only to catalyze new contributions and more efficient delivery of goods and services without at the same time addressing and rejecting those strategies and factors known to undermine SDG targets and the overarching aim of the Agenda.

1.2.4 Uncritical reliance on the private sector

At the core of each of these vices in the 2030 Agenda is the positioning of the private sector as, invariably, the protagonist. One of the most important critiques of the 2030 Agenda from a human rights perspective has been its increased push for private sector involvement (Heller 2020). This was a significant point of contention of civil society in the negotiations and early implementation of the 2030 Agenda (Mining Working Group 2017). As Donald (2020, p. 378) observes, both in the actual design of the Agenda on paper as well as the way it is presented publicly, 'the private sector is seen as an uncomplicated positive actor, with none of the nuance or safeguards that would be necessary from the human rights perspective'.

The corollary of this approach is that the central role of the state in achieving the SDGs and guaranteeing rights is eroded, with private actors emerging as the only ones with capacity and solutions. The role of the state is focused more on creating a conducive environment for businesses than the realization of human rights (Alston 2020).

Beyond the actual negative and/or positive impacts of private actors in particular contexts, the overall trend of an outsized role ceded to the private sector has led to systemic effects that are overwhelmingly negative for the guarantee and realization of human rights: namely corruption, state capture, the closing of space for civic engagement, and a shrinking margin of policy discretion for the state (Young 2020).

The consequence of these interrelated dynamics is that the most transformative openings and aspirations set out by the SDGs have not materialized, as civil society foreshadowed in the negotiations of the Agenda. The failure to make these transformations has contributed to the very structural and unequal vulnerabilities that are multiplying the devastation of the COVID-19 crisis (United Nations 2020a). The 'hard truth' is that the SDGs could have put us on a track to be less vulnerable to crises such as COVID-19 (UN Sustainable Development Group 2020).

Holding the SDGs up as a blueprint for recovery will not automatically translate into just, transformational, and sustainable policies. Yet, the crisis does represent the opening needed to actually advance the kind of transformations that are required to achieve the SDGs, for which there has been little possibility to date. This is the posture assumed by the UN Special Rapporteur on extreme poverty, Olivier de Schutter, who sees in the pandemic 'a once-in-a-generation opportunity to redefine development trajectories in accordance with the Sustainable Development Goals' and to make the necessary transformations to economic, social, and environmental governance (de Schutter 2020b, p. 21). The following section explores dimensions of the crisis that could support and favor this rights-based reorientation.

2 Crisis as catalyst: openings for a more rights-favorable paradigm in the 2030 Agenda and COVID-19 recovery plans

In terms of the proverbial fork in the road, this exceptional moment may present an opportunity to correct course and make previously impossible advances in terms of human rights protection and realization possible. Several interrelated dimensions of the COVID-19 crisis and the responses suggest an opening for advancing a more rights-favorable paradigm in the 2030 Agenda and recovery.

2.1 Traction for a thick, holistic human rights approach

The rights-based claims and analysis coming out of the COVID-19 crises are elevating a 'thick', 'holistic' understanding of human rights in an unprecedented way (Bennoune 2020).

In 1948, the drafters of the Universal Declaration of Human Rights were responding to the post-Second World War context but also to the economic depression of the late 1920s. This is reflected in the integrated (indivisible) vision presented in the Declaration encompassing civil, political, economic, social, and cultural rights – and both negative formulations of the limits on state actions and affirmative guarantees of the rights related to a life lived in dignity (Young 2020; Roberts 2014).

But since that moment, as has been widely observed, the human rights project has operated on two tracks, with civil and political rights on one hand and economic, social, and cultural rights on the other. Although the European and Inter-American systems, organizations in the Global South, and social movements have long applied a more robust version of human rights to economic and social injustices, the dominant perception of human rights, as represented by IFIs, the United States, the Human Rights Council, and organizations in the Global North, has ignored or relegated economic, social, cultural rights to a second plane.

Critics thus have argued that the human rights project overemphasizes a negative rights paradigm aimed at constraining state action, excess, and overreach (Young 2020). This dominant paradigm has mapped onto the advance of a neoliberal economic agenda by 'privileg[ing] legal challenges to governmental interferences while denying access to justice for violations resulting from government neglect, inaction, or failure to regulate private actors' (Dugard et al. eds. 2020).

However, this is not a necessary or inherent bias in the human rights framework. Both positive and negative obligations are captured in the state obligations to respect, protect, and fulfill human rights. Decades of robust engagement from civil society and in the regional systems reveal the dynamic way that the human rights frame can speak to questions of economic and social justice. A well-grounded human rights-based approach incorporates both affirmative and negative state obligations.

While it has always been true, the reality of the 'thick' human rights project seems to be more widely acknowledged now than any other time since the UDHR. In the context of COVID-19, the human rights community has been actively tracking and contesting encroachments on civil and political rights in deep conversation with the contours of state obligations to protect and fulfill the rights related to health, food, housing, social security, and work. Again, this is a staple of a true human rights approach, but for the human rights community itself as well as external observers, the usual practice of maintaining a sharp distinction between different human rights silos seems to be disrupted in a meaningful way.

Additionally, at least in terms of activism, both in concept and in some victories, economic and social rights claims are enjoying a moment. This has much to contribute to a rights-based engagement with the SDGs and the scope of the obligations to protect and fulfill ESC rights. There is an opening in the widespread humanitarian crises to frame the claims in terms of existing entitlements (de Schutter 2020a). The massive mobilization of resources to address the immediate impacts of the pandemic should also be an impetus to ensure long-term resource mobilization aimed at the full and equal enjoyment of human rights (CESCR 2020). Likewise, the shocking exposure of inequalities is an opening to advance rights-based calls for transformations in our national and global economies (Young 2020; Gómez Isa 2020).

2.2 Emphasis on the 'public' and reframing of the essential role of the state as guarantor

This recognized opening for a serious debate and reconsideration of the role of the state as protector and guarantor of human rights in all contexts is a game-changing factor, the likes of which we have not seen since the Great Depression and World War II (Young 2020). As Barbara Adams (2020, p. 82) observed, 'the COVID-19 tragedy has forced governments back into the driver's seat, a role many had relinquished willingly or under pressure'. In many contexts during the pandemic, state action has been critical because of its unique capacity to enact measures for restricting movement and contact, to communicate reliable information to the public, and to get stimulus funds to people on an unprecedented scale. Good government – at all levels – has quite literally meant the difference between life and death, and this provides an opening to reassess what the purpose of the state is (Micklethwait & Wooldridge 2020).

The pandemic has exposed the vulnerability of countries that cannot count on public institutions to swiftly and effectively lead collective responses (Dugard et al. eds. 2020). The crisis has revealed the vulnerability that comes from economic and development models that erode the critical functions of government and public institutions. The connections between expansive privatization at the cost of public services, inequality, and rights of people living in poverty are on display (CESCR 2020). This has raised the visibility of the longstanding claim by advocates of 'the equalising and redistributive power of robust public services' (GI-ESCR 2020).

COVID-19 has created new resonance for longstanding, but often sidelined, demands for governments to actively engage in organizing economies, eradicating inequalities, guaranteeing support for the most vulnerable, and realizing the economic, social, cultural rights of all (Dugard et al. 2020).

Related to this shift in perceived importance of the state is a change in terms of actual influence and ability to alter power dynamics. As Schwab observed in June 2020: '[a]lready and almost overnight, the coronavirus succeeded in altering perceptions about the complex and delicate balance between the private and public realms in favor of the latter' (Schwab & Malleret 2020). He predicted that governments will most likely 'decide that it's in the best interest of society to rewrite some of the rules of the game and permanently increase their role' (Schwab & Malleret 2020).

This is particularly evident in the need for public relief for the private sector (Micklethwait & Wooldridge 2020). This may be an opening to increase the visibility of the many ways the public subsidizes the operations of the private sector. Civil society and academic observers have been emphatic in calling for clear and enforceable conditions on aid to private actors tied to workers' rights, tax justice, and accountability for environmental and climate degradation and human rights abuses (CSRG 2020, p. 12). The crisis has undoubtedly increased the bargaining power of states (Young 2020; Micklethwait & Wooldridge 2020; Mohamadieh 2020), but whether this will be leverage for actual transformation is not clear.

2.3 Recognition of the need for multilateralism and international solidarity and cooperation

As Julian Coman (2020) noted in his look at the growing number of COVID-19 reflections that call for a reaffirmation of liberal values and institutions, '[t]he collective pronoun is back in fashion'. This has played out on many levels, but globally it can be seen in a renewed affirmation of multilateralism – not just any multilateralism but a 'substantive, rights-based multilateralism' (Adams 2020, p. 82). The Civil Society Network has called COVID-19 a 'global wake-up call' for international solidarity and cooperation (CSRG 2020, p. 12). The Human Rights Council (2020) recognized this with its July 2020 resolution on 'The central role of the State in responding to pandemics and other health emergencies, and the socioeconomic consequences thereof in advancing sustainable development and the realization of all human rights'. The pandemic has made the obvious need for coordinated, global responses to global crises visible and urgent in a new way.

The 2030 Agenda is premised on this very principle – global responses to global crises. Thus, the pandemic could have important leverage value to build up key multilateral institutions and practices that are also needed to address protracted global crises such as systemic poverty, inequality, and the climate emergency. As noted by Yamin and Habibi (2020), '[t]his crisis may provide an opportunity to see the value of truth and trust in democracy and multilateralism, and the starkly dystopian reality we face without them'.

As Barbara Adams (2020, p. 82) has emphasized, '[t]he UN should be the standard bearer at the global level, not a neutral convenor of public and private engagement'. For this to be more than aspirational, the international multilateral system must count on public resources, the mobilization of which requires addressing key questions of tax justice and curbing illicit financial flows. The pandemic hit at a moment of vulnerability for the UN human rights system and other important multilateral spaces, during a crisis of political legitimacy and funding. The visible and pressing need for global cooperation and solidarity is also a chance to address this pre-existing disinvestment.

3 Trends that will aggravate vices in the 2030 Agenda

Yet, the disruption caused by COVID-19 could just as likely serve as an opening for the consolidation of approaches that would limit the space and capacity to protect and promote human rights in the COVID-19 recovery efforts. This section highlights two likely trends that would map onto existing vices in the 2030 Agenda in problematic ways: the anticipated push for austerity measures and cuts to public spending, and increased corporate capture through the advance of 'stakeholder capitalism'.

3.1 Austerity measures

As the immediate health risks recede and public health measures are lifted, the economic consequences will likely lead to strong pushes for austerity – namely, efforts to address deficits by cutting public spending or increasing tax revenue, or a combination. In the past, the prescription has been to cut spending on public services and to prioritize economic growth as the path to increase the tax revenue. The human rights framework is not neutral vis-à-vis these pressures and proposals.

The mobilization of resources to fund public services is required by human rights law, and the role of public goods and social services in terms of mitigating inequality is widely recognized (CESCR 2020). Important guidance can be found in the CESCR's General Comment 24 on business activities and economic, social, cultural rights, as well as the UN Guiding Principles for Human Rights Impact Assessments for Economic Reform Policies. In terms of COVID-19, advocates are prioritizing reclaiming public management and direction of recovery funds, progressive taxation or 'tax justice', tackling inequality through redistribution, and international assistance to support public services (GI-ESCR & CESR 2020; CSRG 2020, p. 12).

The measures adopted in response to the global financial recession of 2008 illustrate how pressure on states to adopt austerity measures quickly eclipsed human rights-based calls for welfare investments (Young 2020). It is precisely these disinvestments in essential rights-related goods and services that have added layers of vulnerability exacerbating the devastating and discriminatory effects of the pandemic (CESCR 2020). Constrained and weakened by austerity policies, many national and local governments lacked the mandate, resources, and administrative capacities to effectively address the pandemic (Alston 2020).

A corollary of the cutting of public services has been expansive privatization, the 'process through which the private sector becomes increasingly, or entirely, responsible for activities traditionally performed by government, including many explicitly designed to ensure the realization of human rights' (Alston 2018, p. 4). A generally accepted stance in the international human rights framework has been that privatization is not *per se* incompatible with a states' human rights obligations (CESCR 2017). However, this has incorrectly 'opened the door for the acritical idea that public or private provision are equivalent in terms of human rights compliance' (Heller 2020, p. 4).

In fact, there is increasing evidence and consensus that widespread privatization is incompatible with states' human rights obligations. While the manifestations of privatization vary by country, context, and sector, a survey of human rights analyses of privatization suggests six categories of systemic negative impacts in terms of important human rights benchmarks: affordability problems with people living in poverty excluded or exploited; discrimination that maps onto historic marginalization and vulnerabilities; insufficient quality as defined by human rights standards; unsustainability, as investments last only as long as profitable; a lack of accountability both in terms of the guarantee of participation and access to remedy; and the long-term diversion of funds, undermining public provision (Nolan 2018; Alston 2018).

Previously, much of the human rights focus on privatization has been on the state obligation to protect economic, social, and cultural rights from abuses by private actors (CESCR 2017). However, the duty to fulfill is a major concern: the prospects of guaranteeing accountability for the participation of private actors in the delivery of public services and goods is undermined by the trends of eroding the power of the state vis-à-vis the power of the private sector. As a coalition of current and former Special Rapporteurs recently alerted in the context of privatization: 'If human rights are to be taken seriously, the old construct of states taking a back seat to private companies must be abandoned' (Farha et al. 2020). The paradigm shift that is needed is a 'fundamental shift in the relation between States and corporations, and a demonstration of willingness by States to utilize policy, institutional and legal tools that could allow a balancing in the power relations' between the private sector on one hand and states and rights-holders on the other (Mohamadieh 2020).

Yet, the next generation of post-pandemic austerity policies will likely accelerate 'the dramatic transfer of economic and political power to the wealthy elites that has characterized the past forty years' (Alston 2020, p. 9). A human rights-based approach then is not only focused on accountability for private actors in a particular context, but more broadly on ensuring a balance of power that empowers people as rights-holders and their governments as guarantors.

2.2 Corporate capture through 'stakeholder capitalism' and mulitstakeholderism

In terms of global policymaking and agenda-setting, there are pronounced trends in terms of the erosion of multilateralism compared to the rise of multistakerholderism (Transnational Institute 2019) and 'philantrolaterialism' (Seitz & Martens 2017). Corporate power has translated into political power in terms of agenda-setting at the UN.

In 2019, the UN and the WEF signed a memorandum of understanding, generating significant concern from civil society (Lyons & Christiancy 2021). The World Economic Forum is the 'international organization for public-private partnerships' and has an increasingly dominant role in UN agenda-setting.

The 2030 Agenda has been an important vehicle for expanding public-private partnerships, broadly understood, at the global and national levels. The WEF has been particularly visible in convening global business leaders and states around the framework of the 2030 Agenda and has centered the SDGs in its new calls for the Great Reset in the COVID-19 recovery.

The specific aim of the Great Reset is to consolidate the paradigm of stakeholder capitalism – contrasted with 'shareholder capitalism' and 'state capitalism'. While much has been written on the definition of stakeholder capitalism, the January 2020 Davos Manifesto offers a relevant summary of the shift in purpose that this concept proposes:

> The purpose of a company is to engage all its stakeholders in shared and sustained value creation. In creating such value, a company serves not only its shareholders, but all its stakeholders – employees, customers, suppliers, local communities and society at large. The best way to understand and harmonize the divergent interests of all stakeholders is through a shared commitment to policies and decisions that strengthen the long-term prosperity of a company.
>
> *(Schwab 2019)*

The consolidation of stakeholder capitalism as the dominant new model has been called the 'silver lining' of the pandemic (Georgescu 2020). Yet, it had secured a solid footing prior to the pandemic: in 2019, the Business Roundtable made a pivotal statement on the new purpose of corporations, widely regarded as launching a new moment in corporate social responsibility (BRT 2019). This watershed statement also led to the theme of the January 2020 Davos Conference: 'Stakeholders for a Cohesive and Sustainable World'.

The WEF has set out its stakeholder principles for the COVID Era (WEF 2020d). These reference the 2030 Agenda but only on environmental sustainability (WEF 2020d, p. 1). The WEF has issued its own ESG metrics for corporate reporting that are loosely linked to UN Guiding Principles and the SDGs and in September 2020 conformed a Global Future Council on Human Rights with the mandate to 'help shape the new corporate human rights agenda' and 'explore the shift needed for business to take a leading role in protecting universal human rights'.

While full consideration of this question is outside the scope of this chapter, the threats that come from a parallel system of agenda-setting and meaning are numerous. These fora have in many ways supplanted the multilateral spaces. These spaces are largely inaccessible to civil society and are completely disconnected from important accountability mechanisms that have special meaning for marginalized groups, namely the UN human rights mechanisms. The massive communicative capacity of the WEF far surpasses other actors, states and UN agencies included, and the influence in shaping the narrative of the SDGs is unmatched. Because of the direct impact on policy and practice, this further distances decision-making about sustainable development from those most affected.

In the COVID-19 recovery efforts, we must prioritize the reaffirmation and building up of critical, multilateral spaces. For this, we 'must start with bending the arc of governance back again – from viewing people as shareholders – to stakeholders – to rights holders' (Adams 2020, p. 82).

4 Conclusion: Build Back Better – but better for whom?

In terms of advancing human rights aims, the 2030 Agenda presents both opportunities and threats (Donald 2020). The SDGs are only up to task of serving as a blueprint for transformative recovery from the pandemic if the vices of the Agenda, as well as the threats emerging from the crisis, are confronted. The COVID-19 crisis could lead to a paradigm shift in terms of sustainable development policies at the national and global levels – we could see a consolidation of space ceded to 'stakeholder capitalism', with the private sector in the driver's seat, or a course correction in terms of a more rights-favorable adjustment in the power dynamics between the public and the private sector, with a renewed primary focus on people as rights-holders.

The crisis has brought new visibility to the importance of a holistic human rights-based approach integrating limits on state action from negative obligations to respect, but also a clarity and emphasis on the affirmative obligations on states to take actions to protect rights-holders vis-à-vis private actors and to take concrete measures to fulfill human rights. Relatedly, there is momentum for recognizing the central role of the public – the state at the local and national level and multilateral cooperation and solidarity at the global level.

While the crisis presents an opportunity to advance on those fronts, simultaneously we can anticipate that the disruption will also intensify pressure for austerity measures, including privatization, as well as corporate capture of key policymaking spaces under the banner of 'stakeholder capitalism' and multistakeholderism.

The chapter concludes that for the 2030 Agenda and its 17 SDGs to overcome existing vices and truly serve as a guide for just and transformative global and national COVID-19 recovery efforts, the Agenda must be anchored in human rights. This requires a robust human rights approach that is both pragmatic and stubborn – engaging in the 'nitty gritty' (Sharp 2018) of policymaking that addresses the root causes of human rights violations and deprivations but also stubbornly insisting on and reaffirming the role of the formal human rights framework: an approach based on human rights and Human Rights (Hopgood 2013).

References

Adams, B 2020, 'Re-inventing Multilateral Solidarity: Rhetoric, Reaction or Realignment of Power?', in *Spotlight on Sustainable Development 2020*, Social Watch, Montevideo, viewed 30 December 2020, pp. 81–82, www.2030spotlight.org/sites/default/files/download/Spotlight_Innenteil_2020_web_re-invent.pdf

Alston, P 2018, *Report of the Special Rapporteur on Extreme Poverty and Human Rights on Privatization*, UN Doc. A/73/396, viewed 30 December 2020, https://undocs.org/A/73/396

Alston, P 2020, *The Parlous State of Poverty Eradication*, Report of the Special Rapporteur on Extreme Poverty and Human Rights, UN Doc. A/HRC/44/40, viewed 30 December 2020, www.ohchr.org/EN/HRBodies/HRC/RegularSessions/Session44/Documents/A_HRC_44_40_AUV.docx

Bennoune, K 2020, '"Lest We Should Sleep": COVID-19 and Human Rights', *American Journal of International Law*, vol. 114, no. 4, pp. 666–676.

Bergman, MM 2020, 'The World after COVID', *World 2020*, vol. 1, no. 1, pp. 45–48.

Business Roundtable (BRT) 2019, Statement on the Purpose of a Corporation, https://s3.amazonaws.com/brt.org/BRT-StatementonthePurposeofaCorporationOctober2020.pdf

Civil Society Reflection Group on the 2030 Agenda for Sustainable Development (CSRG) (ed.) 2017, *Reclaiming Policies for the Public*, Social Watch, Montevideo, viewed 30 December 2020, www.2030spotlight.org/sites/default/files/download/spotlight_170626_final_web.pdf

Civil Society Reflection Group on the 2030 Agenda for Sustainable Development (CSRG) (ed.) 2020, *Spotlight on Sustainable Development 2020*, Social Watch, Montevideo, viewed 30 December 2020, www.2030spotlight.org/sites/default/files/Spotlight_Innenteil_2020_web_gesamt_.pdf

Coman, J 2020, 'Let Us Dream by Pope Francis Review – The Holy Father of Fraternity', *The Guardian*, 29 November, viewed 30 December 2020, www.theguardian.com/books/2020/nov/29/let-us-dream-by-pope-francis-review-the-holy-father-of-fraternity

Committee on Economic and Social Rights (CESCR) 2020, *Statement on the Covid-19 Pandemic and Economic, Social and Cultural Rights*, E/C.12/2020/1, viewed 30 December 2020, https://undocs.org/E/C.12/2020/1

Committee on Economic and Social Rights (CESCR) 2017, *General Comment No. 24: State Obligations under the International Covenant on Economic, Social and Cultural Rights in the*

Context of Business Activities, E./C.12/GC/24, viewed 30 December 2020, https://digitallibrary.un.org/record/1304491?ln=en

Committee on Economic and Social Rights (CESCR) 2019, *The Pledge to Leave No One Behind: The ICESCR and the 2030 Agenda for Sustainable Development*, E/C.12/2019/1, viewed 30 December 2020, https://undocs.org/E/C.12/2019/1

de Schutter, O 2020a, *Looking Back to Look Ahead: A Rights-based Approach to Social Protection in the Post-COVID-19 Economic Recovery*, Report of the Special Rapporteur on Extreme Poverty and Human Rights, viewed 30 December 2020, www.ohchr.org/Documents/Issues/Poverty/covid19.pdf

de Schutter, O 2020b, *The "Just Transition" in the Economic Recovery: Eradicating Poverty within Planetary Boundaries*, UN Doc. A/75/181, Report of the Special Rapporteur on Extreme Poverty and Human Rights, viewed 30 December 2020, https://undocs.org/A/75/181

Donald, K 2020, 'The 2030 Agenda for Sustainable Development: Opportunity or Threat for Economic, Social and Cultural Rights?', in J Dugard, B Porter, D Ikawa, & L Chenwi, *Research Handbook on Economic, Social and Cultural Rights as Human Rights*, Edward Elgar, Cheltenham, pp. 367–386.

Dugard, J, Porter, B, Ikawa, D, & Chenwi, L (eds.) 2020, 'Introduction', in *Research Handbook on Economic, Social and Cultural Rights as Human Rights*, Edward Elgar, Cheltenham, pp. xviii–xxvii.

Farha L, Bohoslavsky, JP, Boly Barry, K, Heller, L, de Schutter, O, & Sepúlveda Carmona, M 2020, 'Covid-19 Has Exposed the Catastrophic Impact of Privatizing Vital Services', *The Guardian*, 19 October, viewed 30 December 2020, www.theguardian.com/society/2020/oct/19/covid-19-exposed-catastrophic-impact-privatising-vital-services

Georgescu, P 2020, 'Can Stakeholder Capitalism Be a Silver Lining of Covid-19', *Forbes*, viewed 30 December 2020, www.forbes.com/sites/justcapital/2020/06/29/could-covid-19-be-good-for-us/?sh=15d2aa4d12b7

Global Initiative for Economic, Social, and Cultural Rights (GI-ESCR) & Center for Economic and Social Rights (CESR) 2020, 'Topic 11: Public Financing of Public Services', *COVID-19: Recovering Rights Series*, Center for Economic and Social Rights, viewed 30 December 2020, www.cesr.org/sites/default/files/Public%20financing%20of%20public%20services%20-%20FINAL_0.pdf

Gómez Isa, F 2020, 'Economic, Social and Political Costs of the (Non-) Realization of Human Rights: Towards a New Social Contract', in J Wouters, K Lemmens, T Van Poecke, & M Bourguignon (eds.), *Can We Still Afford Human Rights?*, Edward Elgar, Cheltenham, pp. 220–240.

Guterres, A 2020, 'World Has Moral Obligation to Ensure Future Generations Not Burdened by Mountain of Debt on Broken Planet, Secretary-General Tells G20 Summit', *United Nations*, viewed 30 December 2020, www.un.org/press/en/2020/sgsm20440.doc.htm

Hawkes C (2020). Five Steps towards a Global Reset: Lessons from COVID-19. Global Sustainability 3, e30, 1–8. https:// doi.org/10.1017/sus.2020.24

Heller, L 2020, *Human Rights and the Privatization of Water and Sanitation Services*, Report of the Special Rapporteur on Human Rights to Water and Sanitation, UN Doc. A/75/208, viewed 30 December 2020, https://undocs.org/a/75/208

Hopgood, S 2013, *The End Times of Human Rights*, Cornell University Press, Ithaca.

Human Rights Council 2020, 'The Central Role of the State in Responding to Pandemics and Other Health Emergencies, and the Socioeconomic Consequences Thereof in Advancing Sustainable Development and the Realization of All Human Rights: Draft resolution, UN Doc. A.HRC/44/L.23/Rev.1', *United Nations*, viewed 30 December 2020, https://undocs.org/A/HRC/44/L.23/Rev.1

Jain, N 2020, 'Pandemics as Rights-Generators', *American Journal of International Law*, vol. 114, no. 4, pp. 677–686.
Jensen, L (ed.) 2020, *The Sustainable Development Goals Report 2020*, United Nations, New York.
Klein, N 2020, 'The Great Reset Conspiracy', *The Intercept*, viewed 30 December 2020, https://theintercept.com/2020/12/08/great-reset-conspiracy/
Lewis, S 2020, 'Stakeholder Capitalism and the Pandemic Recovery', *Harvard Law School Forum on Corporate Governance*, viewed 30 December 2020, https://corpgov.law.harvard.edu/2020/06/08/stakeholder-capitalism-and-the-pandemic-recovery/
Lyons, A & Christiancy, C 2021, 'Reclaiming the Human Rights Foundations of the UN Standards of Conduct for Business on Tackling Discrimination against LGBTI People', *Business and Human Rights Journal* (under review 2021).
MacNaughton, G 2017, 'Vertical Inequalities: Are the SDGs and Human Rights Up to the Challenges?', *International Journal of Human Rights*, vol. 21, no. 8, pp. 1052–1056.
Micklethwait, J & Wooldridge A 2020, 'The Virus Should Wake Up the West', *Bloomberg*, viewed 30 December 2020, www.bloomberg.com/opinion/articles/2020-04-13/coronavirus-pandemic-is-wake-up-call-to-reinvent-the-state
Mining Working Group 2015, A Rights-based Approach to Natural Resource Extraction in the Pursuit of Sustainable Development, https://miningwg.files.wordpress.com/2014/05/advocacy-brief.pdf
Mining Working Group 2017, Water and Sanitation: A Peoples' Guide to SDG 6 – A Rights-based Approach to Implementation, https://sacredheartattheun.org/sites/default/files/attachments/water-guide-final-pdf.pdf
Mohamadieh, K 2020, 'Corporate Power and States' (In)action in Response to the COVID-19 Crisis', *Third World Network Briefing Paper*, Third World Network, viewed 30 December 2020, https://twn.my/title2/resurgence/2020/343-344/cover13.htm
Niewenkamp, R 2017, 'Ever Heard of SDG Washing? The Urgency of SDG Due Diligence', *OECD Development Matters*, viewed 30 December 2020, https://oecd-development-matters.org/2017/09/25/ever-heard-of-sdg-washing-the-urgency-of-sdg-due-diligence/
Nolan, A 2018, 'Privatization and Economic and Social Rights', *Human Rights Quarterly*, vol. 40, no. 4, pp. 815–858.
Roberts, C 2014, *The Contentious History of Human Rights*, Cambridge.
Saiz, I, & Donald, K, 2017 'Tackling Inequality through the Sustainable Development Goals: Human Rights in Practice, *The International Journal of Human Rights*, vol. 21, no. 8, pp. 1029–1049
Santos-Carrillo, F, Fernández-Portillo, LA, & Sianes, A 2020, 'Rethinking the Governance of the 2030 Agenda for Sustainable Development in the COVID-19 Era', *Sustainability 2020*, vol. 12, no. 18, pp. 7680–7704.
Schwab, K 2019, 'Davos Manifesto 2020: The Universal Purpose of a Company in the Fourth Industrial Revolution', *World Economic Forum*, viewed 30 December 2020, www.weforum.org/agenda/2019/12/davos-manifesto-2020-the-universal-purpose-of-a-company-in-the-fourth-industrial-revolution/
Schwab, K & Malleret, T 2020, *COVID-19: The Great Reset*, Forum Publishing, New York.
Seitz, K & Martens, J 2017, 'Philanthrolateralism: Private Funding and Corporate Influence in the United Nations', *Global Policy*, vol. 8, no. S5, pp. 46–50.
Sepúlveda Carmona, M 2021, 'From Stigma to Rights: Uncovering the Hidden Dimension of Poverty', in MF Davis, M Kjaerum & A Lyons (eds.), *Research Handbook on Human Rights and Poverty*, Edward Elgar, Cheltenham.
Sharp, DN 2018, 'Pragmatism and Multidimensionality in Human Rights Advocacy', *Human Rights Quarterly*, vol. 40, no. 3, pp. 499–520.

Transnational Institute 2019, *Multistakeholderism: A Critical Look*, Amsterdam.

United Nations 2020a, *A UN Framework for the Immediate Socio-economic Response to COVID-19*, United Nations, Geneva, viewed 30 December 2020, https://unsdg.un.org/sites/default/files/2020-04/UN-framework-for-the-immediate-socio-economic-response-to-COVID-19.pdf

United Nations 2020b, 'Summary by the President of the Economic and Social Council of the High-level Political Forum on Sustainable Development Convened under the Auspices of the Council at its 2020 Session', United Nations, viewed 30 December 2020, https://sustainabledevelopment.un.org/content/documents/269252020_HLPF_Presidents_summary.pdf

UN Sustainable Development Group 2020, 'Shared Responsibility, Global Solidarity: Responding to the Socio-Economic Impacts of COVID-19', United Nations, viewed 30 December 2020, https://unsdg.un.org/sites/default/files/2020-03/SG-Report-Socio-Economic-Impact-of-Covid19.pdf

UN Department of Economic and Social Affairs 2020a, 'Impact of COVID-19: Perspective from Voluntary National Reviews', *Policy Brief #85*, UN/DESA, viewed 30 December 2020, www.un.org/development/desa/dpad/publication/un-desa-policy-brief-85-impact-of-covid-19-perspective-from-voluntary-national-reviews/

UN Department of Economic and Social Affairs 2020b, 'Achieving SDGs in the Wake of COVID-19: Scenarios for Policymakers', *Policy Brief #84*, UN/DESA, viewed 30 December 2020, www.un.org/development/desa/dpad/publication/un-desa-policy-brief-84-achieving-sdgs-in-the-wake-of-covid-19-scenarios-for-policymakers/

Winkler, I & Williams, C 2017, The Sustainable Development Goals and human rights: a critical early review, *The International Journal of Human Rights*, vol. 21, no. 8, pp. 1023–1028.

World Economic Forum (WEF) 2020a, 'Global Future Councils', *World Economic Forum*, viewed 30 December 2020, www.weforum.org/communities/global-future-councils

World Economic Forum (WEF) 2020b, 'Global Future Council on Human Rights', *World Economic Forum*, viewed 30 December 2020, www.weforum.org/communities/gfc-on-human-rights

World Economic Forum (WEF) 2020c, 'Measuring Stakeholder Capitalism Towards Common Metrics and Consistent Reporting of Sustainable Value Creation', *White Paper*, World Economic Forum, viewed 30 December 2020, www3.weforum.org/docs/WEF_IBC_Measuring_Stakeholder_Capitalism_Report_2020.pdf

World Economic Forum (WEF) 2020d, 'Stakeholder Principles in the COVID Era', *World Economic Forum*, viewed 30 December 2020, www3.weforum.org/docs/WEF_Stakeholder_Principles_COVID_Era.pdf

Yamin, AE & Habibi, R 2020, 'Human Rights and Coronavirus: What's at Stake for Truth, Trust, and Democracy?', *Health and Human Rights Journal*, viewed 30 December 2020, www.hhrjournal.org/2020/03/human-rights-and-coronavirus-whats-at-stake-for-truth-trust-and-democracy/

Young, K 2020, 'The Idea of a Human Rights-Based Economic Recovery after COVID-19', *Legal Studies Research Paper No. 538*, Boston College Law School, viewed 30 December 2020, http://dx.doi.org/10.2139/ssrn.3680094

12

THE HUMAN RIGHT TO FOOD

Lessons learned toward food systems transformation

Ana María Suárez Franco

The health crisis generated by COVID-19 and the related lockdown measures prompted international organizations to announce a looming global food crisis in early 2020. In March 2020 the Committee on World Food Security (CFS) launched a call to diverse actors to prevent the health crisis from becoming a food crisis (CFS 2020). With other international organizations, the Food and Agriculture Organization (FAO) recognized in July 2020 that 'the COVID-19 pandemic is intensifying the vulnerabilities and inadequacies of global food systems' (FAO 2020b). That report estimated that while it is too soon to assess the full impact, 'at a minimum, another 83 million people, and possibly as many as 132 million, may go hungry in 2020 as a result of the economic recession triggered by COVID-19' (FAO 2020b).

Affected communities and advocacy organizations working for the right to food have emphasized the role that the dominant agro-industrial food system has played in making our societies more vulnerable to the pandemic. The industry's influence over governmental responses and recovery measures has led to neglect of and discrimination against small food producers. The adverse impact on small food producers increases the risks to the enjoyment of the right to food more generally, since small family farms supply around 80 percent of food needed in the world (FAO & IFAD 2019).

In this context, in 2020 the Committee on World Food Security (CFS) negotiated the Guidelines on Food Systems and Nutrition. Despite an apparent agreement on the need for food systems transformation, the process showed a clear dispute between the supporters of the powerful agro-industrial sector and those representing small food producers as to what the transformation should be and how it should be achieved.

The COVID-19 crisis, together with the existing state obligations to protect and fulfill the right to food are key to proposing an alternative that can guide the way in which the dispute around food systems transformation should be solved, in line with the UN Charter and international human rights law.

This chapter presents (1) an introduction to the right to food, and its relation to the concepts of food sovereignty, food security, and food systems; (2) a description of the main impacts of the pandemic on the right to food and other human rights in the food system; (3) an analysis of the different responses, including those by civil society, human rights bodies, FAO and other relevant Rome-based organizations, and the agro-industry; (4) the strengths and promises of the rural movements' proposal; and finally, (5) conclusions and recommendations. This chapter draws primarily on reports from civil society collected as part of FIAN International's tracking of the effects of COVID-19 on the right to food, giving the first overview of the impacts on and responses of specific communities in the Global North and Global South, as well as social movements.

1 Introduction to the concepts of the human right to food

After the Second World War, the debates on the right to food were present in the *travaux preparatoires* of the Universal Declaration on Human Rights (UDHR). The right to food was included in Article 25 of the UDHR under the right to an adequate standard of living. Later, a more explicit reference was included in Article 11 of the International Covenant on Economic, Social and Cultural Rights (ICESCR). Since then, diverse international bodies have established a *corpus juris* guiding states on how to implement the right to food (Suárez Franco 2020).

The Committee on Economic, Social and Cultural Rights (CESCR) has established that:

> The right to adequate food is realized when every man, woman and child, alone or in community with others, have physical and economic access at all times to adequate food or means for its procurement. The right to adequate food shall therefore not be interpreted in a narrow or restrictive sense, which equates it with a minimum package of calories, proteins and other specific nutrients. The right to adequate food will have to be realized progressively. However, States have a core obligation to take the necessary action to mitigate and alleviate hunger as provided for in paragraph 2 of article 11, even in times of natural or other disasters.
>
> *(CESCR 1999, p. 2)*

The CESCR has defined the central legal content of the right in terms of adequacy, access, availability, and sustainability. This chapter focuses on the first three elements. *Adequacy* means that food shall be sufficient in quantity and quality, does not contain biologic or chemical components making it unsafe, respects the culture of the right holders, covers rights holders' nutritional needs according to their age, gender and activity, and is biodiverse. *Access* means that rights holders shall have the capacity to physically and economically acquire food and/or the resources to produce it. *Availability* means that productive land and other natural resources and well-functioning distribution, processing, and market systems that move food from the place of provision to the place of demand shall be obtainable (CESCR 1999).

The concept of the right to food is related to the concept of food security. The CFS states that food security exists 'when all people, at all times have physical, social and economic access to sufficient, safe and nutritious food that meets their dietary needs and food preferences for an active and healthy life' (CFS 2017). This does not refer to the human rights obligations of states but establishes a goal for public policies. This concept is widely used, including by the FAO, the Committee on World Food Security, and other related Rome-based organizations.

Also relevant is the concept of 'food sovereignty', developed by the peasants' movement La Via Campesina (LVC) as a political project based on the rights of peoples to define their own food systems and to develop policies on how food is produced, distributed, and consumed. With small-scale food producers at the center, food sovereignty is grounded in processes of empowerment and the generation of knowledge, supporting collective construction of alternatives that reinforce peasant economies.

The concept of food sovereignty has been included in international human rights standards, including General Recommendation 34 of the Committee on the Elimination of all forms of Discrimination against Women (CEDAW), the UN Guiding Principles on Extreme Poverty and Human Rights, the reports of the Special Rapporteur on the right to food, and the 2018 UN Declaration on the Rights of Peasants and other People Working in Rural Areas (UNDROP) (United Nations General Assembly 2018).

Moreover, in 2015, SDG 2 set up the prime goal to 'end hunger and ensure access by all people, in particular the poor and people in vulnerable situations, including infants, to safe, nutritious and sufficient food all year round', by 2030. Specifically target 2.4 aims to 'ensure sustainable food production systems by the same year'. In the debates about SDG 2 achievement as well as in the CFS, the concept of 'food systems' has gained currency.

Food systems 'gather all the elements (environment, people, inputs, processes, infrastructures, institutions, etc.) and activities that relate to the production, processing, distribution, preparation and consumption of food, and the output of these activities, including socio-economic and environmental outcomes' (High Level Panel of Experts on Food Security and Nutrition 2014). The concept is useful because it recognizes the plurality of food systems and includes social, cultural, environmental, gender, and other dimensions, beyond economic aspects. Nonetheless, there is the risk that this concept could be narrowed to the agro-industrial food system, ignoring a human rights approach.

The concept of food as a human right is a key tool to guide state responses to COVID-19. In contrast to the concept of food security, the rights-based framing sees each person (or community) as a rights-holder and not just as a passive beneficiary. Instead of a charity approach, it requires states to focus policy priorities on the most disadvantaged and marginalized communities. In the asymmetric relation between agro-industrial food production and small-scale food production, food sovereignty is indispensable for the realization of the right to adequate food and nutrition, especially for those in peasant and Indigenous peoples' food systems, as well as for consumers.

The debate around food systems transformation is contentious and centers around assertions promoted by the food industry and some governments that food governance should move towards more digitalized and commoditized food systems, pushing aside human rights and food sovereignty. On the other side of the debate, many CSOs and others argue that the lessons learned through the COVID-19 crisis should guide decision makers to advance healthier, more just, and sustainable food systems for present and future generations (CSM 2020).

2 The main impacts of the COVID-19 pandemic on the realization of the right to food and nutrition

Since March 2020, FIAN International, as secretariat of the Global Network on the Right to Food and Nutrition (GNRTFN), has received information from communities and other non-governmental organizations (NGOs) denouncing the multiple food crises in various regions of the world. FIAN International produced two global reports on COVID-19 (FIAN 2020a; 2020b) based on testimonies and analysis by the members of the GNRTFN, media reports, analysis by the Civil Society Mechanism of the Committee on World Food Security, and the national reports of FIAN sections in several countries. This global, grassroots reporting, as well as the statements of the Rome-based organizations and the human rights system, are summarized below.

2.1 Pre-existing conditions of fragility – indivisibility of rights

Diverse grassroots communities close to the GNRTFN and their advocates have emphasized the need to analyze the impact of COVID-19 on the right to food in the light of the pre-existing food-related crises and structural problems identified as causes of the food systems' fragility, including:

- land grabbing, as a cause of the transmission of diseases from animals to humans (zoonosis), created by the rupture of natural frontiers between ecosystems;
- extensive use of pesticides weakening peasants' and consumers' health;
- policies prioritizing agro-industrial food production through globalized food chains, making food systems vulnerable to lockdowns;
- standardized diets of ultra-processed edible products, increasing health vulnerability; and
- digitalization of food, i.e. using digital technologies to trade food and related resources, which excludes people living in poverty.

Other structural factors have compounded the crisis in terms of access to food during the pandemic, including:

- dismantling of social security, which reduces income possibilities in cases of loss of work or increased health costs;
- reduction of labor protection standards, affecting people's access to unemployment insurance or other related services;
- inequalities and discrimination, making marginalized communities more vulnerable to right to food violations in times of crisis;
- gender inequality and violence affecting women in their access to food;
- repression and criminalization, impeding people from denouncing irregularities in access to public services connected to the right to food during the pandemic; and
- conflict, occupation, and war, which have destroyed people's capacity to feed themselves before the pandemic and in many cases have made them dependent on fluctuating food aid.

2.2 Impacts on the right to food, in light of its legal elements

The ways that COVID-19 and lockdown measures have affected the right to food are complex and the different elements of the right are generally impacted simultaneously. However, to facilitate analysis this section describes the COVID-19 pandemic's distinct impacts on each of the three elements of the right to food: accessibility, adequacy, and availability.

2.2.1 Food accessibility

COVID-19 has reduced children's access to food due to the closing or suspension of school feeding programs (FIAN 2020a, p.6). Closure of charity centers, soup kitchens, and food assistance services has left marginalized people and grassroots communities without access to food in many cities, including in the Global North (FIAN 2020a, p. 6). This, together with the digitalization of public services and supply services, has affected people without access to the internet or the required technology, with a particular impact on elderly people. Digital payments might reduce the risk of contagion, but they make access to food more difficult for people without access to financial products (e.g. bank accounts) or people lacking needed knowledge and equipment such as computers or smartphones.

At the beginning of the pandemic, several countries, including Italy, Spain, and Switzerland, ordered the closure of farmers' markets (FIAN 2020a, p. 6). The weekly distribution by agriculture cooperatives was restricted, while supermarkets remained open. Shelves were empty in supermarkets due to panic buying, restricting consumers' access to adequate food. Yet peasants had to pile up fresh, good quality food and see it perish.

As a result, peasants' income was reduced, undermining their own economic access to adequate food. In Ecuador, Uganda, South Africa, France, and El Salvador, people reported that price speculation negatively affected their economic access to food (FIAN 2020b, p. 14). Several countries introduced measures that outlaw informal markets and the selling of goods by street vendors (FIAN 2020a, p. 7). This led to loss of income for marginalized and poor households, putting them at risk of food and nutrition insecurity.

Food accessibility has been negatively impacted worldwide due to the loss or reduction of income (FIAN 2020b, p. 14). In Colombia, people suffering from hunger hung shirts (Pardo 2020) and rags (Oquendo 2020) in their windows as a call for help. Likewise, the media reported cases of hunger and imminent starvation in Argentina (Agencia AP 2020), Indonesia (Savitri 2020), and India (Dave 2020). More people have resorted to food banks in even richer and 'developed' nations like Spain (Viejo 2020), the United States (CNN 2020), and Switzerland.

2.2.2 Food adequacy

Food adequacy has also worsened, especially for the poorest sectors of the society, since the cheapest and most available food at supermarkets are ultra-processed edible products, while food produced agroecologically is not available due to the lockdown measures imposed on farmers, fishers, and other small-scale food producers. School children have been particularly affected due to the distribution of ultra-processed edible products to fill the gap created by the suspension of school feeding programs. Unhealthy and innutritious food provided by school feeding programs often had to feed entire families (FIAN 2020b, p. 3). Elderly people may also be unable to access sufficient and adequate food due to confinement and mobility problems (Goger 2020).

2.2.3 Food availability

The availability of food has been threatened due to a lack of seasonal workforce, as was the case in Germany and India. In March and April seasonal agricultural workers – often migrant workers – were not able to carry out the work due to the closure of borders and other measures that restricted free movement (FIAN 2020b, p. 8).

The decisions of some states such as Romania, Russia, Kazakhstan, and Vietnam to limit exports of rice and wheat and to stockpile food have further increased the risk of food speculation (Yamashita 2020). There are reports that food shortages have caused social unrest (BBC 2020).

These impacts have been well-recognized by international actors. On 20 March 2020, Maximo Torero, chief economist of the FAO, indicated that transport restrictions and quarantine measures were likely to impede farmers' access to input and output markets, curbing productive capacities and denying a point of sale for produce (2020, p. 4). He further explained how labor shortages could disrupt the production and processing of food, especially for labor-intensive crops, and how blockages to transport routes would be particularly obstructed for fresh food supply chains, increasing levels of food loss and waste. The CESCR (2020) also recognized the pandemic's devastating impacts on food production and availability.

2.3 Differential impacts on specific population groups

The impacts of COVID and lockdown measures are uneven. The deepest impacts are on the most marginalized and disadvantaged groups of society and especially to those living in poverty (CESCR 2020, p. 2). This section describes some of the differential impacts on specific groups, as reported by FIAN International (2020b).

2.3.1 Women and LGBTQ persons

COVID-19 has revealed and exacerbated gender inequalities. Women play a key role in producing and providing food for their families, yet paradoxically, they constitute around 60 percent of undernourished people in the world (Merckel 2016). The impact on women is intersectional, aggravated by diverse conditions of vulnerability – for example being a woman and Indigenous, or a woman and peasant. Having to dedicate more time to care work, women often sacrifice their jobs and income. Women's reduced capacity for working negatively affects their contribution to food systems and consequently the enjoyment of the right to food and nutrition of their families and of many others. Domestic violence can cause women to eat less, to be the last to eat, or not to eat at all.

In Africa, the majority of women and girls work in the informal sector. They are self-employed or work as daily wage laborers (FIAN 2020b, p. 7). Strict confinement measures with no alternative safety nets have compelled women to eat last and less. In Uganda, for example, women in small-scale fishing communities have faced enormous pressure due to the closure of fish markets, struggling to put food on the table.

In Latin America, organizations reported a drastic increase of working hours for women. While men have taken on more household chores, women were still overburdened (Requena Aguilar 2020). In Mexico, people worry that this 'new normal' will affect women negatively since schools will remain closed, and women will have to continue with unpaid care work. In Ecuador, Indigenous women highlighted the anxiety and stress created by the lockdown since they cannot sell their agricultural products and feed their families.

In Spain, Coordinación Baladere raised concerns regarding the inability to access information about the situation of women working in red-fruit plantations and under confinement. It was feared that women, mostly from Morocco, would be sent home without the required precautions at the end of the harvest season. Reports from India point out how women working in the sex industry are struggling for survival and starving due to the lockdown (Chakraborty & Ramaprasad 2020).

LGBTIQ+ populations also suffer disproportionately from the impact of lockdown measures based on pervasive gender discrimination. In Peru, Colombia, and Panama, men and women were allowed to leave their homes on alternate days. Such discriminatory measures have endangered the lives of transgender, non-binary, and queer people who face harassment or violence for going out according to their gender identity and not necessarily their biological sex (Libardi 2020). These discriminatory measures impact the lives of LGBTIQ+ people in myriad ways, including their ability to access food.

2.3.2 Agricultural workers in the industrial sector

Agriculture workers have been hit by the measures taken in the pandemic. La Via Campesina in Europe has denounced the harsh effects of border closures and COVID-19 containment measures on agricultural workers' incomes and livelihoods (ECVC 2020, p. 2). For example, at the beginning of the lockdown in Germany the entry of migrant agricultural workers was barred, affecting their income.

The pandemic has exacerbated the appalling working and living conditions of seasonal workers. In India, the nationwide lockdown has forced millions of stranded migrant workers to travel back to their home villages. Of those wage laborers interviewed by Stranded Workers Action Network (2020, p. 14) in April, around 82 percent out of 12,248 had not received rations from the government and 68 percent had not received any cooked food during the previous 32 days. Seasonal agricultural workers belong predominantly to the most deprived strata of the rural hierarchy. Moreover, female migrant workers (many of whom are daily wage laborers) and agricultural workers are bearing the brunt of this pandemic having lost their jobs and incomes and now finding themselves unable to purchase or access essential supplies such as menstrual hygiene products.

The COVID-19 pandemic has also exposed the extremely precarious condition of food workers, especially those working in industrial meat production. Several industrial slaughterhouses and meat processing factories in Europe and the United States have become hotspots for coronavirus infections (FIAN 2020b, p. 9).

2.3.3 Peasant and fisher communities

Impacts on small food producers are doubly relevant, since the majority of hungry and malnourished people live in rural areas but family farming supplies the majority of healthy food. Obstacles faced by peasants in the realization of their right to food have an impact on the availability of adequate food in urban areas (El Tiempo 2020).

Subsidies to offset the effects of the crisis have been mainly aimed at the agro-industrial sector, while small and medium-sized cooperatives and peasant enterprises received negligible amounts (Camargo 2020). At the same time, intermediaries were using the crisis as an excuse to pay less to peasants.

The lockdown restrictions have prevented small-scale food producers from activities that enable them to provide nutritious food for themselves and their communities and ensure that they earn income for necessities such as electricity and other utilities and expenses. This has forced small-scale food producers to rely on social grants and food parcels; in other words, they have gone from being able to feed themselves to needing to be fed. In Ecuador, Colombia, Zimbabwe, Senegal, Mozambique, and the United States, peasants and other small-scale farmers were adversely impacted by dumping, denial of access to markets, and being left with no choice but to destroy their crops and euthanize livestock (FIAN 2020b)

Small-scale fishers and fish workers have also suffered from the impact of COVID-19. In India, 100,000 fishers and migrant fish workers were stranded in their fishing boats on March 24 as a nationwide lockdown was declared (Jamwal 2020). The country's 1,547 fish landing centers were closed with no transport facilities, ice for storage, sellers, or markets. Unable to fish, small-scale fishers experienced reduced access to adequate food for themselves and their families. The National Fishworkers Forum expressed its disappointment over the economic stimulus package announced by the central government for the fisheries sector (The Hindu 2020). Instead of providing emergency support to fishers trying to make ends meet, the government was focused on measures to promote prawn farming and fisheries exports.

As small-scale fishing is highly seasonal, many fishers have had to resort to non-fishing activities to earn an additional income. Most of these activities have come to a standstill because of the pandemic, threatening the ability to generate supplementary incomes. Tourism, which provides additional income opportunities for coastal fishing communities, has also been hard hit.

2.3.4 Indigenous peoples

Indigenous peoples have been disparately affected by the pandemic. Amazonian Indigenous peoples in Ecuador have decried the inadequacy of food kits distributed to respond to the crisis. Several organizations of Amazonian Indigenous Peoples wrote to the UN Special Rapporteur on the rights of Indigenous people regarding their concerns about food kits arriving in Indigenous and Afro-Ecuadorian communities: 'These were to supply a family of six to eight members for fifteen days. They contained food that perished in one day and were mostly culturally inappropriate' (FIAN Ecuador 2020).

This overview shows how the impact of COVID-19 on the right to food of diverse groups requires specific and differentiated responses from policy makers at all levels, from the local to the international, to conform to states' human rights obligations.

3 A survey of responses and recommendations

The crisis has generated diverse recommendations from communities and national and international authorities. This section surveys the main responses by right to food defenders, states, corporations, and UN actors relevant to the right to food.

3.1 The responses by affected communities, social movements, and civil society organizations

While immediately responding to COVID-19 crises with short-term solidarity solutions, affected communities have also taken action to hold authorities accountable in the short- and medium-term and have formulated clear proposals on how to transform food systems to address the vulnerability to pandemics and other disasters in the long term. These proposals show that social movements were not just asking for a state response, but came with concrete proposals in line with the right to food and nutrition. They also show how important it is for state authorities to apply participative approaches in developing recovery measures in line with their human rights obligations.

For example, the Brazilian Forum for Food Sovereignty and Food and Nutritional Security (FBSSAN) recommended the establishment of the 'Emergency Committees Against Hunger' and measures that include controlling food storage and prices, as well as the introduction of a universal basic income (FIAN 2020a). Responding to farmers' markets closure in France, Romania, and Switzerland, peasant organizations' advocacy led to government guidelines clarifying that local food markets should remain open under specific biosecurity conditions (Ziare 2020; Confédération Paysanne 2020). Communities also used litigation in Chiapas/ Mexico, Nepal, and Uganda (FIAN 2020b, p. 17).

In African countries, the Committee of Municipalities in Action (Committee de Villes en action) mobilized to research and implement solutions to respond to the cumulative crises, including COVID-19, which have affected people's right to food. It also sought to foster engagement and mobilization, recovery of productive capacities, and better social and economic development models. In the United States, Why Hunger has shed light on the challenging interconnection between the agricultural sector and food banks during the crisis. (These transformational proposals are explored in more depth in Section 4).

3.2 Responses by national decision makers

Governmental measures have been mostly focused on the short term. Monitoring by the GNRTFN (FIAN 2020b, p. 12) revealed that a number of governments have channeled their support to the agri-food industry, leaving small food producers with weak support or simply at the mercy of the market. Governmental measures have included monitoring cash transfers, regulations to ensure access to food, and measures focused on supporting the agri-food industrial sector.

For example, in India, the central government has conducted a survey among the most vulnerable sections of society to determine the effectiveness of existing schemes, such as food rations, scholarships, and pensions (Sharma 2020). In South Africa the government announced a $27 billion USD economic stimulus package to assist municipalities in providing water, sanitation, food, and shelter to the homeless (FIAN 2020b, p. 3). In Italy the government approved a decree to allow temporary work permits for migrants to work on farms, while Portugal granted temporary citizenship rights to all migrants waiting for a residence permit, thus ensuring their access to health, social security, employment stability, and housing (FIAN 2020b, p. 4).

Some examples of pro-agri-food-business measures include the case of Colombia, where the government approved regulations suspending import taxes for soy, corn, and sorghum (Forbes 2020), with a foreseeable impact on local producers. In Bolivia, the government approved the use of genetically modified seeds (Mundubat 2020), which are commercialized by corporations. In Ecuador, communities denounced how the government favors the distribution of edible products from the agro-industries while peasants do not receive comparable support to sell their products (FIAN Ecuador 2020).

Despite that general trend, other states have reacted to possible abuse of the dominant position and power in the market by corporations. For instance, Denmark and Poland decided not to give financial aid to companies registered in offshore tax havens (Bostock 2020). The African Commission on Human and Peoples' Rights (2020) adopted a resolution on the need to develop norms on states' obligations to regulate private actors involved in the provision of social services. Facing speculation by intermediaries, the governments of Argentina and Colombia introduced measures regulating prices of essential products in order to protect economic access by consumers (President of the Argentinian Nation 2020; President of the Republic of Colombia 2020).

3.3 *Some responses by the corporate sector*

Before the COVID-19 crisis, agri-food corporations established an industrialized food system (Bello 2020) in which small-scale food producers are marginalized from policy development and victimized by systematic abuses and discrimination. These same corporations push for a corporate-led diet, which weakens health and makes the rights holders' bodies vulnerable to communicable diseases such as COVID-19 (FIAN 2020b).

In the wake of the pandemic, civil society and media have reported how powerful enterprises are using the health crisis to their advantage, with tactics including pushing governments to delay or derogate from regulations protecting the citizens while lobbying for approval of corporate-friendly laws (Hourticq 2020). Agro-industries have been denounced for oligopolistic behavior and exploiting workers in the meat sector. Equally concerning is the danger of companies using the crisis to impose digital technologies, artificial intelligence, and the elimination of cash, affecting the social and cultural aspects of the right to food and dismantling in-person human interactions. This disrupts the social fabric of our societies and excludes those without access to technologies (FIAN 2020b, p. 13).

3.4 *Responses of international human rights institutions*

Several UN human rights system mandates have issued pronouncements related to the right to food. While the CESCR has primarily focused on short-term measures, the UN Special Rapporteurs on the right to food and on extreme poverty have called for a transformation of the current economic model.

The CESCR focused on measures addressing the most marginalized groups, ensuring mobility for agricultural workers and financial support and access to credit, markets, and agricultural inputs for small-scale farmers, especially women. The Committee reiterated the state obligation to use maximum available resources in responding to the pandemic, for example through social relief and income-support programs to ensure food and income security to all those in need (CESCR 2020, p. 3).

Regarding access to food, the Committee recommended the adoption of regulatory measures to prevent profiteering on foodstuffs. Additionally, it suggested lifting all value-added taxes and subsidizing the cost of essential foodstuffs and hygiene products to ensure that they are affordable for people living in poverty. Moreover, CESCR recalled states' extraterritorial obligations, reaffirmed states' obligation to cooperate in seeking solutions, and emphasized that states should ensure that unilateral border measures do not hinder the flow of necessary and essential goods, including staple foods (CESCR 2020, p. 4).

In his report to the UN General Assembly, the Special Rapporteur on the right to food expressed the need for economic transformation. He highlighted the need to rethink the political economy of food and hunger, noting that the global concentration of market power in the hands of a few corporations has led to volatile prices. He explained how availability, adequacy, and accessibility require that people control the production, distribution, and consumption of their food and that all these steps remain open to democratic dialogue and re-creation according to the evolving circumstances (Fakhri 2020, p.19).

The Special Rapporteur on extreme poverty and human rights has also proposed structural economic and social transformation. He called for a development model that places social inclusion and ecological sustainability at the heart of public policies, deconstructing the belief that economic growth is the key to solve all human ills. For the Special Rapporteur the promotion of equality must be the priority (De Schutter 2020).

4 The strengths and promises of the rural movements' proposal

The COVID-19 crisis has exacerbated hunger and malnutrition and made highly impossible the achievement of SDG 2 by 2030. It has also revealed the range of medium- and long-term solutions that policy makers could adopt. On the one side, the agri-food industrial sector and governments defend profit-centered solutions, while on the other side, the UN human rights mandates and social movements agree on the need for food systems transformations that put people and their human rights, as well as the planet, over profit through a democratic process.

The power of those espousing the 'industrialized solution' provides more visibility to 'commoditized' solutions. The proposals of rural movements, those who feed the world, are less visible. Nonetheless, solutions proposed by the rural movements and their supporters are arguably more suitable from a human rights perspective when facing COVID-19 and similar disasters for present and future generations.

The following paragraphs present the key elements of the proposals developed by rural social movements and their supporters based on the views of the organizations composing the Civil Society and Indigenous Peoples' Mechanism (CSM) of the CFS (CSM 2020b).

Members of CSM hold that human rights should guide food systems transformation. Rights holders should be entitled to hold their states accountable for their obligations under the right to food. Human dignity should have priority over commercial interests. Public policies should prioritize disadvantaged and vulnerable populations. Processes towards policy implementation in the field shall comply with the principles of participation, accountability, non-discrimination, transparency, empowerment, and the rule of law (including the primacy of human rights). Furthermore, fair food systems require the recognition and support of small food producers, including of Indigenous peoples and peasant food systems through the implementation of the UNDRIP and UNDROP, as well as the ILO Conventions. States are called on to jointly and individually strengthen food governance based on cooperation as a state obligation under article 2.1 of the ICESCR.

Rights holders most affected by food insecurity and malnutrition must be able to meaningfully participate, collectively or individually, in the determination of public priorities and the development of strategies, policies, legislation, and other measures within food systems. Food governance shall put food sovereignty into practice.

For social movements, the transformation of food systems requires a holistic, systemic approach that goes beyond agricultural productivism, food fortifications, and decisions based on data. Instead, the transformation of food systems must consider the interrelations and complexity of food systems. This includes considering the social, cultural, and environmental aspects of the right to food and not reducing it only to its mere economic dimension. A holistic approach reclaims food systems as public goods and food as commons and not as commodities. The realization of the right to food and nutrition cannot be left to market-based solutions only, but requires public policies to correct perverse impacts of market forces on the right to food to put rights holders' wellbeing and the planet at the center. To be just, food systems shall recognize the role and contribution of women to the enjoyment of the right to food, including through the redistribution of care work.

States shall reaffirm the primacy of the public sphere (vis-à-vis multistakeholder approaches). This includes the autonomy, self-governance, and self-determination of rural and urban local communities, grassroots social movements and their organizations, and Indigenous peoples. Moreover, to ensure that power imbalances in food systems are corrected, states must adopt and implement binding regulations for corporate legal accountability to prevent and remedy corporate conduct undermining or nullifying rights holders' enjoyment of the right to food and nutrition. States jointly or individually must adopt strong regulations against conflicts of interests to prevent undue corporate influence or corporate capture.

The support of local and territorial markets is key to ensuring more resilient food systems (instead of subsidizing global value chains, which are vulnerable to lockdown measures adopted in the context of pandemics such as COVID-19). Becoming more sensitive to local populations and ecosystems can help to prevent forced migration and reduce vulnerability during future pandemics. In short, the transformation of food systems to better align with human rights requires the redistribution of wealth and correction of inequalities.

5 Conclusion

The agro-industrial food system dominating our societies together with pre-existing crises have made humanity extremely vulnerable to the pandemic; the impacts on the right to food have been evident. This fragility is connected to the reliance of our societies on agro-industrial value chains for food availability. The dominant system is based on forms of food production that negatively impact the ecosystems, enable zoonotic processes, destroy food diversity, and promote the consumption of edible food products that weaken our bodies' capacity to respond to pandemics like COVID-19. The agro-industrial corporate sector influences governance decisions and recovery measures, leading governments to systematically neglect small producers, despite the fact that they produce around 80 percent of food worldwide. This interference in governance spaces also affects consumers, for instance through the quality of food assistance provided or the imposition of digital technologies to access to food.

While international organizations identified a looming global food crisis, communities promptly reported multiple local crises in diverse regions both in the Global South and North. These crises have had and will have a negative impact on the enjoyment of the right to adequate food by marginalized and disadvantaged communities and especially on women.

Local communities, organizations, and some governments reacted quickly to support the most adversely affected, but the recession caused by the pandemic and the lockdown measures will have a long-term impact on the capacity of people to feed themselves and their families, making it highly unlikely to achieve SDG 2 by 2030. To respond to the long-term effects of COVID-19 on the right to food and related rights and to better respond to future epidemics, a transformation of the dominant food system is needed. The social movements of the CSM affirm that transformation including a human rights approach. States have the duty to ensure the meaningful participation of such movements and to consider their proposals in order to ensure the right to food to present and future generations.

References

African Commission on Human and Peoples' Rights 2020, *434 Resolution on the Need to Develop Norms on States' Obligations to Regulate Private Actors Involved in the Provision of Social Services*, ACHPR/Res. 434, viewed 29 December 2020, www.achpr.org/sessions/resolutions?id=465

Agencia AP 2020, 'Pandemia alimentaria. Terrorífica cifra de la ONU: podrían morir de hambre 300.000 personas por día', *Clarín*, 22 April, viewed 29 December 2020, www.clarin.com/viste/terrorifica-cifra-onu-podrian-morir-hambre-300-000-personas-dia_0_E2LBkq8QO.html

BBC 2020, 'Coronavirus: Chile Protesters Clash with Police over Lockdown', 19 May, viewed 29 December 2020, www.bbc.com/news/world-latin-america-52717402?fbclid=IwAR0jFTfCm2mhZWwmMVrGwdkWoUBQCAp6PuGVDssNPLZBHF-62geouV6mZqs

Bello, W 2020, 'The Corporate Food System Is Making the Coronavirus Crisis Worse', *Foreign Policy in Focus*, 22 April, viewed 29 December 2020, https://fpif.org/the-corporate-food-system-is-making-the-coronavirus-crisis-worse/?fbclid=IwAR1739odzfxQdL7vKlvgv9MPyJeL3zZfsHbketd7OQ4jl23mi-4eAOosbRM

Bertsch, M 2020, 'Covid-19: la chaîne alimentaire sur le fil du rasoir', *France 24*, 11 May, viewed 29 December 2020, www.france24.com/fr/plan%C3%A8te/20200511-covid-19-la-cha%C3%AEne-alimentaire-sur-le-fil-du-rasoir?fbclid=IwAR1WRjhcTXEEmnfYA6eUQJ8Lri_a7Pg23YR0d36P0iRDzy2DsLe7uP_zHHw

Bostock, B 2020, 'Denmark and Poland Are Refusing to Bail out Companies Registered in Offshore Tax Havens', *Business Insider*, 20 April, viewed 29 December 2020, www.businessinsider.com/coronavirus-companies-tax-havens-banned-denmark-poland-bailout-2020-4?r=US&IR=T

Brazilian Forum for Food Sovereignty and Food and Nutritional Security 2020a, 'Human Right to Food in Times of COVID-19', 27 March, viewed 29 December 2020, https://fbssan.org.br/2020/03/human-right-to-food-in-times-o-covid-19/

Brazilian Forum for Food Sovereignty and Food and Nutritional Security 2020b, 'Guia para alimentação escolar em tempos de Covid-19', 5 May, viewed 29 December 2020, https://fbssan.org.br/2020/05/guia-para-alimentacao-escolar-em-tempos-de-covid-19/

Camargo, J 2020, 'Lamentable: créditos para campesinos colombianos estarían manos de Multinacionales', *Soy Campesino*, 18 April, viewed 29 December 2020, https://soycampesino.org/2020/04/18/lamentable-creditos-para-campesinos-colombianos-estarian-manos-de-multinacionales/

CFS 2020, 'Interim Issue Paper on the Impact of COVID-19 on Food Security and Nutrition', viewed 29 December 2020, www.fao.org/fileadmin/templates/cfs/Docs1920/Chair/CFS_Chair_Statement_HLPE_COVID.pdf

Chakraborty, R & Ramaprasad, H 2020, '"They Are Starving": Women in India's Sex Industry Struggle for Survival', *The Guardian*, 29 April, viewed 29 December 2020, www.theguardian.com/global-development/2020/apr/29/they-are-starving-women-in-indias-sex-industry-struggle-for-survival?CMP=Share_AndroidApp_WhatsApp

Civil Society and Indigenous Peoples' Mechanism for the Relations with the CFS (CSM) 2020a, 'Open Call for Civil Society and Indigenous Peoples' Engagement to Respond to the UN Food Systems Summit', viewed 29 December 2020, www.csm4cfs.org/wp-content/uploads/2020/10/EN-Open-Call-on-UN-Food-Systems-Summit-12-October-2020-1.pdf

Civil Society and Indigenous Peoples' Mechanism for the Relations with the CFS (CSM) 2020b, 'Voices from the Ground: from COVID-19 to Radical Transformation of our Food Systems', viewed 29 December 2020, www.csm4cfs.org/wp-content/uploads/2020/10/EN-COVID_FULL_REPORT-2020.pdf

Civil Society Mechanism to the Committee on World Food Security, Voices from the ground from covid-19 to radical transformation of our food systems, 2020, viewed 16 March 2021, www.csm4cfs.org/wp-content/uploads/2020/12/EN-COVID_FULL_REPORT-2020.pdf

Committee on Economic, Social and Cultural Rights (CESCR), General Comment 12, 1999, UN Doc E/C.12/1999/5), viewed 16 March 2021, www.refworld.org/pdfid/4538838c11.pdf

Committee on Economic, Social and Cultural Rights (CESCR) 2020, *Statement on the Coronavirus Disease (COVID-19) Pandemic and Economic, Social and Cultural Rights*, UN Doc. E/C.12/2020/1.

Committee on World Food Security (CFS) 2017, 'Global Strategic Framework for Food Security and Nutrition', *FAO*, viewed 29 December 2020, www.fao.org/cfs/OnlineGSF/en/

Confédération Paysanne 2020, 'Lettre ouverte aux citoyennes. Coronavirus: la nécessaire refondation de nos systèmes agricoles et alimentaires', 20 March, viewed 29 December 2020, www.confederationpaysanne.fr/actu.php?id=9885&PHPSESSID=fllago79tqmb3163v6vc8gmi62

CNN 2020, 'Food Bank Demand Skyrockets as Supplies Dwindle', viewed 29 December 2020, https://edition.cnn.com/videos/business/2020/04/29/food-bank-shortage-demand-high-carroll-dnt-newday-vpx.cnn

Dave, N 2020, '"Give Us Food or Kill Us NOW": Over 200 Daily Wagers Say They Haven't Had a Morsel to Eat for Past Four Says', *Ahmedabad Mirror*, 11 May, viewed 29 December 2020, https://ahmedabadmirror.indiatimes.com/ahmedabad/others/give-us-food-or-kill-us-now/articleshow/75665931.cms?utm_source=contentofinterest&utm_medium=text&utm_campaign=cppst

de Schutter, Olivier 2020, 'UN Poverty Expert: Promotion of Equality Must be Our Priority', viewed 29 December 2020, www.un.org/en/coronavirus/un-poverty-expert-promotion-equality-must-be-our-priority

El Tiempo, 'Drama en el campo: no hay quien compre y las cosechas se pierden', 30 May, viewed 29 December 2020, www.eltiempo.com/colombia/otras-ciudades/cultivos-en-colombia-durante-la-pandemia-por-coronavirus-499102

European Coordination Via Campesina 2020, 'Open Letter to the European Commission and European Parliament on Urgent and Necessary Measures in Europe for Rural Workers in the Context of COVID-19', 30 April, viewed 29 December 2020, www.eurovia.org/wp-content/uploads/2020/04/WEB_with_signatories_Open_letter_migrant_workers_FINAL_EN.pdf

Fakhri, M 2020, 'The Right to Food in the Context of International Trade Law and Policy', UN Doc No. A/75/219.

Food and Agricultural Organization of the United Nations (FAO) 2007, *Declaration of Nyeleni*.

FAO 2020a, 'Coronavirus Food Supply Chain Under Strain: What to do?', 24 March, www.fao.org/3/ca8308en/ca8308en.pdf

FAO 2020b, 'As More Go Hungry and Malnutrition Persists, Achieving Zero Hunger by 2030 in Doubt, UN Report Warns', 13 July 2020, viewed 29 December 2020, www.fao.org/news/story/en/item/1297810/icode/

FAO & IFAD 2019, 'United Nations Decade of Family Farming 2019–2028. Global Action Plan', viewed 29 December 2020, www.fao.org/3/ca4672en/ca4672en.pdf

FIAN 2019, https://www.fian.org/files/files/Suarez_Franco___RTFN_article_IIDH.pdf

FIAN 2020a, 'Impact of COVID-19 on the Human Right to Food and Nutrition', *FIAN International*, viewed 29 December 2020, https://fian.org/files/files/Preliminary_monitoring_report_-_Impact_of_COVID19_on_the_HRtFN_EN(1).pdf

FIAN 2020b, 'Monitoring Report on the Right to Food and Nutrition during COVID-19', viewed 29 December 2020, www.fian.org/files/files/Covid_Monitoring_Report_-Template_EN(1).pdf

FIAN Ecuador 2020, '¿Crisis alimentaria en Ecuador?: nuestro derecho a la alimentación en los tiempos de COVID-19', viewed 29 December 2020, www.fian.org/en/publication/article/food-crisis-in-ecuador-our-right-to-food-in-times-of-covid-19-2606

Forbes 2020, 'Colombia suspende aranceles al maíz, soya y sorgo', 9 April, viewed 29 December 2020, https://forbes.co/2020/04/09/actualidad/colombia-suspende-aranceles-al-maiz-soya-y-sorgo

Goger, A 2020, 'For Millions of Low-income Seniors, Coronavirus is a Food-Security Issue', *Brookings Institution*, 16 March, viewed 29 December 2020, www.brookings.edu/blog/the-avenue/2020/03/16/for-millions-of-low-income-seniors-coronavirus-is-a-food-security-issue/

High Level Panel of Experts on Food Security and Nutrition, Extract from the Report Food Losses and Waste in the Context of Sustainable Food Systems Summary and Recommendations P2.Parr8, 2014, viewed 16 March 2021, www.fao.org/fileadmin/user_upload/hlpe/hlpe_documents/HLPE_S_and_R/HLPE_2014_Food_Losses_and_Waste_Summary_EN.pdf

Himalayan News Service 2020, 'PIL Filed Seeking Relief', *The Himalayn Times*, 13 April, viewed 29 December 2020, https://thehimalayantimes.com/kathmandu/public-interest-litigation-filed-seeking-relief/?fbclid=IwAR1M9rFyB2PNRHvQfUnqBmcui_X7BXGH_vdalwq83FeCiMgEsRtW02XZzBE

Hourticq, B 2020, 'Behind Their Current Display of Charity, It's Business as Usual for Multinationals', *Equal Times*, 14 May, viewed 29 December 2020, www.equaltimes.org/behind-their-current-display-of?lang=en#.X9LtbWhKjIX

Hughlett, M & Spencer J 2020, 'With Farmers Pressed by Plant Closing, JBS Worthington Begins Killing Pigs without Processing Them', *Star Tribune*, 30 April, viewed 29 December 2020, www.startribune.com/with-farmers-pressed-by-plant-closing-jbs-worthington-begins-killing-pigs-without-processing-them/570053952/?refresh=true

Jamwal, N 2020, 'Lockdown Enforced When They Were at Sea – so more Than a Lakh of Fishers Now Wait in Deep Waters', *GaonConnection*, 2 April, viewed 29 December 2020, https://en.gaonconnection.com/lockdown-enforced-when-they-were-at-sea-so-lakhs-of-fishers-now-wait-in-deep-waters/

Libardi, M 2020, 'El peligro de ser transgénero en América Latina en tiempos de cuarentena', *Open Democracy*, 21 April, viewed 29 December 2020, www.opendemocracy.net/es/el-peligro-de-ser-transgenero-en-america-latina-en-tiempos-de-cuarentena/

Merckel, K 2016, 'Women and Hunger Facts', *World Hunger Education Service*, 22 February, viewed 29 December 2020, www.worldhunger.org/women-and-hunger-facts/

Monjane, B, Ntauzazi, C, & Zamchiya, P 2020, 'The Four Immediate Impacts of Covid-19 Regulations on the Mozambican Farmers', *Future Agricultures*, 27 April, viewed 29 December 2020, www.future-agricultures.org/blog/the-four-immediate-impacts-of-covid-19-regulations-on-the-mozambican-farmers/

Mundubat 2020, 'El gobierno de facto en Bolivia aprueba un decreto que autoriza el uso de semillas transgénicas', viewed 29 December 2020, www.mundubat.org/el-gobierno-de-facto-en-bolivia-aprueba-un-decreto-que-autoriza-el-uso-de-semillas-transgenicas/

Office of the Hight Commissioner (OHCHR) 2020, 'COVID-19 Guidance', viewed 29 December 2020, www.ohchr.org/EN/NewsEvents/Pages/COVID19Guidance.aspx

Oquendo, C 2020, 'El hambre como bandera', *El País*, 17 April, viewed 29 December 2020, https://elpais.com/sociedad/2020-04-17/el-hambre-como-bandera.html

Pardo, D 2020, 'Por qué tantos colombianos han colgado trapos rojos en sus casas en medio de la cuarentena por la pandemia', *BBC Mundo*, 20 April, viewed 29 December 2020, www.bbc.com/mundo/noticias-america-latina-52349231

President of the Argentinian Nation 2020, *Decree 100*, viewed 29 December 2020, www.boletinoficial.gob.ar/detalleAviso/primera/224921/20200129

President of the Republic of Colombia 2020, *Decree 507*, viewed 29 December 2020, https://dapre.presidencia.gov.co/normativa/normativa/DECRETO%20507%20DEL%201%20DE%20ABRIL%20DE%202020.pdf

Requena Aguilar, A 2020, 'Más hombres haciendo la compra pero más carga de cuidados sobre las mujeres: la pandemia refuerza la brecha de género', *El Diario.Es*, 27 April, viewed 29 December 2020, www.eldiario.es/economia/hombres-haciendo-cuidados-mujeres-pandemia_1_5916227.html

Savitri, L 2020, 'Die from Starvation or Die from Illness? Pandemic in the Data Crisis Country', *Fian Indonesia*, 28 April, viewed 28 December 2020, http://fian-indonesia.org/die-from-starvation-or-die-from-illness-pandemic-in-the-data-crisis-country/

Sharma, N 2020, 'Ahead of Lockdown 2.0, Government Does Survey of Poor', *The Economic Times*, 13 April, viewed 29 December 2020, https://economictimes.indiatimes.com/news/politics-and-nation/ahead-of-lockdown-2-0-government-does-survey-of-poor/articleshow/75130411.cms

Stranded Workers Action Network 2020, '32 Days and Counting: COVID-19 Lockdown, Migrant Workers, and the Inadequacy of Welfare Measures in India', viewed 29 December 2020, https://covid19socialsecurity.files.wordpress.com/2020/05/32-days-and-counting_swan.pdf

Suárez Franco, AM 2020, 'The Right to Food', *FIAN*, viewed 29 December 2020, https://www.fian.org/files/files/Suarez_Franco___RTFN_article_IIDH.pdf

The Hindu 2020, 'Fishers Fume over Stimulus Package', 16 May, viewed 29 December 2020, www.thehindu.com/news/national/kerala/fishers-fume-over-stimulus-package/article31602900.ece

Torero, M 2020, 'Coronavirus Food Supply Chain Under Strain What To Do?', *FAO*, 24 March, viewed 29 December 2020, www.fao.org/3/ca8308en/ca8308en.pdf

UN General Assembly, UN Declaration on the Rights of Peasants and other People Working in Rural Areas A/HRC/RES/39/12, https://undocs.org/A/HRC/RES/39/12

Viejo, M 2020, 'Las colas del hambre y la pobreza inician su escalada en Madrid: "cada día viene más gente nueva"', *El País*, 23 April, viewed 29 December 2020, https://elpais.com/espana/madrid/2020-04-23/la-pobreza-inicia-su-escalada-cada-dia-viene-gente-nueva-las-colas-son-larguisimas-para-pedir-comida.html?fbclid=IwAR3L9WiT9x1kmzsMvgVcr8TX7vmfPzLXZ3nWe0TaiE0E8YlZLUjwdccPWrU

Yamashita, K 2020, 'Will the COVID-19 Pandemic Cause a Food Crisis?', *The Japan Times*, 17 April, viewed 29 December 2020, www.japantimes.co.jp/opinion/2020/04/17/commentary/japan-commentary/will-covid-19-pandemic-cause-food-crisis/#.Xs5HxExuI2x

Ziare 2020, Pietele raman deschise. Ministrul Agriculturii: Samsarii, speculantii si falsii producatori sa nu aiba acces aici!', 23 March, viewed 29 December 2020, https://ziare.com/economie/agricultura/pietele-raman-deschise-ministrul-agriculturii-samsarii-speculantii-si-falsii-producatori-sa-nu-aiba-acces-aici-1602940

13

COVID-19 AND THE HUMAN RIGHTS TO WATER AND SANITATION

Pedi Obani

Experiences with the coronavirus pandemic illustrate the crucial importance of access to water and sanitation as basic human rights and as necessities for the realization of health, education, food, gender equality, and other human rights (United Nations 2020). Emergent issues include the high public health risks associated with lack of water and sanitation and the disproportionate burden borne by women and girls, transgendered people, people living in informal settlements, people living with disabilities, the urban poor, migrant workers, workers in the informal sector, people who are sick or living with underlying health conditions, the elderly, school-aged children, and other groups living in vulnerable situations (Banerji 2020; Tan 2020; UNESCO n.d.). These highlight intersecting layers of inequalities in different situations of vulnerability and the interconnectedness of human rights. The pandemic has also demonstrated the imperative of leaving no one behind and ensuring universal access to water and sanitation to achieve sustainable development. From Africa to the Pan-European region, it is a similar picture: there are remarkable inequities in access to water and sanitation based on whether people live in urban or rural areas, whether people are rich or poor, and whether they have any special circumstances which render them vulnerable (Local Burden of Disease WaSH Collaborators 2020; Wang et al. 2019; World Health Organization & UN-Water 2019; United Nations 2020). Furthermore, because of the pandemic, several assumptions and modes of service delivery need to be reexamined to ensure continued suitability for promoting universal access to water and sanitation. It is in light of these realizations that this chapter examines the question: How has COVID-19 influenced water, sanitation, and hygiene services and how can the rights to water and sanitation strengthen resilience in health pandemics? This question is addressed from the perspective of inclusive development theory which emphasizes the need to address the social, relational, and ecological aspects of human development (Gupta, Pouw, & Ros-Tonen 2015).

1 Evolution of the rights to water and sanitation over the past decade

The past decade represents a significant milestone in the evolution of water and sanitation as human rights within the United Nations (UN) system. The General Assembly in July 2010 adopted Resolution 64/292 recognizing 'the right to safe and clean drinking water and sanitation as a human right that is essential for the full enjoyment of life and all human rights' (General Assembly 2010a, para. 1). The Resolution was adopted with 122 votes in favor and 41 abstentions, while 29 countries were absent (General Assembly 2010b). The lack of opposing votes and the largely political and procedural reservations expressed by the countries voting on the Resolution was an indication of the widespread appreciation of the important human rights status of water and sanitation, particularly at the international level (Obani & Gupta 2015). The Human Rights Council affirmed in October 2010, in its Resolution 15/9 on *Human Rights and Access to Safe Drinking Water and Sanitation*,

> that the human right to safe drinking water and sanitation is derived from the right to an adequate standard of living and inextricably related to the right to the highest attainable standard of physical and mental health, as well as the right to life and human dignity.
>
> *(Human Rights Council 2010, para. 1)*

Both resolutions are remarkable for establishing the legal basis for recognizing water and sanitation as international human rights, despite the lack of explicit mention in the International Bill of Rights.[1] Treaty bodies such as the Committee on Economic, Social and Cultural Rights (CESCR) have also recognized that the right to water is essential for realization of the right to an adequate standard of living in article 11(1) of the International Covenant on Economic, Social and Cultural Rights and other economic, social, and cultural rights. Instances can be found in General Comment No. 6 of 1995 on the economic, social, and cultural rights of older persons and in General Comment No. 15 of 2002 on the right to water, which links the right to water to an adequate standard of living, the highest attainable standard of health, adequate housing and food, life and human dignity. Similarly, the Human Rights Committee, the monitoring body for the International Covenant on Civil and Political Rights has specified in its General Comment No. 36 of 2018 on the right to life, para. 26, that water is essential for guaranteeing the right to life. States parties have a duty to take appropriate measures to address direct threats to life or conditions which will prevent the enjoyment of the right to life with dignity.[2]

While the rights to water and sanitation have evolved closely in international human rights law and water and sanitation services are often combined in the international development agenda, the distinctiveness of the right to sanitation from the right to water and the need for their separate consideration in some contexts was earlier recognized by the CESCR in its 2010 statement on the right to sanitation.

The distinctiveness of the right to sanitation was also recognized in the General Assembly Resolution 70/169 in 2015, which signaled the recognition of the right to sanitation as an independent right. This is in line with scholarly arguments for delinking water and sanitation in policy and practice to promote the normative development and progressive realization of the latter right especially (Ellis & Feris 2014; Obani & Gupta 2015).

The past decade has witnessed a greater impetus for universal access to water and sanitation as part of the international development agenda. This is a testament to the growing influence of the human rights to water and sanitation in policy and practice. For instance, the Sustainable Development Goals (SDGs) prioritize achieving by 2030 'universal and equitable access to safe and affordable drinking water for all' (SDG 6.1) and 'access to adequate and equitable sanitation and hygiene for all and end open defecation, paying special attention to the needs of women and girls and those in vulnerable situations' (SDG 6.2). In contrast, the earlier UN Millennium Declaration adopted in September 2000 and the Plan of Implementation of the World Summit on Sustainable Development focused on halving by 2015 the proportion of people without access to an improved drinking water source and/or to improved sanitation, particularly in developing countries (Fukuda, Noda & Oki 2019; Obani 2020). The past decade has also witnessed an increase in the promotion of the rights to water and sanitation, both implicitly and expressly, through national constitutions, domestic laws, judicial decisions, and domestic human rights institutions (WaterLex 2014a; WaterLex 2014b). There has been significant progress in the normative development of the rights to water and sanitation over the past decade and significant progress in understanding best practices for progressive realization.

Remarkably, there is growing emphasis on addressing inherent limitations of the rights which affect utility value (Feris 2015; Hall, Van Koppen, & Van Houweling 2014) and on improving the synergies and interrelations between the rights to water and sanitation, water governance broadly, and other related rights to reduce tensions and improve mutual gains in practice (Water Supply & Sanitation Collaborative Council (WSSCC) & United Nations Human Rights Office of the High Commissioner (OHCHR) 2020; Obani & Gupta 2014; Barry 2020; Viñuales 2019). Concerns also remain around the drivers of lack of access (Sinharoy, Pittluck, & Clasen 2019); the role of States and other actors (including the private sector, development partners, implementing partners, and others involved in the water and sanitation sectors) towards promoting the realization of the rights to water and sanitation (Alston 2018); limitations of a purely technocratic approach to implementing the rights to water and sanitation (Birkenholtz 2016); and best practices for ensuring inclusive access to and allocation of water and sanitation and promoting the accountability of all relevant stakeholders, particularly for the most vulnerable and marginalized groups that are characteristically left behind and excluded from accessing water and sanitation services (World Health Organization, UN-Water 2019; Heller 2018; Joshi 2017; WSSCC 2020).

The impact of environmental disasters, climate change, public health crises, and (financial, natural, and other) resource constraints also continue to drive interest in improving the resilience of water and sanitation infrastructure and governance systems (McGranahan 2015; Johannessen et al. 2014). Against this background, the normative content of the rights to water and sanitation – namely, availability; accessibility; safety; affordability; and acceptability – offer a basis for assessing the quality of service delivery and promoting continuous and reliable access for everyone, during and post-crisis.

2 Impacts of COVID-19 on water and sanitation services

Infection prevention and control during the pandemic requires continuous and reliable access to water, sanitation, and hygiene (WASH) services, including sufficient residual chlorine in water supplies, among other recommended measures. There are also concerns about the risks of contamination of the water cycle and the need for environmental sanitation management to prevent COVID-19 transmission and environmental degradation generally (Patrício Silva et al. 2021; Vardoulakis et al. 2020). Moreover, there are indications that wastewater surveillance can contribute to the management of COVID-19 (World Health Organization 2020; Street et al. 2020; Daughton 2020; Bogler et al. 2020). Recognizing the importance of water and hygiene for the control of transmission and management of COVID-19, there has been an increasing focus on ensuring continuous, safe, and reliable basic water and hygiene services in many countries. Overall, the COVID-19 pandemic has impacted the rights to water and sanitation in at least three ways: (a) availability of services; (b) affordability and other economic impacts on consumers and operators; and (c) impacts on governance and regulation of services.

2.1 Availability of services

With most people confined to their homes during lockdowns, there was significant increase in domestic demand for water. Jordan recorded an increase of 40 percent in domestic demand for water supply during the early stages of the pandemic (Jordan 2020). People could increasingly resort to open defecation due to the inaccessibility of public toilets or fear of infection from using shared toilets during the pandemic. In countries such as the United Kingdom, for instance, the closure of public lavatories during the early lockdown was shown to have reduced the availability of WASH facilities (Khan 2020; Brown 2020). There are also reports of healthcare facilities and quarantine centers in several countries that were operating without adequate WASH services, thereby increasing the risk of infection among populations in vulnerable situations (Kumari & Pisharody 2020; Human Rights Watch 2020). The negative impacts of the pandemic on availability, coupled with increased demand for WASH services, are likely to impede progress with access to improved water sources and the eradication of open defecation.

The widespread closure of borders and ensuing global supply chain disruptions at the beginning of the pandemic also resulted in shortages of menstrual hygiene materials and other hygiene supplies in some countries, exacerbating period poverty and hygiene-related health risks to women and girls (Plan International 2020; Ortman 2020). Household sanitation and hygiene supplies such as toilet rolls and hand sanitizers were often among the items which consumers hoarded at the beginning of the lockdowns, leading to temporary scarcity and significant price hikes in several countries (Mao 2020; Mullen 2020; Agence France-Presse 2020). Under such circumstances, people are forced to resort to unhygienic alternatives and practices which endanger their health and increase the risk of environmental degradation.

2.2 Affordability and other economic impacts on consumers and operators

The loss of income and the economic downturn during the pandemic has affected the ability of some persons to pay their bills and/or access basic WASH services, particularly for consumers who rely on private service providers (Gout & Kelly 2020; Carman & Nataraj 2020). A recent report of the immediate past Special Rapporteur on the human rights to safe drinking water and sanitation, Léo Heller (2020), focused on human rights and the privatization of water and sanitation services, and draws from experiences during pandemics in South Africa, Spain, and Brazil. He hints at the distinct approaches to service delivery by the private sector, concerned with the economic sustainability of their operations and the right to disconnect customers for non-payment of bills, and the public sector and civil society organizations, concerned with universal access irrespective of consumers' economic ability. The report highlights that:

> [T]he coronavirus disease (COVID-19) pandemic in 2020 … mak[es] clear the need for States to intervene in the water sector by suspending payments of water bills, temporarily prohibiting disconnections and reconnecting people to services in order to ensure sufficient water for handwashing.
>
> *(Heller 2020, para. 11)*

The COVID-19 pandemic-related measures have also increased or at least altered the means and related cost of providing basic services, particularly for vulnerable groups, with the potential effect of eroding the progress made so far with advancing national, regional, and global development goals such as the SDGs. Utilities have incurred additional costs related to either adapting their operations to the crisis or implementing the regulatory requirements for ensuring the safety of their operations, sourcing materials and services for their operations, and other general challenges with keeping their businesses running during the pandemic (Butler et al. 2020). They are also exposed to billing losses and reduced revenues linked to

COVID-19 related measures (Butler et al. 2020), while some who are reliant on foreign loans, equipment, and materials have sustained losses due to fluctuations in the value of the dollar. Utilities may not have recorded any significant increase in water consumption because the shutdown of many businesses and public places during the lockdowns would have offset any additional demand for water by residential consumers. However, the closure of commercial buildings and industries during the periods of lockdowns may have negatively affected the cross-subsidy systems, due to the loss of earnings from higher paying commercial consumers. Conversely, households are likely to have recorded significant increase in consumption (Kalbusch 2020), at a time when consumers without stable sources of income or savings may be unable to afford tariffs for basic services.

On the flip side, experiences with the pandemic have increased attention to alternative ways of improving the efficiency of the water and sanitation sector in crisis situations, particularly through digitization and automation of processes. This is mainly beneficial to utilities that have the resources to transition to the requirements of the 'new normal' without compromising the quality of service delivery in the process.

2.3 COVID-19 and the governance and regulation of services

In the wake of the pandemic, national and subnational governments around the world have enacted laws imposing quarantine, physical distancing, curfews, and other similar measures with implications for the governance of organizations, regulation of services, and related human rights. Although operators of water and sanitation services have often been exempted from closure due to the essential nature of their services for preserving human life and wellbeing during the COVID-19 pandemic, the sector is not immune from the broader impacts of COVID-19 response measures. For instance, the initial disruptions to global supply chains due to border closures may have affected access to water treatment chemicals and hygiene materials for operators depending on imported chemicals (Chau et al. 2020). Also, physical distancing obligations and health concerns among the workforce may have limited the ability of service providers and even regulatory agencies to work at their full capacity (Chau et al. 2020).

The fast pace of regulatory changes and developments with the pandemic require coordination with various stakeholders, including various levels of government responsible for the regulation of water, sanitation, health and emergencies, service providers, consumers, and other key stakeholders. In the case of Brazil, water and sanitation services fall under the regulatory competence of the municipal government (Werneck 2020). Nonetheless, over 50 regulatory instruments affecting water and sanitation have been passed during the COVID-19 pandemic, by other levels of government as well, often without prior technical support and interaction between the various levels. The lack of coordination between government agencies and other stakeholders in the water and sanitation sector, particularly operators, negatively affects regulatory efficiency and outcomes in practice (Obani & Gupta 2014). In one instance in Brazil, the legislative assembly of one federal district passed an emergency regulation providing that everyone consuming less than 10 cubic meters of water per month should be entitled to free services (Werneck 2020). This amounted to 60–70 percent of the total number of consumers in that federal district; subsequent consultations with the regulatory agency revealed that the regulation would result in around $20 million in revenue loss (Werneck 2020). This realization led to a review of the regulation so that only those consuming less than 10 cubic meters of water per month and registered as a low-income household would be entitled to the free services, thereby reducing the revenue loss reduced to around $6 million (Werneck 2020).

The fast pace of changes during the COVID-19 pandemic also has implications for the number of enquiries, demands, or complaints from consumers, increasing the workload for service providers and regulators (Chau et al. 2020). Furthermore, there has been widespread reprioritizing of scheduled activities of operators and regulators, to refocus attention on the immediate needs during the pandemic (Chau et al. 2020). In some cases, the COVID-19 pandemic has affected the quality of data available for planning purposes as regulators face constraints in conducting new surveys during the pandemic (Chau et al. 2020).

3 Human rights implications of measures adopted for water and sanitation services during the pandemic

3.1 Affordability and flexible payment options

Extension of free or subsidized services to existing consumers, cash-based interventions for households, and price control mechanisms are some of the policies so far adopted for ensuring affordability of WASH services during the COVID-19 pandemic (Capodeferro & Smiderle 2020). Other interventions adopted by several countries, particularly during the early months of the pandemic, include targeted tariff reduction strategy for specified consumers, reconnection of consumers, suspension of service disconnections due to non-payment of tariffs and other similar changes in billing methods, suspension of procedures for payment defaults including fines and interests on late payments and the listing of consumers owing tariffs in public debtors' lists (Capodeferro & Smiderle 2020; UNICEF 2020). Such interventions are often mainly beneficial to consumers who are already linked to the network and may inadvertently widen the service gap between the served and the un/underserved in the absence of deliberate efforts for service expansion during the pandemic. Considering this, policies for affordability ought to be combined with the deliberate expansion of services to vulnerable populations and those without piped connections, including through the adoption of emergency solutions and alternative supply options, repair of leakages, and promotion of conservation and behavioral change to support the efficient use of available WASH services.

The availability of financial support from the government to the water and sanitation sector in some countries may have cushioned operators from significant increases in operation cost, thereby ensuring that tariffs remained stable for consumers. While it is not yet clear how much of COVID-19 recovery funds from government and other stakeholders are invested in the WASH sector, the human rights framework requires the application of maximum available resources for the progressive realization of universal access. Legal and systemic barriers to the progressive realization of universal access to water and sanitation ought to be removed, including through legal reform to formally recognize the obligations of the government relating to water and sanitation services. In practice, progressive realization requires improvements in the number of persons served, as well as the quality of service which they access (Heller 2015). This would require monitoring and disaggregation of the data on access and service levels, to understand the intersecting drivers of access and identify persons who need the most assistance with affordability measures and other forms of support to improve their access levels.

3.2 Physical accessibility

Governments, development partners, and other key stakeholders have adopted several approaches for ensuring the accessibility of WASH services during the pandemic, including promoting widespread local production and direct distribution of hygiene materials, provision of WASH services in public settings, and utilities increasing water supply volumes and service hours to meet surge in demand (UNICEF 2020). The courts have also played a key role in compelling the executive arm of government to respect the rights to basic services during the COVID-19 pandemic, for instance in Zimbabwe where the right to water is recognized in the national constitution (Tapfumaneyi 2020).

Whereas the human rights framework does not prescribe technical guidelines for availability, accessibility, or any other normative content, it is important that as a minimum, the design and quality of the infrastructure, materials, and services do not compromise the safety of users or the environment. The COVID-19 pandemic makes it more critical to ensure proper education on the operation and maintenance of the infrastructure. Furthermore, the number of functional water service points and sanitation facilities should be sufficient to encourage proper use and physical distancing while also minimizing the waiting time for users and crowds around the service points and facilities, in order to reduce the risk of community transmission. It is also necessary to carefully consider precautionary public health measures and options for service delivery with minimal physical contact between the operators and consumers, including suspension of field visits except for handling urgent complaints and repairs and equipping the workers with sufficient personal protective equipment (PPE) and hygiene supplies.

The exigencies of the COVID-19 pandemic hindered the full implementation of drinking water quality control and solid management plans, especially during the start of the pandemic (Chau et al. 2020). This required the identification of regulatory measures to safeguard reliable supply of services, including the adoption of some degree of flexibility by utilities and service providers in meeting service requirements. Utilities are also inclined to increase digitalization and automation of their processes, where possible, to improve the resilience of their operations and risk preparedness (Chau et al. 2020). Notwithstanding, such flexibility must not compromise the safety of users and the workers involved in the delivery of the WASH services. Neither should there be an overreliance on digital solutions and automation of processes resulting in a relapse into a technocratic approach to the delivery of WASH services at the expense of the rights and wellbeing of the public.

3.3 Access to information, participation, and accountability

With the COVID-19 pandemic, major concerns at the onset were access to information about the disease and government response measures and expectations of the citizens (Human Rights Watch 2020). In addition to access to service points and facilities for infection prevention and control, information about the proper use of the facilities and compliance measures for COVID-19 prevention and control are also critical for ensuring good health outcomes. Over time, many countries, development partners, and other key stakeholders have adopted various approaches for improving access to information about COVID-19 (including proper handwashing, hygiene, proper use of infrastructure, proper use and disposal of personal protective equipment and face masks, and how to comply with infection prevention and control measures to ensure effectiveness) and public access to figures on confirmed COVID-19 cases, recoveries, and fatalities (UNICEF 2020). Many countries, such as Nigeria, Ghana, the United Kingdom, Brazil, and China, are maintaining ongoing communication with the public, including through dedicated webpages with official information on COVID-19 and helplines for the public to contact about COVID-19 symptoms or related concerns.

Improved access to information has been important for empowering the population to cope better with COVID-19, protect themselves against infection and seek health assistance from the proper channels, and strengthen their health outcomes overall. Access to information about governments' financial, economic, and social policy responses to the COVID-19 pandemic has also facilitated requests for accountability over the decision making and implementation of the relevant policies by the government and other key stakeholders charged with managing the COVID-19 pandemic (Arce & Forti 2020). There have also been efforts to facilitate the participation of key stakeholders and left-behind groups in the promotion of infection prevention and control and compliance monitoring within the population. Approaches adopted for this include partnering with the representatives of key stakeholders and left-behind groups to disseminate COVID-19 information, context-specific communication materials, and targeted behavior change and hygiene messaging. For instance, in the Middle East and North Africa (MENA) region, UNICEF adopted the approach of training religious leaders on COVID-19 information to reach millions of local people with information about good handwashing and hygiene practices and engaged with the Child Advisory Council of the Supreme Council for Women and Childhood in the United Arab Emirates on issues of misinformation over COVID-19 (UNICEF 2020). Similarly, in Egypt, the IOM engaged leaders of the migrant community through 'communication corridors' designed to facilitate constant circular exchanges (UNICEF 2020).

4 Towards sustainability of the rights to water and sanitation

Overall, the COVID-19 pandemic has produced contrary impacts on the rights to water and sanitation. On the one hand, the pandemic has significantly raised the importance of universal access to continuous, safe, and reliable water, sanitation, and hygiene services within households and in public places, as a key infection prevention and control measure. The difficulties experienced by vulnerable groups, particularly at the beginning of the pandemic and during the lockdowns, have highlighted the disproportionate burden of multidimensional risks which they face during crisis, largely due to poor access to basic services. Notwithstanding, the lack of reliable, sufficiently disaggregated official population data remains a major impediment to planning, implementing, and monitoring specific progress in the access and use of WASH and other essential services by those furthest behind. This reinforces the need for progressive implementation of the rights to water and sanitation and the monitoring of progress for various groups within the population, both as a legal obligation of the government and as an important component of risk preparedness.

On the other hand, the COVID-19 pandemic threatens to cause retrogression in the progress made with the eradication of open defecation and access to improved water and sanitation due to the difficulties of accessing basic services because of lockdowns, loss of income, or supply chain disruptions among other factors. To minimize the negative impacts, it is important to ensure that vulnerable groups are prioritized in policies for continuous and reliable supply of safe drinking water, sanitation, and hygiene during the pandemic. This is in line with the human rights principle of the progressive realization of access and requires the use of maximum available resources for this purpose. The resilience of critical supply chains for products required for basic WASH services should also be strengthened as part of risk preparedness, to ensure that relevant products remain locally available during crisis and the recovery phases.

An analysis of the approaches adopted for the provision of WASH services during the COVID-19 pandemic highlight important lessons for the realization of the rights to water and sanitation, particularly during health pandemics. First, approaches which focus on averages without disaggregating the special needs of vulnerable groups at risk of limited or no access to WASH services will exacerbate inequities in access and raise public health risks. Second, providing access to WASH services during the pandemic may require some degree of flexibility with technical and regulatory standards and increased digitalization of processes. There may also be a need to adapt emergency solutions and alternative temporary approaches for service provision to ensure coverage expansion during the pandemic. These should be deployed in ways that safeguard the health and safety of consumers and service providers. Strengthening institutional governance processes, data integrity and adaptability of institutions should also be part of risk preparedness strategy.

In addition, most of the interventions for improving access to WASH during the pandemic, particularly for vulnerable groups who would otherwise have been left without basic services, have involved partnerships between government and other stakeholders such as development partners, UN agencies, civil society, faith-based organizations, media, and the private sector. Each of these stakeholders strengthened the WASH interventions through their respective attributes, such as their public interest values, financial capacity, legitimacy and motivational qualities, strong grassroots networks, or historical rootedness. This underscores the need for inclusive and participatory governance processes in the WASH sector and the risks of corporate capture. The capacity of various stakeholders who are either directly involved in the delivery of WASH services or whose actions impact the rights to water and sanitations in any way should be strengthened to promote the progressive realization of the rights and improve coordination within the sector.

Beyond addressing the immediate concerns of the COVID-19 pandemic, it is important to prioritize approaches which can support long-term risk reduction and preparedness and can be consolidated beyond the pandemic. Multi-stakeholder partnerships for promoting universal access to water and sanitation that have been active in the pandemic response should be assessed for responsiveness to various drivers of vulnerability. The partnerships should also be designed with the active participation of the public, bearing in mind spatial, social, cultural, and legal barriers to effective participation of groups in vulnerable situations. It is important for the population, as rightsholders, to be empowered to contribute to operationalizing disaster preparedness and response plans, participatory governance processes, and to generally demonstrate agency in support of the progressive realization of the rights to water and sanitation for all during the next decade.

Furthermore, it is important for utilities to align their emergency response measures with human rights standards. Utilities should also prioritize safe exit strategies from their emergency COVID-19 operations which do not compromise progressive realization of universal and equitable access in the recovery phase. This would entail not only paying attention to technical standards for drinking water safety, for instance, considering that the quality of the stagnant water in building pipelines may have deteriorated during lockdowns, but prioritizing the progressive realization of the rights to water and sanitation including through the adoption of measures that guarantee access to basic services for vulnerable users according to their circumstances and needs. Utilities may also need additional financial or other forms of support from the government and other stakeholders to improve their capacity to mitigate any negative impacts on their operations caused by the pandemic and the duty to expand services to vulnerable groups.

Overall, COVID-19 has triggered the active engagement of the public and private sector, including multiple stakeholder and grassroots social networks, in efforts to limit the spread of the pandemic and mitigate the resulting social and economic disruptions and other environmental problems (Kanda & Kivimaa 2020; Shorfuzzaman, Hossain, & Alhamid 2021; Rume & Islam 2020). COVID-19 has significantly influenced the behaviors of individuals and the operations of businesses, particularly in relation to sustainable consumption and environmental awareness (Severo, De Guimarães, & Dellarmelin 2020). Also, the impacts of the pandemic are likely to last into the recovery phase and beyond (Rowan & Laffey 2021). The evidence highlights the potential of COVID-19 to elicit sustainability transitions in diverse sectors (Karmaker et al. 2021; Wells, Abouarghoub, Pettit, & Beresford 2020). As regards water and sanitation, the pandemic could similarly shape a transition to inclusive service delivery models and be used in collective demands and claims by social groups requesting national and local authorities to respect, protect, and fulfill the human rights to water and sanitation (Parikh, Diep, Gupte, & Lakhanpaul 2020).

Notes

1 Beyond the International Bill of Rights, the rights to water and sanitation have been recognized in a variety of human rights treaties and international declarations and standards. See for instance, Article 14, paragraph 2, of the Convention on the Elimination of All Forms of Discrimination Against Women, which stipulates that States parties shall ensure to women the right to 'enjoy adequate living conditions, particularly in relation to … water supply'. Article 24, paragraph 2, of the Convention on the Rights of the Child requires States parties to combat disease and malnutrition 'through the provision of adequate nutritious foods and clean drinking water'.

2 It is debatable whether the right to life can form the legal basis for the recognition of the right to water (cf. Kiefer & Brölmann 2005). Obani & Gupta (2015) consider some of the limitations that are associated with implying the rights to water and sanitation from other substantive rights rather than explicit recognition of water and sanitation as independent rights.

References

Action Against Hunger 2020, 'Quarantine and Isolation Center Alert', July 2020, viewed 2 October 2020, www.actioncontrelafaim.org/wp-content/uploads/2020/07/ACF-Quarantine-Center-Alert-V3.pdf

Agence France-Presse 2020, 'Toilet Rolls, Hand Sanitisers, Masks Fly Off Shelves Amid Coronavirus Fears', NDTV, 5 March 2020, viewed 5 October 2020, www.ndtv.com/world-news/toilet-rolls-hand-sanitisers-masks-fly-off-shelves-amid-coronavirus-fears-2190143

Alston, P 2018, *Extreme Poverty and Human Rights*, United Nations General Assembly A/73/39.

Amankwah-Amoah, J 2020, 'Stepping Up and Stepping Out of COVID-19: New Challenges for Environmental Sustainability Policies in the Global Airline Industry', *Journal of Cleaner Production*, vol. 271, p. 123000 https://doi.org/10.1016/j.jclepro.2020.123000

Arce, S & Forti, J 2020, 'Open Government Approaches to Tackling COVID-19', *Open Government Partnership*, 12 May 2020, viewed 5 October 2020, www.opengovpartnership.org/stories/open-government-approaches-to-tackling-covid-19/

Banerji, A 2020, 'Coronavirus and Stigma among Priorities for India's new Transgender Council', *Reuters*, viewed 25 September 2020, www.reuters.com/article/us-india-lgbt-council-idUSKBN25L1V1

Barry, KB 2020, *Right to Education*, United Nations General Assembly A/75/178.
Bhowmick, GD, Dhar, D, & Nath, D et al. 2020, 'Coronavirus Disease 2019 (COVID-19) Outbreak: Some Serious Consequences with Urban and Rural Water Cycle', npj *Clean Water*, vol. 3, 32.
Birkenholtz T 2016, 'Drinking Water' in P Jackson, W Spiess, & F Sultana (eds), Eating, Drinking: Surviving, Springer, Cham, pp. 23–30.
Bogler, A, Packman, A, Furman, A, Gross, A, Kushmaro, A, Ronen, A et al. 2020, 'Rethinking Wastewater Risks and Monitoring in Light of the COVID-19 Pandemic', *Nature Sustainability*. https://doi.org/10.1038/s41893-020-00605-2.
Brown, A 2020, 'The Pandemic Has Closed Public Restrooms, and Many Have Nowhere to Go', *PEW*, 23 July, viewed 2 October 2020, www.pewtrusts.org/en/research-and-analysis/blogs/stateline/2020/07/23/the-pandemic-has-closed-public-restrooms-and-many-have-nowhere-to-go
Butler, G, Pilotto RG, HongY, & Mutambatsere E, 2020, The Impact of COVID-19 on the Water and Sanitation Sector, IFC World Bank Group, viewed 5 October 2020, www.ifc.org/wps/wcm/connect/126b1a18-23d9-46f3-beb7-047c20885bf6/The+Impact+of+COVID_Water%26Sanitation_final_web.pdf?MOD=AJPERES&CVID=ncaG-hA
Capodeferro, MW & Smiderle, JJ 2020, 'The Brazilian Sanitation Sector's Response to COVID-19', *Revista de Administração Pública*, vol. 54, no. 4, pp. 1022–1036.
Carman, KJ & Nataraj, S 2020, *How are Americans Paying Their Bills during the COVID-19 Pandemic?*, Rand Corporation, viewed 5 October 2020, www.rand.org/pubs/research_reports/RRA308-3.html
Chau, S, Albuquerque, A, Guerrini, A, & Werneck, J 2020, 'COVID-19: The Regulators' Response in Brazil', 29 April, online video, viewed 5 October 2020, https://iwa-network.org/learn/covid-19-a-regulators-response/
Daughton, CD 2020, 'Wastewater Surveillance for Population-wide Covid-19: The Present and Future', vol. 736, p. 139631.
Ellis, K & Feris, L 2014, 'The Right to Sanitation: Time to Delink from the Right to Water', *Human Rights Quarterly: A Comparative and International Journal of the Social Sciences, Philosophy, and Law*, vol. 36, no. 3, pp. 607–629.
Feris, L 2015, 'The Human Right to Sanitation: A Critique on the Absence of Environmental Considerations', *Review of European, Comparative & International Environmental Law*, vol. 24, no. 1, pp. 16–26.
Fukuda, S, Noda, K, & Oki, T 2019, 'How Global Targets on Drinking Water Were Developed and Achieved', *Nature Sustainability*, vol. 2, no. 5, pp. 429–434.
General Assembly 2010a, *Resolution Adopted by the General Assembly on 28 July 2010 64/292: The Human Right to Water and Sanitation*, United Nations General Assembly A/RES/64/292.
General Assembly 2010b, *General Assembly Adopts Resolution Recognizing Access to Clean Water, Sanitation as Human Right, by Recorded Vote of 122 in Favour, None Against, 41 Abstentions*, United Nations, viewed 1 October 2020, www.un.org/press/en/2010/ga10967.doc.htm
Gout, E & Kelly, C 2020, 'Bridging the Water Access Gap Through COVID-19 Relief', *Center for American Progress*, 5 August, viewed 2 October 2020, //www.americanprogress.org/issues/green/news/2020/08/05/488705/bridging-water-access-gap-covid-19-relief/.
Gupta, J, Pouw, N, & Ros-Tonen, M 2015, 'Towards an Elaborated Theory of Inclusive Development', *European Journal of Development Research*, vol. 27, pp. 541–559. https://doi.org/10.1057/ejdr.2015.30.
Hall RP, Van Koppen B, & Van Houweling E 2014, 'The Human Right to Water: the Importance of Domestic and Productive Water Rights', *Science and Engineering Ethics*, vol. 20, no. 4, pp. 849–868. doi:10.1007/s11948-013-9499-3.

Heller, L 2015, *Different Levels and Types of Services and the Human Rights to Water and Sanitation*, United Nations General Assembly A/70/203.

Heller, L 2018, Expert Consultation on the Human Rights to Water and Sanitation of Forcibly Displaced People in Need of Humanitarian Assistance – Organized by the UN Special Rapporteur on the Human Rights to Safe Drinking Water and Sanitation, Léo Heller, held on 16–17 May 2018, Geneva.

Heller, L 2020, *Human Rights and the Privatization of Water and Sanitation Services*, United Nations General Assembly A/75/208.

Human Rights Council 2010, *Resolution Adopted by the Human Rights Council 15/9: Human Rights and Access to Safe Drinking Water and Sanitation*, United Nations Human Rights Council A/HRC/RES/15/9.

Human Rights Watch 2020, 'Human Rights Dimension of COVID-19 Response', *Human Rights Watch*, 19 March, viewed 2 October 2020, www.hrw.org/news/2020/03/19/human-rights-dimensions-covid-19-response

Jafri, AA 2020, 'No Food, Water, or Even Soap: Migrant Workers in Quarantine Desperate to Return Home', *News Click*, 17 April, viewed 2 October 2020, www.newsclick.in/Uttar-Pradesh-Migrant-Workers-Quarantine-Conditions-COVID-19

Johannessen, A, Rosemarin, A, Thomalla, F, Swartling, AG, Stenström, TA, Vulturius, G 2014, 'Strategies for Building Resilience to Hazards in Water, Sanitation and Hygiene (WASH) Systems: The Role of Public Private Partnerships', *International Journal of Disaster Risk Reduction*, vol. 10, no. A, pp. 102–115. https://doi.org/10.1016/j.ijdrr.2014.07.002.

Jordan – Socio-economic Framework for COVID-19 Response, viewed 5 October 2020, https://reliefweb.int/sites/reliefweb.int/files/resources/JOR_Socioeconomic-Response-Plan_2020.pdf

Joshi, N 2017, 'Low-income Women's Right to Sanitation Services in City Public Spaces: A Study of Waste Picker Women in Pune', *Environment & Urbanization*, vol. 30, no. 1, pp. 249–264. DOI: 10.1177/0956247817744932.

Kalbusch A, Henning E, Brikalski MP, Luca FV, & Konrath AC 2020, 'Impact of Coronavirus (COVID-19) Spread-prevention Actions on Urban Water Consumption', *Resource, Conservation, and Recycling*, vol. 163, p. 105098. doi:10.1016/j.resconrec.2020.105098.

Kanda, W & Kivimaa, P 2020, 'What Opportunities Could the COVID-19 Outbreak Offer for Sustainability Transitions Research on Electricity and mobility'?, *Energy Research & Social Science*, vol. 68, p. 101666 https://doi.org/10.1016/j.erss.2020.101666

Karmaker, CL et al. 2021, 'Improving Supply Chain Sustainability in the Context of COVID-19 Pandemic in an Emerging Economy: Exploring Drivers Using an Integrated Model', *Sustainable Production and Consumption*, vol. 26, pp. 411–427 https://doi.org/10.1016/j.spc.2020.09.019.

Khan, C 2020, 'Public Inconvenience: How Lockdown Caused a Loo Crisis', *The Guardian*, 9 June, viewed 2 October 2020, www.theguardian.com/society/2020/jun/09/public-inconvenience-lockdown-loo-crisis-restrictions-easing-uk-no-public-toilets

Kiefer, T & Brölmann, C 2005, 'Beyond State Sovereignty: The Human Right to Water', *Non-State Actors and International Law*, vol. 5, no. 3, pp. 183–208.

Kumari, N & Pisharody, A 2020, *Bangalore Quarantine Centres: No Food, No Water and no Hygiene*, Gauri Lankesh News, 4 June, viewed 2 October 2020, https://gaurilankeshnews.com/bangalore-quarantine-centres-no-food-no-water-and-no-hygiene/

Local Burden of Disease WaSH Collaborators 2020, 'Mapping Geographical Inequalities in Access to Drinking Water and Sanitation Facilities in Low-income and Middle-income Countries, 2000–17', *Lancet Glob Health*, vol. 8, pp. e1162– e1185.

Mao, F 2020, 'Coronavirus Panic: Why Are People Stockpiling Toilet Paper?', *BBC News*,, 4 March 2020, viewed 5 October 2020, https://www.bbc.com/news/world-australia-51731422

McGranahan, G 2015, 'Realizing the Right to Sanitation in Deprived Urban Communities: Meeting the Challenges of Collective Action, Coproduction, Affordability, and Housing Tenure', *World Development*, vol. 68, pp. 242–253.

Mullen, C 2020, 'Toilet Paper's back, but These Items Have Become Hard to Find', *The Business Journals*, 20 July, viewed 5 October 2020, https://www.bizjournals.com/bizwomen/news/latest-news/2020/07/toilet-papers-back-these-items-hard-to-find.html?page=all

Obani, P 2020, 'SDG 6.2 and the Right to Sanitation: Exploring the Complementarities and Incoherence', *UNIPORT Journal of International and Comparative Law*, vol. 1, no. 1, pp. 1–17.

Obani, P & Gupta, J 2014, 'Legal Pluralism in the Area of Human Rights: Water and Sanitation', *Current Opinion in Environmental Sustainability*, vol. 11, pp. 63–70.

Obani, P & Gupta, J 2015, 'The Evolution of the Right to Water and Sanitation: Differentiating the Implications', *Review of European, Comparative & International Environmental Law*, vol. 24, no. 1, pp. 27–39. doi:10.1111/reel.12095.

Ortman E 2020, 'Women Struggle to Access Menstrual products during COVID-19 Pandemic', *Society for Women's Health Research*, 27 May 2020, viewed 2 October 2020, https://swhr.org/women-struggle-to-access-menstrual-products-during-covid-19-pandemic/

Parikh, P, Diep, L, Gupte, J, & Lakhanpaul, M 2020, 'COVID-19 Challenges and WASH in Informal Settlements: integrated Action Supported by the Sustainable Development Goals', *Cities*, vol. 107, p. 102871 https://doi.org/10.1016/j.cities.2020.102871.

Patrício Silva, A. L., Prata, J. C., Walker, T. R., Duarte, A. C., Ouyang, W., Barcelò, D., & Rocha-Santos, T. (2021). 'Increased Plastic Pollution Due to COVID-19 Pandemic: Challenges and Recommendations'. *Chemical Engineering Journal* (Lausanne, Switzerland: 1996), vol. 405, p. 126683. https://doi.org/10.1016/j.cej.2020.126683

Plan International 2020, *Coronavirus is Making Periods Worse for Girls and Women*, 28 May 2020, viewed 2 October 2020, https://plan-international.org/news/2020-05-28-coronavirus-making-periods-worse-girls-and-women

Rowan, NJ & Laffey, JG 2021, 'Unlocking the Surge in Demand for Personal and Protective Equipment (PPE) and Improvised Face Coverings Arising from Coronavirus Disease (COVID-19) Pandemic – Implications for Efficacy, Re-use and Sustainable Waste Management', *Science of The Total Environment*, vol. 752, p. 142259, https://doi.org/10.1016/j.scitotenv.2020.142259

Rume, T & Didar-Ul Islam, SM 2020, 'Environmental Effects of COVID-19 Pandemic and Potential Strategies of Sustainability', *Heliyon*, vol. 6, no. 9, p. e04965 https://doi.org/10.1016/j.heliyon.2020.e04965

Severo, EA, De Guimarães, GCF, & Dellarmelin, ML 2020, 'Impact of the COVID-19 Pandemic on Environmental Awareness, Sustainable Consumption and Social Responsibility: Evidence from Generations in Brazil and Portugal', *Journal of Cleaner Production*, https://doi.org/10.1016/j.jclepro.2020.124947

Shorfuzzaman, M, Hossain, MS, &Alhamid, MF 2021, 'Towards the Sustainable Development of Smart Cities through Mass Video Surveillance: A Response to the COVID-19 Pandemic', *Sustainable Cities and Society*, vol. 64, p.102582 https://doi.org/10.1016/j.scs.2020.102582

Sinharoy, SS, Pittluck, R, & Clasen, T 2019, 'Review of Drivers and Barriers of Water and Sanitation Policies for Urban Informal Settlements in Low-income and Middle-income Countries', *Utilities Policy*, vol. 60, p. 100957. https://doi.org/10.1016/j.jup.2019.100957

Street, R, Malemaa, S, Mahlangenia, N, & Mathee, A 2020, 'Wastewater Surveillance for Covid-19: An African Perspective', *Science of the Total Environment*, vol. 743, p. 140719.

Tan, Y 2020, 'Covid-19 Singapore: A 'Pandemic of Inequality' Exposed', *BBC News*, viewed 25 September 2020, www.bbc.com/news/world-asia-54082861

Tapfumaneyi, R 2020, 'Residents' Victory as Court Orders Harare City to Deliver Clean Water Daily', *New Zimbabwe*, 2 April, viewed 22 September 2020, www.newzimbabwe.com/residents-victory-as-court-orders-harare-city-to-deliver-clean-water-daily/

Tonne, C 2020, 'Lessons from the COVID-19 Pandemic for Accelerating Sustainable Development', *Environmental Research*, p. 110482 https://doi.org/10.1016/j.envres.2020.110482

UNESCO n.d., *Education: From Disruption to Recovery*, viewed 25 September 2020, https://en.unesco.org/covid19/educationresponse

United Nations 2020, *The Sustainable Development Goals Report 2020*, United Nations, New York.

United Nations Children's Fund (UNICEF) 2020, UNICEF COVID-19 WASH Response C/3/2020: *COVID-19 WASH Responses by Governments, Water Utilities and Stakeholders in Middle East and North Africa (MENA) Countries*, UNICEF, New York.

UNICEF & World Health Organization (WHO) 2020, *Progress on Drinking Water, Sanitation and Hygiene in Schools: Special Focus on COVID-19*, UNICEF and WHO, New York.

Vardoulakis, S, Sheel M, Lal, A, & Gray, D 2020, 'COVID-19 Environmental Transmission and Preventive Public Health Measures', *Australian and New Zealand Journal of Public Health*, online. doi: 10.1111/1753-6405.13033.

Viñuales, JE 2019, 'The Protocol on Water and Health as a Strategy for Global Water Governance Integration', *International & Comparative Law Quarterly*, vol. 68, no. 1, pp. 175–192. doi:10.1017/S0020589318000362

Wang, C, Pan, J, Yaya, S, Yadav, RB, & Yao, D 2019, 'Geographic Inequalities in Accessing Improved Water and Sanitation Facilities in Nepal', *International Journal of Environmental Research and Public Health*, vol. 16, no. 7, pp. 1269–1281. https://doi.org/10.3390/ijerph16071269

WaterLex 2014a, *The Human Rights to Water and Sanitation in Courts Worldwide: A Selection of National, Regional, and International Case Law*, WaterLex, Geneva.

WaterLex 2014b, *National Human Rights Institutions and Water Governance: Compilation of Good Practices*, WaterLex, Geneva.

Water Supply & Sanitation Collaborative Council (WSSCC) 2020, *Report on Leave No One Behind*, WSSCC, Geneva.

Water Supply & Sanitation Collaborative Council (WSSCC) & United Nations Human Rights Office of the High Commissioner (OHCHR) 2020, *Interdependencies between Water and Sanitation and Other Human Rights. Strengthening Accountability of States and Partners through the Human Rights Council and Voluntary National Review Processes to Leave No One Behind in SDG 6 – Roundtable Report*, WSSCC, Geneva.

Wells, P, Abouarghoub, W, Pettit, S, & Beresford, A 2020, 'A Socio-Technical Transitions Perspective for Assessing Future Sustainability Following the COVID-19 Pandemic', *Sustainability: Science, Practice and Policy*, vol. 16, no. 1, pp. 29–36.

Werneck, J 2020, COVID-19: The Regulators' Response in Brazil, 29 April, online video, viewed 5 October 2020, https://iwa-network.org/learn/covid-19-a-regulators-response/

World Health Organization (WHO) 2020, *Status of Environmental Surveillance for SARS-CoV-2 virus*, Scientific Brief, WHO, Geneva. WHO/2019-nCoV/Sci_Brief/EnvironmentalSampling/2020.1

World Health Organization, UN-Water 2019, *National Systems to Support Drinking-Water, Sanitation and Hygiene: Global Status Report 2019*. UN-Water Global Analysis and Assessment of Sanitation and Drinking Water (GLAAS) 2019 Report, World Health Organization, Geneva.

14

LAND RIGHTS IN CRISIS

Juliana Nnoko-Mewanu

Governments and business enterprises, including national elites, are taking advantage of the current global health crisis, containment measures, and weakened government and civil society scrutiny to 'grab' land.[1]

Land deals that are illegal – contested or without government authorization – or that lack community buy-in, have long resulted in forced evictions, human rights abuses, and conflicts, particularly in countries with weak land governance frameworks (Cotula & Berger 2017). These land deals and consequent land-related developments involve changes in the control of land (often changed property regimes) and exploitation of natural resources such as water, trees, and forest products, to the detriment of interests held by Indigenous peoples and local communities (Gilbert 2018). Indigenous peoples' culture, way of life, and survival have come under attack from business enterprises illegally expanding their operations onto Indigenous territories without their free, prior, and informed consent (AIPP 2020).

Large-scale land deals that are backed by government officials and strongly contested by local individuals and communities who would lose access to land, water, and food resources are not new (Dell'Angelo et al. 2017). These investments raise complex issues across various dimensions – legal, economic, social, environmental, ethical, and cultural (Gilbert 2018). Risks for local communities include the loss of customary or legal control over land that they use, deepening inequalities in access to land, as well as environmental degradation (Kugelman & Levenstein 2013). Yet, some governments seem willing to disregard the evidence of such risks. They fail to mitigate future harm to affected communities through meaningful consultation with the full participation of everyone who might be impacted (El Tiempo 2020).

Government and private sector initiatives to undermine access to and control of land used by communities, including Indigenous peoples, are not an accidental by-product of the current health crisis (Szoke-Burke 2020; Cotula 2020). These types of badly executed land-related developments are run-of-the-mill in countries with weak legal frameworks and weak democracies, but they are also more likely to occur during or after a crisis, such as an armed conflict (Westerman 2020), a natural disaster (Uson 2017), a health crisis (Global Witness 2015), or folded within supposedly well-intentioned development and conservation agendas (Bayrak & Marafa 2016).

In the months following the World Health Organization's declaration of a global coronavirus pandemic, attention to land governance, including policy reform and funding, seemed to vanish. Like many other sectors not explicitly related to health, health-related emergency responses have superseded concerns about land rights as the novel coronavirus ravaged across the world, crippling healthcare systems and economies (Wieckardt, van der Haar, & van Westen 2020). Governments raced to close borders, restrict movement, and shut down non-essential services in a bid to curb infection rates. Government agencies, including land governance offices and non-government entities specialized in monitoring and mediating land conflicts, temporarily closed (KTV News Kenya 2020; Daily Monitor Uganda 2020). In many countries, the activities of the judiciary were also temporarily suspended.

This suspension of 'non-essential' branches of government resulted in what Cotula (2020) termed 'policy grabs' by national governments, elites, and business enterprises. As regulators have turned their attention away from land and watchdog groups have been locked down or constrained, land 'grabbers' have been on the move (Szoke-Burke 2020; Cotula 2020). In some cases, authorities have facilitated this (Cotula 2021; HRW 2020a; OHCHR 2020a; Earthworks et al. 2020).

This chapter describes reported incidents of land rights violations by government and non-state actors within the context of the COVID-19 pandemic. Section 1 of the chapter briefly introduces the human rights-based approach based on existing international laws and standards related to land and property rights. Section 2 discusses how crises influence public policy, specifically highlighting Naomi Klein's (2007) 'disaster capitalism' narrative. For example, land rights have been violated during previous crises, such as Liberia's Ebola crisis, and other non-health crises such as natural disasters, wars, and internal conflicts. Section 3 examines how, with government oversight and enforcement mechanisms under strain, private individuals and business enterprises have pushed to dispossess communities and Indigenous people of land, exacerbating poverty and other vulnerabilities. Section 4 assesses government failures to protect land rights, and how some governments weakened key protections, including on meaningful public consultations relevant to land proceedings. Section 5 describes new policies to restrict social activism and criminalize the actions of activists as they work to protect their land and document intimidation and violence experienced during the pandemic. The chapter concludes by outlining basic interventions that governments can take to protect rights for communities, Indigenous peoples, and particularly women, and ensure transparency within the land sector.

1 Human rights and land: a rights-based approach

International and regional human rights treaties establish standards relevant to land use, agricultural development, and the rights of affected individuals and communities (OHCHR 2015). International law protects rights related to land and security of tenure, including the rights to an adequate standard of living, rights related to property, and prohibitions on forced evictions (UDHR 1948). Land rights specific to Indigenous peoples are protected within international law (UNDRIP 2007). Businesses also have responsibilities to conduct human rights due diligence to identify actual and potential adverse human rights impacts, avoid or mitigate causing or contributing to human rights abuses through their operations, and remediate harm when it occurs (UN Guiding Principles 2011).

Importantly, neither international nor regional human rights protections on housing or property hinge on individuals holding formal title to land or property. The UN Committee on Economic, Social and Cultural Rights (CESCR) emphasizes that rights protections apply whether or not individuals hold formal title. The CESCR notes in its General Comment No. 4 that legal security of tenure 'takes a variety of forms, including … occupation of land or property. Notwithstanding the type of tenure, all persons should possess a degree of security of tenure which guarantees legal protection against forced eviction, harassment and other threats' (CESCR 1991).

Land governance based on human rights standards promotes more equitable and secure tenure and advances a human rights-centered development (Wisborg 2013).

2 'Shock strategy' and land rights in a crisis

Governments, companies, and national elites use their access to information and socio-political clout to forcibly acquire land even in cases where the land is claimed or managed under customary or Indigenous systems (Nnoko-Mewanu 2016). Previous research has highlighted how these actors take advantage of crisis, including non-health crises such as natural disasters, wars, and internal conflicts, to acquire land (Uson 2017; Klein 2007).

Naomi Klein (2007) used the term 'disaster capitalism' to describe how post-disaster governments and corporate alliances, with help from international financial institutions (IFIs), take advantage of devastation to create market opportunities that tend to disadvantage the poorest groups in society. Land-related development planning is often ongoing while those seeking to acquire or exploit land wait for the right time – namely a disaster or crisis – to push forward. Since the food crisis of 2008 unprecedented amounts of capital have been invested in land, especially farmland, as security for financial instruments and traded on global markets (Fairbarn 2015). Reports on farmlandgrab.org highlight that these deals are ongoing in the first months of the COVID-19 pandemic. According to Klein, a crisis presents the perfect window of opportunity to transfer ownership or to jump-start or expand operations. She aptly coined the term 'shock doctrine' to 'describe the brutal tactic of using the public's disorientation following a collective shock – wars, coups, terrorist attacks, market crashes or natural disasters – to push through radical pro-corporate measures' (Klein 2007, 2017).

Thus the current particularities of dispossession and policy grabs during the COVID-19 crisis are not unique, especially in a context dominated by insecure property rights or land tenure insecurities and weak democracies. But shoddy land acquisitions take on an especially sinister cloak when viewed in the context of a health crisis. In 2015 Global Witness reported how business enterprises, with the help of government officials, more than doubled their land holdings during the Ebola crisis in Liberia by encouraging local community members, who were devastated by the spread of the virus and countless deaths, to sign over their land (Global Witness 2015).

According to Klein's logic, the current global health, social, and economic challenges create the shock that governments and corporate interests could use to push through policies that benefit their interests at the expense of communities. The difference from past examples lies in the scale, as governments across the world take a page out of the 'disaster capitalism' playbook.

3 Government oversight and enforcement mechanisms under strain due to the pandemic

Land governance in many countries in the Global South has been secretive and covert, resulting in calls for transparency from civil society actors (Transparency International 2020). According to international obligations, governments ought to oversee land transactions and regulate land-based investments, keeping all players in line and ensuring that local communities are not made worse off by land-related developments. Authorities should be transparent about licenses, permits, leases, regulatory decisions, and other actions that impact land. Unfortunately, that was rarely the case before the pandemic. And with all eyes focused on the coronavirus health crisis, land transparency is poised to get even worse.

At the onset of the pandemic, governments were faced with enormous uncertainties regarding the trajectory, impacts, and responses. After the World Health Organization (WHO) declared the coronavirus to be a pandemic, governments quickly implemented containment measures, temporarily shutting down non-essential services, restricting movement, and requiring 'social distancing'.

Government officials, including those working in the land sector, stayed home. They were unsure when they would resume work and were often incapable of performing key monitoring functions remotely. Services halted at ministries of land, environment, and the judiciary, while field enforcement agents were hemmed in by quickly implemented shelter-in-place measures (Gross et al. 2020). In Kenya, for example, the Ministry of Lands and Physical Planning closed its operations for about two months following government directives to shut down non-essential services (Mwagae 2020).

In Brazil, the operations of government environment agents charged with monitoring illegal activity within the Amazon forest ground to a halt (Pearshouse

& Werneck 2020). Brazil decreed environmental protection an 'essential service' during the pandemic, but in practice, under the lockdown and facing risk of infection, environmental authorities have less capacity to fulfill their enforcement roles (Spring 2020). Illegal forest fire activity increased during the pandemic, with more fire hotspots compared to the same months in 2019 (Programa Queimadas). Illegal land-grabbing, mining, logging, and poaching in the Brazilian Amazon appeared to continue at full steam, with criminals using the pandemic period to ramp up deforestation in the region. According to the National Institute of Space Research's (INPE) real-time deforestation detection system, alerts of deforestation in the Amazon increased 64 percent in April 2020, compared to the same month in 2019 (The Brazilian Report 2020; Jordan 2020). Data from multiple sources paint a similar picture across Asia and Africa as well (Gross et al. 2020).

As months of these lockdown restrictions wore on, some governments cut back financial and human resources in the land governance sector, focusing instead on the healthcare sector while managing the economic downturn resulting from the pandemic (Spring 2020). For example, Ecuador and Mexico announced cuts in most government ministries, including environment and land-related agencies, which would impact resources allocated to monitoring (Lopez-Feldman et al. 2020). This is further exacerbated when the government is redirecting funding from the land sector, seriously hampering the monitoring of illegal activity (Spring 2020).

The reduced scrutiny, oversight, and funding in the land governance sector creates the opening for interests that have long been seeking to acquire swaths of land, expand operations to more land, or activate previous land concession contracts that are fiercely contested and have been dormant.

4 Government failures to protect land are exacerbating inequality and poverty

The reports of government failures to protect land that is owned or used traditionally in rural communities and Indigenous territories from dispossession, including criminalization of the actions of environment and land rights defenders, highlight how the vulnerabilities of poorer and disadvantaged groups are exacerbated during the pandemic (Cotula 2020). A multitude of players, including government officials, elites, and national and multinational businesses, are involved in numerous incidences of evictions, demolitions, and land dispossessions that have occurred during the pandemic (The Brazilian Report 2020; Chandran 2020). Reports of lapses in land governance across several countries highlight how national elites are profiting from diminished government oversight and accountability to seize lands (Chandran 2020).

Some countries have set in motion processes to weaken protections over land and the environment (AIPP 2020). For example, Indonesia adopted a contested mining law during the pandemic without adequate public participation, according to media reporting (Harsono 2020). The law removes previous limits on the land concession size that can be awarded by the government and allows for automatic contract renewal by mining companies, limiting oversight and accountability possibilities (Harsono 2020). In October 2020, Indonesia also passed an omnibus law that weakens environmental protections with limited public consultation (Amnesty International 2020). The law fast-tracks environmental decisions and business authorizations to exploit land, consequently shrinking the opportunity for community land rights holders to meaningfully participate in processes that would affect their land and livelihood (HRW 2020b). In Colombia, the government announced a plan to hold all consultations for environmental impact assessment processes virtually, even though the poorest or most remote communities would have no or inadequate access to the internet, preventing them from participating fully in these proceedings (El Tiempo 2020). Alda Salomão (2020) provides examples in Mozambique of companies moving consultations online, negatively impacting public participation in land-related decision-making processes. These moves to virtual consultations add another obstacle to communities being able to participate fully in land-related decisions, since all other obstacles to full meaningful participation continue to exist and are exacerbated in the pandemic.

Such opaque and exclusive processes best serve the interests of corrupt and well-positioned elites in the short-term. Even if some affected communities could access these online forums or 'invited spaces', empirical research suggests that the scope for communities to exercise real influence in these spaces will be limited and sometimes mask new forms of control (Cheyns 2011). This is especially true when the agenda is set by particular interests and discussion topics reflect interests of the business operation without allowing discussion of possible impacts and consequences for local communities. All participants need access to sufficient information that allows them to effectively engage in the decision-making process. Procedures for participation and decision-making should explicitly and effectively include the concerns of local people and foster their robust participation in decision-making within any consultative forum.

Not only have some governments weakened policies related to land and shrunk space for public participation; some have fast-tracked land acquisition procedures, reducing opportunities for communities and Indigenous groups to protest, resist, and contest their dispossession (Szoke-Burke 2020). For example, the United States federal government was reported to have accelerated its effort through numerous lawsuits to seize private land along the Rio Grande to build a border wall, while residents sheltered in place, unable to meet with relatives to discuss the government's offers or the lawsuits (Kanno-Youngs 2020).

In some cases, governments have been perpetrators of dispossession, forcibly evicting Indigenous people from their ancestral lands and demolishing urban settlements deemed illegal. In Kenya, not only has the government failed to implement orders from the African Court on Human and Peoples' Rights to reinstate land managed and used by the Ogiek, an Indigenous group, but in July 2020 it allegedly forcibly evicted about 300 families from their homes in the Mau Forest (Lang 2020). Evictions, driven by the Kenyan government's conservation efforts, and backed by international donors and financial institutions, occurred even before the pandemic (HRW 2019). However, in addition to 'conservation evictions' in the Mau Forest, the government carried out a series of forced evictions under the guise of development, also backed by international financial institutions, across multiple cities in Kenya during the pandemic. This exposed evictees to increased risk of infection (HRW 2020c).

5 Intimidation and violence against land and environmental rights defenders

Before and during the pandemic, governments have blacklisted activists and criminalized the actions of environment and land defenders who organize to resist through protests and demonstrations (OHCHR 2020c). During the pandemic some governments have attempted to put in place new rules that criminalize protests and limit freedom of speech and assembly, restricting social activism and penalizing individuals and communities that resist the loss of their land (HRW 2020a). Some governments have deployed security forces to disperse non-violent protests against the expansion of company operations, frequently resulting in the use of excessive force by the police.

With governments exempting some business that they consider 'essential' – in a bid to push economic recovery and to continue operations, particularly in the mining, agricultural, and forestry sectors – some have taken the opportunity to strengthen their claims to land that is contested by local communities, including Indigenous people, who live on, use, and manage the land (Jong 2020). A report jointly produced by a coalition of organizations provides a snapshot of how the mining industry impacted communities' health and environment during the pandemic, including how some mining companies used government-imposed lockdown to advance exploration activities onto Indigenous lands (Earthworks et al. 2020). In Cambodia, rights groups accused a Vietnamese company of clearing land that had been designated for return to an Indigenous group (Nguyen 2020). In some cases, environmental decisions and permits have been granted, facilitating the authorization of new land concessions, even in situations in which these projects were contested by local communities that would be negatively impacted by the project. For example, a mega pipeline expansion project in Canada, which government officials describe as a 'vital interest' to the country, was under construction despite fierce opposition from environmentalists and some Indigenous groups in Canada (Cecco 2020).

Communities and individuals who have publicly protested and organized demonstrations denouncing encroachment on their lands have been arrested by government security forces for violating shelter-in-place policies and some have been threatened with violence in a bid to heavily control or suppress such mobilization. For example, in the United States, several states have signed infrastructure laws that create new felony penalties for protest actions within their states targeting oil and gas facilities during the pandemic (Brown 2020). In Turkey, activists protesting against a mine were violently evicted, with authorities imposing an administrative fine citing non-compliance with COVID-19 measures (Duvar English 2020).

Civil society organizations have reported a heightened threat to environment and land activists across the world (Forst & Taylor 2020; Turkewitz & Villamil 2020). Organizations that advocate for land rights and communities whose lands are impacted have had difficulties communicating, organizing, and mobilizing during the pandemic. In South Africa, an environment and land rights defender was gunned down in her home after her refusal to withdraw legal challenges to existing and future mining operations near her town (HRW 2020d). These threats existed even before the pandemic, but reduced government monitoring, lapses in security details assigned to protect individuals or communities at risk, and stalled judicial processes have heightened the insecurities that activists experience (Daniels 2020). In remote areas where government oversight is weak, the distraction of the pandemic has emboldened the individuals and entities who threaten communities resisting the illegal taking of their land (BBC 2020; Turkewitz & Villamil 2020).

Judicial processes have been stalled due to court closures, resulting in limited access to justice for defenders. This stands in stark contrast to the innovative administrative proceedings that governments implemented relatively quickly to continue consideration of business and land concessions. In some cases, activists who have been arrested are stuck in detention, with pretrial hearings delayed, pending investigation (Nugraha & Marie 2020). Communities may face limited possibilities in terms of obtaining an injunction order suspending business activities that they consider illegal, pending a full investigation by the police (Chandran 2020; Wieckardt, van der Haar, & van Westen 2020). This means that resisting communities are left to do what they can to halt expansion into land they claim, and this sometimes sparks a violent clash between business operators and the community, resulting in police intervention and further arrests.

6 Conclusion

During the first eight months of the pandemic, governments and corporations have used environmental and land-related policies and interventions for their own benefit. The root causes lie in vulnerabilities that existed long before the COVID-19 crisis. The devastating impact of the pandemic on racial and ethnic minorities and the poorest groups highlights the need for changes to avoid 'disaster capitalism' and 'shock tactics' in the future (Klein 2007).

Governments have largely failed to protect people's rights to land and property and, in some cases, have exacerbated vulnerabilities. The chapter has presented patterns of worsened inequality and poverty among people with the least secure rights to land. Given the current economic recession due to the pandemic, governments might rush to deregulate the environment, land, and investment sectors, further weakening protections for local communities, including Indigenous peoples. Any unregulated increases in natural resource exploitation to drive economic growth would result only in short-term benefits and only at the national level (as opposed to local), if at all (Cotula & Schwartz 2020).

In a time of crisis, governments should strengthen rather than weaken land and environmental protections and create effective responses to secure land rights for the most vulnerable (Mwangi, Makelova, & Meinzen-Dick 2012). Human rights experts from the United Nations and the Inter-American Commission for Human Rights issued a statement calling on governments in the Americas to strengthen rather than weaken policies around environmental protections (OHCHR 2020b). For example, while online consultative forums would exclude affected communities and some of the poorest and most vulnerable people, governments can explore technology that can be used in an inclusive manner to empower communities (Cadasta.org).

Land-based investments can generate benefits if they are placed within broader national strategies on rural development that prioritize improving the lives of local farmers and building communities that are resilient to future crises (Szoke-Burke 2020). This fits well within governments' international legal obligations to protect and promote civil and political rights, as well as the progressive realization of economic, social, and cultural rights (OHCHR 2015). Governments must refrain from violating these rights and prevent private companies – such as land-based investment operations – from violating fundamental human rights.

The current situation provides a window of opportunity for governments to put in place viable systems that reflect the cost of monitoring and ensure that people's rights are respected and that businesses comply with national laws, even during a crisis (Cosens et al. 2017). Similarly, during a crisis and with limited oversight options, governments should suspend issuance of permits for land-based development projects and allocation of land for new investments if the necessary resources to enforce national laws and hold businesses accountable for non-compliance are limited. Instead, governments should prioritize finding ways to effectively and responsibly regulate and manage land-related resources during and after the pandemic to protect community rights and wellbeing.

Note

1 'Grab' in this statement refers to the lack of an inclusive process in deciding land allocations/acquisition and environmental protection.

References

Amnesty International 2020, '"Catastrophic" Omnibus Bill on Job Creation Passed into Law', 5 October, viewed 9 November 2020, www.amnesty.id/catastrophic-omnibus-bill-on-job-creation-passed-into-law/

Asia Indigenous Peoples Pact (AIPP) 2020, 'Under the Cover of Covid: New Laws in Asia Favor Business at the Cost of Indigenous Peoples' and Local Communities' Land and Territorial Rights', viewed 17 November 2020, https://aippnet.org/under-cover-covid-new-laws-asia-favor-business-cost-indigenous-peoples-local-communities-land-territorial-rights/

Bayrak, M & Marafa, L 2016, 'Ten Years of REDD+: A Critical Review of the Impact of REDD+ on Forest-Dependent Communities', *Sustainability*, vol. 8, no. 7, pp. 1–22.

BBC 2020, 'Brazil: Amazon Land Defender Zezico Guajajara Shot Dead', *BBC*, 2 April, viewed 8 November 2020, www.bbc.com/news/world-latin-america-52135362

Brown, A 2020, 'A Powerful Petrochemical Lobbying Group Advanced Anti-Protest Legislation in the Midst of the Pandemic', *The Intercept*, 7 June, viewed 29 November, https://theintercept.com/2020/06/07/pipeline-petrochemical-lobbying-group-anti-protest-law/

Cadasta.org, viewed 2 November 2020, https://cadasta.org/use-case/community/

Cecco, L 2020, 'Canada: Minister says Covid-19 Lockdown a "Great Time" to Build Pipeline', *The Guardian*, 26 May, viewed 29 November 2020, www.theguardian.com/world/2020/may/26/canada-coronavirus-alberta-energy-minister-oil-pipeline

Chandran, R 2020, 'Land Conflicts Flare Across Asia during Coronavirus Lockdowns', *Reuters*, 15 May, viewed 5 November 2020, https://uk.reuters.com/article/health-coronavirus-landrights/land-conflicts-flare-across-asia-during-coronavirus-lockdowns-idUKL8N2CN621

Cheyns, E 2011, 'Multi-stakeholder Initiatives for Sustainable Agriculture; Limits of the "Inclusiveness" paradigm', in S Ponte, P Gibbon & J Vestergaard (eds.), *Governing Through Standards: Origins, Drivers and Limitations*, Palgrave Macmillan, Basingstoke.

Cosens, BA, Craig, RK, Hirsch, SL, Arnold, CA, Benson, MH, DeCaro, DA, Garmestani, AS, Gosnell, H, Ruhl, JB, & Schlager, E 2017, 'The Role of Law in Adaptive Governance', *Ecology and Society*, vol. 22, no. 1.

Cotula, L 2020, 'Stopping Land and Policy Grabs in the Shadow of COVID-19', *International Institute for Environment and Development*, viewed 28 October 2020, www.iied.org/stopping-land-policy-grabs-shadow-covid-19

Cotula, L 2021, 'Towards a Political Economy of the COVID-19 Crisis: Reflections on an Agenda for Research and Action', *World Development*, vol. 138.

Cotula, L & Berger, T 2017, *Trends in Global Land Use Investment: Implications for Legal Empowerment*, IIED, London.

Cotula, L & Schwartz, B 2020, 'COVID-19 and Global Economic Ordering: Radical Shift or More of the Same?', *International Institute for Environment and Development*, viewed 6 November 2020, www.iied.org/covid-19-global-economic-ordering-radical-shift-or-more-same

Daily Monitor 2020, 'Uganda: Government Stops All Land Transactions', *Daily Monitor*, 17 April, viewed 9 November 2020, www.monitor.co.ug/News/National/Government-stops-land-transactions-RDCs-DPCs-Kamya-/688334-5527104-7uhbz/index.html

Daniels, J 2020, 'Colombian Death Squads Exploiting Coronavirus Lockdown to Kill Activists', *The Guardian*, 23 March, viewed 12 December 2020, www.theguardian.com/world/2020/mar/23/colombian-groups-exploiting-coronavirus-lockdown-to-kill-activists

Dell'Angelo, J, D'Odorico, P, Rulli, MC, & Marchand, P 2017, 'The Tragedy of the Grabbed Commons: Coercion and Dispossession in the Global Land Rush', *World Development*, vol. 92, pp. 1–12.

Duvar English 2020, 'Environmentalists Protesting Kaz Mountains Mine Imposed a Fine of $8,000', 9 May, viewed 29 November 2020, www.duvarenglish.com/environment/2020/05/09/environmentalists-protesting-kaz-mountains-mine-imposed-a-fine-of-8000

EarthWorks et al. 2020, 'Voices from the Grounds: How the Global Mining Industry is Profitting from the COVID-19 Pandemic', *Earth Works*, 1 June, viewed 26 November 2020, www.earthworks.org/publications/voices-from-the-ground-how-the-global-mining-industry-is-profiting-from-the-covid-19-pandemic/

El Tiempo 2020, 'MinInterior Responde por polémica de las consultas previas virtuales', viewed 8 November 2020, www.eltiempo.com/vida/medio-ambiente/ministerio-del-interior-responde-sobre-las-consultas-previas-virtuales-485312

Fairbairn, M 2015, 'Foreignization, Financialization and Land Grab Regulation', *Journal of Agrarian Change*, vol. 15, no. 4, pp. 581–591.

Forst, M & Taylor, M 2020, 'Land and Environmental Defenders are Sitting Ducks, While World Goes into Lockdown', *Toward Freedom*, viewed 9 November 2020, https://towardfreedom.org/story/land-and-environmental-defenders-are-sitting-ducks-while-world-goes-into-lockdown/

Gilbert, J 2018, *Natural Resources and Human Rights: An Appraisal*, Oxford University Press, New York.

Global Witness 2015, 'The New Snake Oil: Violence, Threats, and False Promises at the Heart of Liberia's Palm Oil Expansion', 23 July, viewed 6 November 2020, www.globalwitness.org/en/campaigns/land-deals/new-snake-oil/

Gross, A, Schipani, A, Palma, S, & Findlay, S 2020, 'Global Deforestation Accelerates During Pandemic', *Financial Times*, 8 August, viewed 2 November 2020, www.ft.com/content/b72e3969-522c-4e83-b431-c0b498754b2d

Harsono, N 2020, 'Explainer: New Rules in Revised Mining Law', *The Jakarta Post*, 14 May, viewed 9 November 2020, www.thejakartapost.com/news/2020/05/14/explainer-new-rules-in-revised-mining-law.html

Human Rights Watch 2020a, 'Peru: Law Protects Abusive Policing', 12 May, viewed 8 November 2020, www.hrw.org/news/2020/05/12/peru-law-protects-abusive-policing#:~:text=On%20March%2027%2C%202020%2C%20Peru's,be%20proportionate% 20to%20the%20threat

Human Rights Watch 2020b, 'Indonesia: New Law Hurts Workers, Indigenous Groups', 15 October 15, viewed 8 November 2020, www.hrw.org/news/2020/10/15/indonesia-new-law-hurts-workers-indigenous-groups

Human Rights Watch 2020c, 'Nairobi Evicts 8,000 People Amidst a Pandemic and Curfew', 10 June, viewed 5 November 2020, www.hrw.org/news/2020/06/10/nairobi-evicts-8000-people-amidst-pandemic-and-curfew

Human Rights Watch 2020d, 'Environmentalists Under Threat in South Africa', 4 November, viewed 30 November 2020, www.hrw.org/news/2020/11/04/environmentalists-under-threat-south-africa

Human Rights Watch 2019, 'Kenya: Mau Forest Evictees' Plight Intensifies', 23 July, viewed 5 November 2020, www.hrw.org/news/2020/07/23/kenya-mau-forest-evictees-plight-intensifies

Jong, HN 2020, 'Land Conflicts Escalate with Spread of COVID-19 in Indonesia', *Mongabay*, 15 April, viewed 9 November 2020, https://news.mongabay.com/2020/04/land-conflicts-escalate-with-spread-of-covid-19-in-indonesia/

Jordan, L 2020, 'Amazonian Deforestation Soaring While Bolsonaro Administration Weakens Safeguards', *UNEARTHED*, 5 August, viewed 2 November 2020, https://unearthed.greenpeace.org/2020/05/08/amazonian-deforestation-soaring-while-bolsonaro-administration-weakens-safeguards/

Kanno-Youngs, Z 2020, 'Border Wall Land Grabs Accelerate as Owners Shelter From Pandemic', *New York Times*, 29 May, viewed 12 December 2020, www.nytimes.com/2020/05/29/us/politics/border-wall-coronavirus.html

Klein, N 2007, *The Shock Doctrine: The Rise of Disaster Capitalism*, Metropolitan Books, New York.

Klein, N 2017, 'How Power Profits from Disaster', *The Guardian*, 6 July, viewed 5 November 2020, www.theguardian.com/us-news/2017/jul/06/naomi-klein-how-power-profits-from-disaster

KTV News Kenya 2020, 'Land Sector Distress: Land Offices Closed Since March 15th', viewed 9 November 2020, www.youtube.com/watch?v=ph607g6KBLM&feature=youtu.be&app=desktop

Kugelman, M & Levenstein, SL (eds.) 2013, *The Global Farms Race: Land Grabs, Agricultural Investments, and the Scramble for Food Security*, Island Press, Washington.

Lang, C 2020, 'Kenya Forest Service Evicts 300 Ogiek Families from their Homes in the Mau Forest', *REDD*, 16 July, viewed 17 November 2020, https://redd-monitor.org/2020/07/16/kenya-forest-service-evicts-300-ogiek-families-from-their-homes-in-the-mau-forest-despite-the-african-court-on-human-and-peoples-rights-2017-ruling-that-the-ogiek-should-not-be-evicted/

Lopez-Feldman, A, Chavez, C, Velez, MA, Bejarano, H, Chimeli, AB, Feres, J, Robalino, J, Salcedo, R, & Viteri, C 2020, 'Environmental Impacts and Policy Responses to COVID-19: A view from Latin America' (Working Paper), *Department of Economics – FEA/USP*.

Mwagae, EW 2020, 'Communities with Insecure Tenure More Vulnerable', *Business Daily*, 14 June, viewed 5 November 2020, www.businessdailyafrica.com/analysis/columnists/Communities-with-insecure-tenure-more-vulnerable/4259356-5576326-y8jv8n/index.html

Mwangi, E, Markelova, H, & Meinzen-Dick, R (eds.) 2012, *Collective Action and Property Rights for Poverty Reduction: Insights from Africa and Asia*, University of Pennsylvania Press, Philadelphia.

Nguyen, S 2020, 'Vietnam Firm with World Bank Links Accused of Bulldozing Indigenous Land in Cambodia', *This Week in Asia*, 29 May, viewed 29 November 2020, www.scmp.com/week-asia/health-environment/article/3086758/vietnam-firm-world-bank-links-accused-bulldozing

Nnoko-Mewanu, JM 2016, 'Who Is Not at the Table: Land Deal Negotiations in Southwestern Cameroon', *Iowa State Graduate Theses and Dissertations*, viewed 6 November 2020, https://lib.dr.iastate.edu/etd/15781

Nugraha, I & Marie, Y 2020, 'Palm Oil Firm has Farmers Jailed for Harvesting from Land it Stole from them', *Mongabay*, 17 March, viewed 6 November 2020, https://news.mongabay.com/2020/03/indonesia-palm-oil-land-dispute-kalimantan-indigenous-hmbp/

OHCHR 2020a, 'COVID-19 is Devastating Indigenous Communities Worldwide, and It's not Only about Health', viewed 8 November 2020, www.ohchr.org/EN/NewsEvents/Pages/DisplayNews.aspx?NewsID=25893&LangID=E

OHCHR 2020b, 'The Americas: Governments Should Strengthen, not Weaken, Environmental Protection during COVID-19 Pandemic', viewed 8 November 2020, www.ohchr.org/EN/NewsEvents/Pages/DisplayNews.aspx?NewsID=26165&LangID=E

OHCHR 2020c, 'Philippines: UN Human Rights Experts Renew Call for an On-the-Ground Independent, Impartial Investigation', viewed 29 November 2020, www.ohchr.org/EN/NewsEvents/Pages/DisplayNews.aspx?NewsID=25999&LangID=E

OHCHR 2015, 'Land and Human Rights: Standards and Applications', HR/PUB/15/5/Add.1, viewed 16 November 2020, www.ohchr.org/Documents/Publications/Land_HR-StandardsApplications.pdf

Pearshouse, R & Werneck, J 2020, 'Land Seizures and Covid-19: The Twin Threats to Brazil's Indigenous Peoples', *Amnesty International*, 6 April, viewed 9 November 2020, www.amnesty.org/en/latest/news/2020/04/land-seizures-and-covid-19-the-twin-threats-to-brazils-indigenous-peoples/

Programa Queimadas 2020, 'Monitoramento dos focos ativos por estado', viewed 5 August 2020, http://queimadas.dgi.inpe.br/queimadas/portal-static/estatisticas_estados/

Salomão, A 2020, 'The Impact of Covid-19 on the Land Sector in Mozambique', *LANDac*, 10 June, viewed 29 November 2020, www.landgovernance.org/online-hub-land-governance-and-the-covid-19-pandemic/online-hub-land-governance-and-the-covid-19-pandemic-blogs/20191-2/

Spring, J 2020, 'Exclusive: Brazil Scales Back Environmental Enforcement Amid Coronavirus', *Reuters*, 27 March, viewed 8 November 2020, https://uk.reuters.com/article/uk-health-coronavirus-brazil-environment/exclusive-brazil-scales-back-environmental-enforcement-amid-coronavirus-idUKKBN21E15V

Szoke-Burke, S 2020, 'Land and Resource Investment Consultations in the Time of COVID-19: The Hazards of Pressing on, Columbia Center on Sustainable Investments', *Thomson Reuters Foundation News*, 24 May, viewed 12 December 2020, https://news.trust.org/item/20200524095046-4fhrd

The Brazilian Report 2020, 'Deforestation and Land-Grabbing in the Amazon During COVID-19', *Think Brazil*, 23 June, viewed 2 November 2020, www.wilsoncenter.org/blog-post/deforestation-and-land-grabbing-amazon-during-covid-19

Transparency International 2020, 'Land Corruption and Urban Land Governance', viewed 6 November 2020, www.transparency.org/en/projects/urban-land-governance#

Turkewitz, J, & Villamil, S 2020, 'Indigenous Colombian, Facing New Wave of Brutality, Demand Government Action', *New York Times*, 24 October, viewed 8 November 2020, www.nytimes.com/2020/10/24/world/americas/colombia-violence-indigenous-protest.html

UN Committee on Economic, Social and Cultural Rights (CESCR) 1991, *General Comment 4. The Right to Adequate Housing*, U.N. Doc. E/1992/23, annex III, art. 114.

United Nations General Assembly, *UN Declaration on the Rights of Indigenous Peoples* (UNDRIP), G.A. Res. 61/295, U.N. Doc. A/RES/47/1.

United Nations General Assembly, *Universal Declaration of Human Rights* (UDHR), G.A. Res. 217A(III), U.N. Doc. A/810 at 71.

United Nations Human Rights Council 2011, 'UN Guiding Principles on Business and Human Rights: Implementing the "Protect, Respect and Remedy" Framework', A/HRC/17/31.

Uson, M 2017, 'Natural Disasters and Land Grabs: The Politics of their Intersection in the Philippines Following Super Typhoon Haiyan', *Canadian Journal of Development Studies / Revue Canadienne d'Études du Développement*, vol. 38, no. 3, pp. 414–430.

Westerman, A 2020, 'Over 120,000 People Remain Displaced 3 Years After Philippines' Marawi Battle', *NPR*, 23 October, viewed 12 December 2020, www.npr.org/2020/10/23/925316298/over-120-000-people-remain-displaced-3-years-after-philippines-marawi-battle

Wieckardt, C, van der Haar, G, & van Westen, G 2020, 'Land Administration, Land Governance Institutions and COVID-19', *New America*, viewed 9 November 2020, www.newamerica.org/future-property-rights/reports/land-housing-and-covid-19/land-administration-land-governance-institutions-and-covid-19/

Wisborg, P 2013, 'Human Rights Against Land Grabbing? A Reflection on Norms, Policies, and Power', *Journal of Agricultural and Environmental Ethics*, vol. 26, no. 6, pp. 1199–1222.

15

HOW THE PANDEMIC HAS IMPACTED THE VARIOUS LAYERS OF THE GLOBAL GARMENT SUPPLY CHAIN

Sanchita Banerjee Saxena, Harpreet Kaur, and Salil Tripathi

The complex world of global supply chains, linking thousands of factories across multiple cultural and political boundaries, has provided countries in the Global South with investment, employment, technology, and access to international markets. At the same time, workers who manufacture these goods are at the bottom of these supply chains. They often work in precarious conditions that adversely affect their mental and physical health, and in some cases, even cost them their lives. The dispersion of manufacturing across multiple countries has created new sites of production made possible by the abundant availability of workers willing to accept salaries considerably below those in the developed world. Rapidly declining shipping costs, the development of leaner distribution networks, and efficiencies in inventory management have hastened the dispersion of manufacturing. The new production sites, beyond the jurisdiction of the governments of the Global North, often escape not only their regulatory framework, but also lack adequate social protections for the workers. This happens because some governments in the Global South often lack the capacity or the will to fully provide social safety nets or require adherence to international standards. This situation results in many factories falling into a 'regulatory void' where working conditions are precarious, labor rights deteriorate, and workers lack basic benefits.

The COVID-19 pandemic has shaken the world's economy and supply chains worldwide, and the global garment industry is certainly no exception. Garment retailers with globalized operations, particularly ones relying on Chinese inputs for production, suffered the initial supply chain disruption due to COVID-19 (UNCTAD 2020). Production closure in China caused initial disruption, which increased with lockdowns in other countries. For example, with fewer people leaving their homes and many people working from home, global demand for certain kinds of apparel[1] declined steeply.

This was perhaps not surprising. Global supply chains today show hyper-flexibility, lack of transparency, and unequal power dynamics (Reinecke et al. 2019), which are seen as essential features for these complex networks to function. However, these characteristics are not likely to promote – and may in fact undermine – respect for human rights and labor rights. For decades, many global brands and buyers have been able to use the unequal distribution of bargaining power within these supply chains to require their suppliers to meet the competitive pressures within the industry by producing smaller batches of increasing varieties of products more rapidly and at decreasing prices. The emergence of 'fast fashion' – cheap clothing produced quickly and distributed rapidly around the world capturing every shift in fashion trends – accentuated some of these inherent problems. During the pandemic, already difficult conditions have been made even more precarious for the millions who depend on these jobs for their livelihoods. This pandemic has put a spotlight on many of the inequalities and unequal power dynamics that were always present in the system.

This chapter draws on the authors' insights from three complimentary projects[2] of primary research involving interviews with senior executives from international brands, suppliers, and more than 1,000 garment workers. Informed by these studies, this chapter will discuss the impact of COVID-19 on garment supply chains in Asia, how the push for change at the source has often been misguided, and the actions taken by global retailers and suppliers during this time. This chapter will demonstrate that these actions negatively impacted workers' livelihoods during this pandemic. Finally, we conclude by envisioning a 'new normal' with respect to global supply chains in the post-COVID-19 era.

1 Compliance programs have done little to change the root causes of labor violations

Despite the complexity, policymakers and brands have focused on placing the responsibility for labor rights and factory improvements at the locus of production – i.e., where the factories are located – and on the owners of those factories. However, critics argue that overseas brands' insistence on lower costs compels local suppliers to cut corners to meet what they describe as demanding and unrealistic expectations of the buyers. In response to the criticism, overseas brands have increased inspections of local factories and evaluated their performance based on standards developed by brands in consultation with international civil society and unions.

Companies in certain cases have examined their own practices. Industry-wide initiatives, which are in some instances multi-stakeholder, have been set up to improve business practices. Their effectiveness deserves further scrutiny. There is a long history of third-party monitoring and corporate social responsibility (CSR) initiatives (Ruggie 2003; Nadvi & Waltring 2004; Vogel 2008; Belal, Cooper, & Khan 2015; Rubenstein 2007). These have been supplemented with the interventions after the 2013 Rana Plaza disaster in Bangladesh (Anner 2018; Schüßler et. al.

2018). Together these have increased scrutiny of the contracting and importing practices of brands in the Global North and the operational practices of suppliers in the Global South, holding both accountable for both the labor violations that occur and for the strategies deployed to mitigate them.

Some authors have critiqued this heavy emphasis on compliance and noted the limitations of CSR programs (Barrientos & Smith 2007; De Neve 2009; Mezzadri 2014; Lund-Thomsen & Lindgreen 2014; Saxena 2020b). Locke (2013) argues that compliance programs have actually done little to change the root causes of poor working conditions. Many of the problems faced in global supply chains, he argues, cannot simply be attributed to unethical factory managers in need of capacity building, auditing, or policing. Much of it is due to the pressures and policies that have been put in place by global brands to maximize profit and minimize risks of not meeting consumer demands in a timely manner. Locke (2013) argues that focus on factories alone is misplaced; recognition of the broader political economy of global supply chains within which these production processes are located is essential. There has been very little discussion around what drives these labor abuses in the first place and how power between the various actors can be redistributed to address these issues in a substantial way. According to the Clean Clothes Campaign (2020, p. 35):

> While the direct employers are legally obligated to pay workers' wages, it is the brands that dictate how profits are made and distributed along their supply chains. Brands choose to base their supply chains in countries with low wages and weak social protections. As workers, unions, and civil society groups have long argued, global supply chains are defined by an acute power imbalance between brands at the top of supply chains and workers employed in factories. Brands' economic power allows them to dictate how profits are made and distributed along their supply chains, including the ever-smaller share available for suppliers to pay their workers decent wages, ensure safe and healthy working conditions, or provide workers with legally mandated benefits upon termination.

A solid body of research has examined the detrimental impacts of current business models and practices. Salient issues include the difficulty that owners and governments have in making substantial gains in the area of improving labor standards (Reinecke et al. 2019), how increasing order volumes and fluctuations in these orders by buyers directly impact increased overtime, the use of sub-standard buildings, and the prevalence of sub-contracting (Anner 2019), as well as how adjustments to these business models could possibly change the incentives of countries to actually improve conditions in the factories (Human Rights Watch 2019; Reinecke et al. 2019). The pandemic has put a spotlight on many of the well-established strategies that have been pursued by global garment retailers for decades. These practices have had a detrimental impact on the livelihoods of millions of workers in the garment sector and have further exacerbated their vulnerable positions in the global value chain.

2 COVID-19 and supply chains: whither the protect-respect-remedy framework

COVID-19 caused a dramatic shift in the demand for apparel worldwide, threatened the viability of many companies, and posed an existential threat to some brands. Without minimizing the significance of these challenges, the human rights discourse is focused on the impact on the most vulnerable. And to that extent, duty-bearers, including companies, have the responsibility to ensure that they assess the human rights impacts of their actions and take steps to mitigate harm.

The UN Guiding Principles on Business and Human Rights (UNGPs) are critical in this respect (OHCHR 2011). The UNGPs call upon States to take appropriate steps to prevent, investigate, and provide redress against abuses by corporations as well as set out expectations that companies 'domiciled in their territory and/or jurisdiction respect human rights throughout their operations' (OHCHR 2011, p. 3). The UNGPs call upon States to ensure that trade and/or investment agreements do not constrain them to meet their human rights obligations.

The UNGPs also call upon all businesses, regardless of their size, to undertake human rights due diligence to identify, mitigate, and address their adverse human rights impacts. This includes four key steps:

- assessing actual and potential human rights impacts;
- integrating and acting on the findings;
- tracking responses; and
- communicating about how impacts are addressed.

This also requires identifying potential remedies, establishing remedies in consultation with affected groups (in this instance, workers), and making continuous improvement.

In the context of the pandemic, according to the UNGPs companies should assess the impact of their business practices on workers and find ways to ensure that workers do not slip into poverty, which may deny them their rights to livelihood, health, and social security. Companies should create mechanisms to ensure that even if laid off, workers have access to resources, including incomes, to maintain an adequate standard of living and continue to have access to healthcare. While human rights law does not guarantee employment, it calls for due process, which means affected workers should be consulted and their meaningful consent obtained before steps are taken that affect their work conditions in any way, in particular if the effects are adverse. This requires recognizing the right to form unions and to engage in collective bargaining, as well as to health and safety. It also means that if and when work resumes at factories, employers have the responsibility to ensure safe and secure working conditions and that workers do not bear a disproportionate burden – financial or otherwise – to protect themselves. In practical terms, it means redesigning factory space to ensure physical distancing, providing personal protection equipment (such as masks and overalls), providing easy access to sanitizers, and redesigning work-flow to minimize the risk of exposure.

With this framework in mind, we look at the impact of the pandemic on the garment supply chain based on the perspectives of workers, suppliers, and overseas brand executives.

3 The impact of COVID-19 on garment supply chains

Three-fifths of the world's garment production occurs in the developing world, and the share in developing Asia is the largest, accounting for 32 percent of the global garment manufacturing (ILO 1996). By 2015, eleven of the world's fifteen largest exporters of garments were in Asia, accounting for nearly two-thirds of global exports in monetary terms (ILO 2017, p. 1). China, Bangladesh, Vietnam, Hong Kong, and India are five of the largest garment exporters in the world. In 2020, the garment industry accounted for 82 percent of Bangladesh's exports and 11 percent of its GDP. At $34.1 billion, Bangladesh accounts for nearly 6 percent of global garment exports, and the industry employs some four million workers, the majority of them being women, many of whom are at the greatest risk of losing their jobs (Leitheiser et al. 2020).

COVID-19 hit Bangladesh hard. By 23 March 2020 reportedly $1.5 billion of orders had been canceled (Devnath 2020), and by April brands had suspended or revoked clothing orders worth $3.2 billion. In June 2020, export orders had fallen by 40–45 percent compared to 2019. According to the international workers' rights organization the Clean Clothes Campaign (2020, p. 7), between March and May 2020 Bangladeshi workers lost nearly 30 percent of their wages, estimated at $502 million.[3] Layoffs and furloughs multiplied: some 2.3 million of the four million workers were out of work. According to Bangladesh Bank Export Earning Data, Bangladesh lost $724 million in apparel exports to the United States between March and June 2020 (Rabbani, Saxena, & Isla 2020). Inflows worth $4.6 billion were lost in total between March and May 2020 (Anner, Nova, & Foxvog 2020).

Lockdown was announced later in Bangladesh than in neighboring India (which went into lockdown in late March), which allowed the Bangladeshi garment industry to service orders for a somewhat longer period of time. Estimates of losses in the Indian garment industry due to the pandemic range from $2 billion (Khan 2020) to $2.86 billion (Stanton 2020). According to the Apparel Exports Promotion Council of India, 83 percent of exporters reported that buyers had wholly or partially canceled orders, and for 72% of those orders exporters were not compensated for materials already purchased (Society for Labour and Development 2020). Campaigning organizations claim that despite government regulations, garment workers received less or no pay from their employers during the lockdown.

Vietnam is the third largest garment exporting country (measured by volume) just behind China and Bangladesh, and the Vietnamese apparel industry accounts for 16 percent of the country's total exports (Fair Labor Association 2019, p. 2). Though Vietnam's economy remained open for most of the time during the pandemic, its clothing production still dropped by 6 percent and its footwear production by 7 percent in the first half of 2020 due to decline in global demand (Russell 2020).

Not only were workers vulnerable to job losses and economic hardship due to the measures described above, but they also have very few rights in these countries across industries. The 2020 ITUC Global Rights Index – which rates countries on a scale from 1 (best) to 5+ (worst) on the degree of respect for workers' rights – rates both Bangladesh and India among the world's ten worst countries for workers. Both are rated at 5, which suggests denial of basic rights. The report rates Vietnam at 4, indicating that workers experience systematic violations of internationally recognized labor rights.

4 Impact of the pandemic on garment workers in Bangladesh

To understand the impact of the pandemic on garment workers, the UC Berkeley-BRAC study interviewed 1,057 workers in mid-2020. Top line results from the survey (Rabbani, Saxena, & Islam 2020) demonstrate how detrimental the COVID-19 crisis has been to workers' physical and mental health and on their livelihoods.

During the pandemic workers' incomes fell significantly: 82 percent of workers said the income they had in April/May 2020 was less than their income in February 2020. But by May, the salary levels had returned to original levels or were higher. This may have been due to the advocacy by workers' organizations and international campaigns and partial resumption of factory work.

The gendered dimension is especially striking when work is broken up by job categories. Entry level positions such as operator and helper (as their assisting subordinates are described in Bangladesh) are often the lowest paid and are primarily held by women. Among the workers surveyed, 70 percent of operators and 82 percent of helpers were women (Rabbani, Saxena, & Islam 2020). These women are trapped in a cycle of poverty due to inadequate wages, lack of job security, and limited opportunities for job mobility within the factory.

Many factories that supply to major brands now have preventive measures in place to protect worker health. Eighty-seven percent of workers surveyed said their factory introduced new precautions against the coronavirus, including giving workers new protective equipment (91 percent), encouraging more hygiene measures (77 percent), sending workers with symptoms home (66 percent), and encouraging distance between workers (75 percent). But workers are still afraid of contracting the virus. Some 59 percent of the workers[4] feel they are 'somewhat likely' or 'very likely' to get infected in their factory, whereas only 29 percent think they will contract it at home.

Protective measures are necessary, but some protocols may be unrealistic. Nearly half the workers said they would not be able to self-isolate at home if they contracted the virus – 54 percent of women and 45 percent of men. If factories continue their operations during this crisis, there needs to be certain contingency plans in place for workers who become sick, including providing places to isolate, healthcare provisions, financial support, and job security (Rabbani, Saxena, & Islam 2020).

Workers reported to be facing enormous hardship. At the time of the survey, 52 percent of the respondents said that they saved less than what they saved in February, the pre-COVID-19 period. Ninety percent said they did not receive any support from the government during this pandemic (Rabbani, Saxena, & Islam 2020, p. 3). More than three-quarters said they found it difficult to feed everyone at home. Families ate less protein and nutritive food, relying on cheaper cereals and pulses. Workers dipped into their savings to pay for household expenses, depleting savings (Rabbani, Saxena, & Islam 2020, p. 2). Four-fifths feared for the future and slightly less felt depressed.

5 Responses to the COVID-19 crisis

5.1 What the brands have done

The power imbalance at the heart of the business model manifested itself in March 2020 when the crisis hit. Many major retailers canceled orders that were under production or had already been produced by factories in the Global South. Some brands also demanded large discounts or rebates in exchange for agreeing to take these orders. As a result, local factories laid off millions of garment workers around the world. Many were let go without pay and many had inadequate savings or safety nets to fall back on. In March 2020 the statistics were shocking:

- 98.1 percent of buyers refused to contribute to the cost of paying the partial wages to furloughed workers that the law required;
- 72.4 percent of furloughed workers were sent home without pay;
- 97.3 percent of buyers refused to contribute to severance pay expenses of dismissed workers;
- 80.4 percent of dismissed workers were sent home without their severance pay (Anner, Nova, & Foxvog 2020, p. 2).

According to Anner, Nova, and Foxvog (2020, p. 1), '[t]his behavior was enabled by the existing payments structure in the apparel industry, under which suppliers bear the up-front cost of production and buyers pay nothing until weeks or months after the factory ships the goods'. Anner, Nova, and Foxvog (2020, p. 2) also estimated that buyers 'in the initial weeks of the crisis, reneged on their financial commitments on roughly USD 40 billion in orders – with devastating implications for suppliers and workers'. This perhaps should not come as a major surprise since, according to one major retailer interviewed in the UC Berkeley-IHRB study, even before this current crisis, brands could and did use their position with suppliers to cancel orders frequently:

> companies … retain the right to invoke cancellation, and it's an open secret, frankly, that cancellations are more common than people think… If a shipment arrives and it doesn't meet any of our quality standards, or if the vendor says the shipment is going to be three months late, [companies] retain the right… to cancel the orders. That is just how the apparel business works.
>
> *(Major brand executive 2020 pers. comm.)*

International advocacy groups, like the Workers' Rights Consortium (WRC 2020), the Clean Clothes Campaign (2020), and Remake's #PayUp campaign (Barenblat & Cline 2020) actively pressured global retailers through social media and consumer activism to honor their commitments. The Business and Human Rights Resource Center (2020) developed the COVID-19 apparel action tracker to monitor company performance.

The authors spoke with ten global retailers to understand their strategies to consider and manage their human rights impact during the pandemic. Retailers who honored their commitments to suppliers had direct relationships with their suppliers or were consolidating their supplier base to deepen relationships. Research has shown that retailers with direct supplier relationships are able to deal with crises better than those with traditional transactional relationships (Reinecke et al. 2019; Baumann-Pauly 2020). The research shows that retailers' interactions with suppliers on COVID-19 included health precautions and modified business processes. Executives interviewed said that their companies had provided factories with advice drawn from credible international standards (to avoid duplication) on worker safety, information on physical distancing, cleaning and disinfecting protocols, tracing COVID-19 positive workers, and isolating those who were unwell. The cost for implementing the changes was borne by local manufacturers (Saxena 2020a).[5]

During interviews several retailers said that they were committed to paying for finished products and, if they had to cancel orders, they honored their contracts and paid for what was already produced. Some brands indicated that if orders were being canceled, it was 'not from corporate malfeasance' but because the company itself was financially vulnerable. To be sure, that did create uncertainty for the local factories. But the brands too faced uncertainty, with retail stores remaining closed and a collapse in global demand. Some retailers partnered with the International Finance Corporation's (IFC) global supply trade finance program to allow vendors to get paid faster. Maintaining liquidity was the key to ensuring that the supplier survived beyond the crisis. According to one senior representative of a major retailer, buyers needed to understand supplier viability as well as what other brands were asking them to do:

> We paid for 100% of our canceled goods during that early time where no one really knew what was going to happen. We worked with our suppliers to figure out how we could be flexible on delivery times after the reopening and really focused on our purchasing practices, and tried to put [in place] realistic timelines, and work with our suppliers so that we were delivering goods in a

> way that allowed those factories to operate safely...We also wanted to understand what they [the suppliers] were being asked to do for others and make sure that we weren't only thinking about the impact of our orders.
>
> *(pers. comm. October 2020)*

Others mentioned working on refining their purchasing practices during the pandemic with the help of ACT (Action Collaboration Transformation), an agreement between 21 global brands and IndustriALL (the global union that represents garment, textile, and footwear workers), to achieve a living wage for workers through collective bargaining, linked to purchasing practices. Some companies also endorsed the Call to Action, an initiative by the International Labour Organization (ILO) and the International Organization of Employers (IOE). They also accepted orders without invoking contractual penalties so that, according to one brand, the factories did not 'shove all the workers [onto] the [factory] floor [in order] to make sure that they [could] catch up with our deadlines' (pers. comm. October 2020) because as another executive said, 'it takes one crisis to destroy (reputation)' (pers. comm. 2020).

Initial findings as of October 2020 from the research study conducted by Behavioral Insights, Architecture and Strategy (BIAS), commissioned by United Nations Development Program's B+HR Asia revealed six stages of the impact of COVID-19 on the garment industry. However, since the situation is still evolving globally, additional stages may appear later.

5.2 What suppliers have done

The suppliers interviewed in the three-country study reiterated the challenges they faced due to orders being canceled, which compelled them to announce layoffs in response to their declining revenues. As explained by a Bangladeshi manufacturer, 'in 2020 garment export was expected to be $35 billion (but) the expectation now is to achieve $15 billion. So you can understand the extent of cancelations of orders' (pers. comm.). Even when lockdowns were lifted, many suppliers reported challenges in managing production levels due to a decline in demand from buyers, labor shortages, and the lack of raw materials. Interviews with suppliers revealed a complex set of responses. Some praised the workers for their flexibility and adaptability to the changing needs and demands, '[Bangladeshi factory owners] are big fighters. We never made medical gowns, PPE, masks in Bangladesh before this, but we started [making them] now', said a Bangladeshi manufacturer during interviews (pers. comm.).

Interestingly, a few suppliers reported difficulty in hiring workers again after the lockdown as government benefits offered to the newly unemployed, in some circumstances as in Vietnam, were sufficient and workers did not wish to return to work.

Then there were some who were concerned about legal action if they failed to comply with government instructions. The suppliers reported confusion about

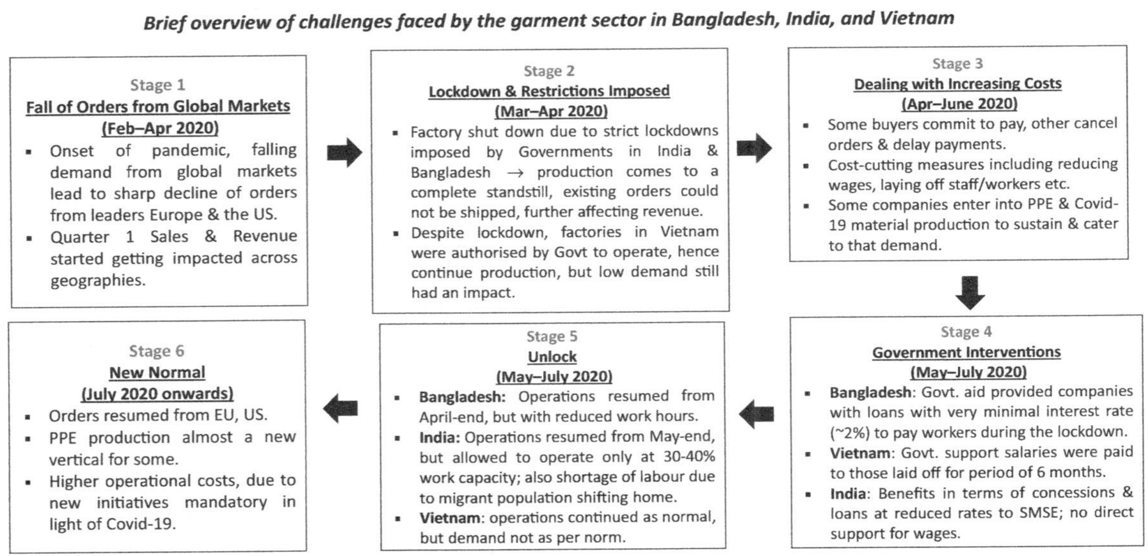

FIGURE 15.1 Impact of COVID-19 on the garment sector

the guidelines issued by governments. In India, factories faced prosecution if the government found infected workers in the factories, but a factory manager said if workers showed no symptoms, how was the management to know? (pers. comm.).

Suppliers undertook various initiatives to ensure access to health and safety for the workers and redesigned shop floors to follow social distancing rules. All the suppliers interviewed across the three countries reported that they checked workers' temperature several times at regular intervals during the day and maintained sanitation facilities and hygiene in the factory. A few suppliers facilitated counseling sessions to address the psychological impact of COVID-19. An Indian supplier (pers. comm.) reported that they

> rearranged the machines to ensure social distancing, and where it wasn't possible – [they] put plastic shields in between, so that there is no direct impact between people. They provided masks and put [hand sanitizer] everywhere. Doctors inspected factories many times and were satisfied.

The same was reported by suppliers in Bangladesh and Vietnam.

6 How do we envision a 'new normal'?

The pandemic has highlighted many of the flaws inherent in the global supply chain. The examples from Bangladesh, India, and Vietnam show the need to examine social safety nets (or their absence); the inadequacy of prevailing wages, which leads to difficulties in accumulating savings; and the skewed gender dynamics present in the system, which creates even greater hardship for women workers.

The right to social security derives from Articles 22 and 25 of the Universal Declaration on Human Rights (United Nations General Assembly 1948), which specify the right to social security at all times including in the event of illness, disability, or unemployment. Furthermore, Articles 9 and 10 of the International Covenant on Economic, Social, and Cultural Rights (ICESCR 1976) elaborate on these rights; the Office of the High Commissioner for Human Rights offers further insight into this connection (OHCHR 2020). Under human rights law, States have the primary obligation to respect, protect, and fulfill rights. As such, governments have a critical role to play in establishing social security. While human rights law does not require the state to be the sole provider of infrastructure that enables the realization of human rights, the state has the obligation to ensure that the rights are realized. This means even if the state is not the provider of benefits it has to ensure the delivery of benefits so that rights are not infringed or undermined.

This includes ensuring access to a safe and secure workplace, grievance mechanisms to address adverse impacts, access to education and technology to protect lives, and making investment in infrastructure to enable that all rights are realized. This may take the form of passing regulations, monitoring performance, establishing insurance schemes, imposing taxation to cover costs, or enabling the establishment of clinics and hospitals.

Brands may not have legal obligations to protect the rights of workers in the supply chain, but under the UN Guiding Principles for business and human rights they have the responsibility to address and mitigate adverse impacts on human rights through their actions and to use their leverage over suppliers and sub-contractors to reduce harm. They can also aid in supporting efforts towards the realization of rights through advocacy and partnering with international organizations as well as channeling their corporate social responsibility efforts. Interviews with local suppliers and global retailers highlight the increased importance of collaboration between brands and suppliers and the necessity of direct or strategic (as opposed to transactional) relationships with suppliers in ensuring the protection of garment workers' human rights.

6.1 Greater collaboration between retailers

The Rana Plaza disaster in Bangladesh in 2013 created an environment for collaboration among retailers. Many brands interviewed indicated that the experience of the Rana Plaza tragedy had prompted them to establish health and safety measures and emergency response mechanisms that prepared them for COVID-19. This helped enforce preventive safety protocols in supplier factories. The years since the tragedy have created an environment that necessitated collaboration between retailers during a time of crisis. As one retailer (pers. comm. October 2020) stated, 'one of the biggest learnings from [Rana Plaza] was that, "okay, you can't win the battle if you're alone," so it's really time to collaborate'. This indicates a slow shift away from isolated efforts by brands towards a more serious examination of how collective actions could affect the industry as a whole because, 'a failing apparel industry anywhere isn't good for anyone' (pers. comm. October 2020).

However, retailers warned that ensuring cooperation among the various global retailers will not be easy, given how diverse the industry is:

> It is unrealistic to think that we are going to operate in the same way… It's been very challenging even to get a common assessment tool for working conditions, [so] imagine when we talk about purely business metrics, and the impacts of changing those practices. I'm not sure if the industry will be able to have [the] common tools to drive it.
>
> *(pers. comm. October 2020)*

While full cooperation among retailers is some way away, the COVID-19 crisis has set the stage for the industry to re-examine its practices to move towards collective and collaborative solutions that can create a new normal.

6.2 Partnerships with suppliers

The perception among companies is that the global supply chain, as it exists, serves a purpose. The global supply chain has kept costs low, ensured the delivery of garments in a timely manner in far-flung markets at prices consumers can afford, and created jobs that earlier did not exist in countries where the factories are located. Such a narrow perspective misses the larger picture: even though the workers have jobs, they do not earn a living wage. The system is efficient but does not serve the needs of the workers.

However, the crisis has forced some rethinking within the industry, including calls for moving centers of production closer to consumption centers and reducing the number of suppliers to a few strategic ones. This can have profound impacts in the Global South.

At the same time, companies that realize the importance of longer-term strategic relationships note that there is a discussion about changing the nature of the brand-supplier relationship: 'COVID-19 has put a light on the importance of resilience and partnerships. If you can't be a good partner to a supplier in times of crisis, how will you convince the supplier in the long-term to do sustainable investments?' said one senior executive during an interview (pers. comm.). Direct and close relationships with fewer suppliers provide brands with more leverage to implement performance measures on social and economic issues; this also allows them to partner closely with their vendors for better risk management, or as one retailer (pers. comm.) put it, 'So I would say that our strategy is not about dating, it's about being married, and that's basically what drives everything.'

7 Conclusions and recommendations

COVID-19 has disrupted all layers of the global supply chain. Several companies have gone bankrupt. The crisis manufacturers face is real: they have had to preserve cash and manage inventories carefully in order to remain in business. And yet, while acknowledging these real difficulties, companies still bear responsibility towards their own workers and those who work in their supply chain. The status quo benefits larger corporations, which are well-resourced, and while some among them have operated responsibly and acted beyond their self-interest during the pandemic, the legal requirements for them to do so remain ambiguous. Companies' voluntary actions are encouraging, and sometimes necessary, but not sufficient. Before closing factories or laying-off workers, businesses need to assess the impact on the most vulnerable workers and examine what they can do to mitigate harm. Towards that end, collective action is necessary. With other companies in similar circumstances and in conjunction with their home governments, overseas brands should explore ways to extend credit, provide liquidity, and protect the supply chain.

This will require enhanced supervision of the entire sector. In all three countries under study, local manufacturers can be divided in two broad categories: those that are part of the global supply chain and those who cater primarily to local markets. In Bangladesh, for example, the garment sector has over 7,000 factories, of which perhaps half are exporters to the major markets. Exporting factories face international scrutiny and many among them implement the changes; others may not and remain outside the purview of this paper as well as the scrutiny of overseas companies and international trade unions or civil society. Government inspectors are unable to monitor all factories regularly for health and safety. Supervisors sometimes overlook infractions, sometimes due to bribery. Workers in factories catering to the domestic market are, at least in theory, operating in riskier environments. Protecting the rights of all workers would require the government to increase the number of supervisors, improve their pay scales, and ensure consistent, regular supervision. A two-tiered structure is good neither for the country, nor for its workers. During a seismic change such as the pandemic, this structure widens inequality and threatens human rights.

Another lever that can influence change is international finance and foreign aid. All three countries receive foreign aid and as a result, donor governments have some influence over decisions. Foreign companies too have some leverage. But neither can monitor adherence to international standards on a permanent or sustained basis. One way forward lies in establishing domestically-owned and domestically-driven multi-stakeholder process. Asian manufacturers, government officials, trade unions, and civil society groups will need to develop a genuine, participative, and inclusive multi-stakeholder process to deal with health and safety, factory conditions, hours of work, wages, access to healthcare, sexual harassment, and violence against unions. A robust, collective domestic process which is inclusive and transparent, where stakeholder consultations are possible, where problems are anticipated and addressed, grievances expressed, and remedies offered, is critical. Greater cooperation and trust-building are becoming essential.

The agency of the workers as rights-holders has eroded the most during the pandemic. Disempowered workers are demoralized. Productivity can fall and attrition levels can be high, raising business costs. Democratically-elected and independent unions that can bargain collectively for all workers are crucial. A united, empowered workforce is good for the society. Business restructuring may become inevitable during the pandemic, but human rights law and local legislation require adequate safety nets, with special focus on women. And if those are absent, or not implemented properly, effective trade unions can negotiate for them. To address their grievances, workers will need access to competent, non-partisan advice, which makes the need for independent legal aid clinics essential, particularly in countries and contexts where labor-management relations are politicized.

While the 'fast fashion' model has made cheap goods available quickly around the world, focus on lean inventories and efficiency has significant costs, which the present crisis has magnified. For many years, advocacy groups, economists, trade unions, and human rights organizations have called for changed purchasing practices. Human rights law takes no view of business philosophies, nor does it prefer one business model over another, and companies need to make profit to remain in business. Profits can be taxed; losses cannot. That said, in reassessing their supply chains and purchasing practices, companies should bear in mind wider social impacts of their planned actions. These include impacts on workers and on environmental sustainability. Timely payment of orders and respect for workers' rights should be at the center of such policies. Social compliance costs, including paying a living wage or paying sufficiently for the goods ordered so that suppliers can pay a living wage to their workers and invest in health and safety and other benefits, should be reflected in the cost structure.[6]

One encouraging sign is that the executives of companies the authors interviewed appear to be in agreement. Another executive (pers. comm.) said: 'Going forward as an industry we need to address social protection'. Other executives spoke of compliance, and making adherence to human rights and environmental norms the bedrock of their program. Responsible sourcing is another term used frequently. Another executive (pers. comm.) said:

> There is finally a realization about that interconnectedness, and I'm personally cautiously optimistic about the idea that consumers are seeing empty shelves and are making that connection back to the fact that that's because factories around the world are unable to operate and there are people who are working in those factories. There is a human element to this.

The pandemic has shown the importance of placing that 'human element' at the center of decisions. This current crisis presents a real opportunity to re-examine and re-imagine the garment industry. The diminishing appetite for fast fashion provides a crucial opportunity to acknowledge the inadequacies of the current model and explore more sustainable approaches consistent with international standards of human and labor rights to recreate a business model that could disrupt the existing unequal power relationships between global retailers, suppliers, and workers. COVID-19 has demonstrated the need to 'build back better', to create a 'new normal', and avoid defaulting to the old normal. The hardworking people in developing economies who clothe the world deserve no less.

Notes

1 Garment manufacturers told the authors of steep decline in purchase of business attire and formal wear.

2 This chapter draws on evidence from three complimentary projects of primary research:
- In the *first study*, the Subir and Malini Chowdhury Center for Bangladesh Studies at the University of California, Berkeley collaborated with the James P. Grant School of Public Health (BRAC JPGSPH) and the Centre for Entrepreneurship Development (CED) at BRAC University in Bangladesh and conducted a rapid response survey of garment workers in order to understand how they have been impacted during this pandemic.
- The *second study*, by Behavioral Insights, Architecture and Strategy (BIAS), supported by B+HR Asia UNDP, was aimed at understanding the impact of COVID-19 on the garment sector in Bangladesh, India and Vietnam, and focused mainly on human rights due diligence.
- In the *third study*, the Subir and Malini Chowdhury Center for Bangladesh Studies at the University of California, Berkeley, in partnership with the Institute of Human Rights and Business, supported by the B+HR Asia and UNDP Bangladesh, focused on

interviews with senior executives from ten companies in Europe and North America which have long-established business relationships with major garment manufacturers in Asia and elsewhere, to better understand their responses to the COVID-19 crisis. The interviews provide qualitative information and the authors have drawn on and consulted other available literature and information accessible publicly. The primary focus of this chapter is on the Bangladesh garment sector, but relevant lessons and examples from India and Vietnam are also included. All interviews in the third study were conducted between October and November 2020 and were conducted confidentially on a non-attribution basis and are on file with the authors.

3 Clean Clothes Campaign (2020, p. 8) estimates global loss of wages to be between $3.19 billion and $5.78 billion.

4 Of these, 68 percent are helpers and 52 percent are in supervisory positions.

5 Saxena (2020a, 2020b) makes a similar point regarding the lack of financial support by global retailers for improvements in Bangladesh's factories post-Rana Plaza.

6 One way to cover some of these expenses is an additional charge levied on freight on board (FOB) prices (Anner 2019). Another is the so-called 'T-shirt Tax' that the Nobel Laureate Muhammad Yunus had proposed at the time of the Rana Plaza disaster, suggesting a small tax of between $1 and $1.50 per garment sold, which could go directly towards improving working conditions.

References

Anner, M 2018, 'Binding Power: The Sourcing Squeeze, Workers' Rights, and Building Safety in Bangladesh Since Rana Plaza', *Penn State Center for Global Workers' Rights*.

Anner, M 2019, 'Squeezing Workers' Rights in Global Supply Chains: Purchasing Practices in the Bangladesh Garment Export Sector in Comparative Perspective', *Review of International Political Economy*, vol. 27, no. 2, pp. 320–347.

Anner, M, Nova, S, & Foxvog, L 2020, 'Unpaid Billions: Trade Data Show Apparel Order Volume and Prices Plummeted through June, Driven by Brands' Refusal to Pay for Goods They Asked Suppliers to Make', *Penn State Center for Global Workers' Rights*, 6 October, viewed 18 December 2020, www.workersrights.org/wp-content/uploads/2020/10/Unpaid-Billions_October-6-2020.pdf

Barenblat, A & Cline, E 2020, 'Introducing Payup Fashion: Why the Future of Any Fashion Sustainability Efforts Must Be Worker-Centric', *Remake*, viewed 18 December 2020, remake.world/stories/news/introducing-payup-fashion-why-the-future-of-any-fashion-sustainability-efforts-must-be-worker-centric/

Barrientos, S & Smith, S 2007, 'Do Workers Benefit from Ethical Trade? Assessing Codes of Labour Practice in Global Production Systems', *Third World Quarterly*, vol. 28 no. 4, pp. 713–729.

Baumann-Pauly, D 2020, 'Beyond COVID-19: The Case for Human Rights in Business', *Saïd Business School*, viewed 29 December 2020, www.youtube.com/watch?v=MhabDpmhVTs

Belal, AR, Cooper, SM, & Khan, NA 2015, 'Corporate Environmental Responsibility and Accountability: What Chance in Vulnerable Bangladesh?', *Critical Perspectives on Accounting*, vol. 33, pp. 44–58.

Business and Human Rights Resource Center 2020, 'COVID-19 Apparel Action Tracker', viewed 18 December 2020, https://covid19.business-humanrights.org/en/tracker/

Clean Clothes Campaign 2020, 'Un(der) Paid in the Pandemic: An Estimate of What the Garment Industry Owes its Workers', viewed 18 December 2020, https://media.business-humanrights.org/media/documents/files/documents/CCC-Report-Web-DEF.pdf de Neve, G 2009, 'Power, Inequality and Corporate Social Responsibility: The Politics of Ethical Compliance in the South Indian Garment Industry', *Economic and Political Weekly*, vol. 44, no. 22, pp. 63–71.

Devnath, A 2020, 'European Retailers Scrap $1.5 Billion of Bangladesh Orders', *Bloomberg*, 22 March, viewed 18 December 2020, www.bloomberg.com/news/articles/2020-03-23/europe-retailers-cancel-1-billion-of-bangladesh-garment-orders

Fair Labor Association 2019, *Towards Fair Wages in Vietnam: Insights on Reaching a Living Wage*, viewed 4 November 2020, www.fairlabor.org/sites/default/files/documents/reports/vietnam_wagereport_final.pdf

Human Rights Watch 2019, '"Paying for a Bus Ticket and Expecting to Fly:" How Apparel Brand Purchasing Practices Drive Labor Abuses', viewed 18 December 2020, www.hrw.org/report/2019/04/24/paying-bus-ticket-and-expecting-fly/how-apparel-brand-purchasing-practices-drive

International Covenant on Economic, Social and Cultural Rights 1976, Opened for Signature on 16 December 1966, 993 UNTS 3.

International Labour Organization (ILO) 1996, 'Globalization Changes the Face of Textile, Clothing and Footwear Industries', viewed 18 December 2020, www.ilo.org/global/about-the-ilo/newsroom/news/WCMS_008075/lang--en/index.htm#:~:text=Asia%20is%20the%20major%20world,of%20the%20world's%20clothing%20exports

International Labour Organization (ILO) 2017, 'From Obligation to Opportunity: A Market Systems Analysis of Working Conditions in Asia's Garment Export Industry', viewed 18 December 2020, www.ilo.org/wcmsp5/groups/public/---ed_emp/---emp_ent/---ifp_seed/documents/publication/wcms_628430.pdf

International Trade Union Confederation (ITUC) 2020, *2020 ITUC Global Rights Index: The World's Worst Countries for Workers*, viewed on 19 December 2020, www.ituc-csi.org/IMG/pdf/ituc_globalrightsindex_2020_en.pdf

Khan, S 2020, 'Covid-19 creates a massive $2 billion hole in India's apparel industry' (*Economic Times* 9 April 2020), viewed 12 March 2021, https://economictimes.indiatimes.com/small-biz/sme-sector/covid-19-creates-a-massive-2-billion-hole-in-indias-apparel-industry/articleshow/75059596.cms

Labowitz S & Baumann-Pauly D 2014, 'Business as Usual is Not an Option: Supply Chains and Sourcing after Rana Plaza', *NYU Stern Center for Business and Human Rights*, viewed 18 December 2020, www.stern.nyu.edu/sites/default/files/assets/documents/con_047408.pdf

Leitheiser, E, Hossain, SN, Sen, S, Tasnim, G, Moon, J, Knudsen, JS, & Rahman, S 2020, 'Early Impacts of Coronavirus on Bangladesh Apparel Supply Chains: Perspectives from a Danida Funded Research Project: The Regulation of International Supply Chains (RISC): Lessons from the Governance of Occupational Health and Safety in the Bangladesh Ready-Made Garment Industry', *Copenhagen Business School*, viewed 18 December 2020, https://research-api.cbs.dk/ws/portalfiles/portal/60550960/Risc_report_impacts_of_coronavirus_on_bangladesh_rmg_1.pdf

Locke, RM 2013, *The Promise and Limits of Private Power: Promoting Labor Standards in a Global Economy*, Cambridge University Press, New York.

Lund-Thomsen, P & Lindgreen, A 2014, 'Corporate Social Responsibility in Global Value Chains: Where Are We Now and Where are We Going?', *Journal of Business Ethics*, vol. 123, no. 1, pp. 11–22.

Mezzadri, A 2014, 'Backshoring, Local Sweatshop Regimes and CSR in India', *Competition and Change*, vol. 18, no. 4, pp. 327–344.

Nadvi, K & Waltring, F 2004, 'Making Sense of Global Standards', in H Schmitz (ed.), *Local Enterprises in the Global Economy: Issues of Governance and Upgrading*, Edward Elgar, Northampton, pp. 53–94.

Rabbani, A, Saxena, SB, & Islam, MF 2020, 'The Impact of COVID-19 on the Lives of Workers in the Bangladesh Garment Industry', *Brac University Centre for Entrepreneurship Development*, viewed 18 December 2020, https://chowdhurycenter.berkeley.edu/sites/default/files/shared/docs/CC-BRAC_Covid.pdf

Reinecke, J, Donaghey, J, Bocken, N, & Lauriano, L 2019, *Business Model and Labour Standards: Making the Connection*, Ethical Trading Initiative, London.

Rubenstein, J 2007, 'Accountability in an Unequal World', *The Journal of Politics*, vol. 69, no. 3, pp. 616–632.

Ruggie, JG 2003, 'Taking Embedded Liberalism Global: The Corporate Connection', in D Held & M Koenig-Archibugi (eds.), *Taming Globalization: Frontiers of Governance*, Polity Press, Cambridge, pp. 93–129.

Russell, M 2020, 'Viet Nam H1 Footwear Exports Down nearly 7%', *Just Style*, viewed on 5 November 2020, www.just-style.com/news/Viet Nam-h1-footwear-exports-down-nearly-7_id139120.aspx

Saxena, SB 2020a, 'Bangladesh's Garment Industry Unraveling', *East Asia Forum*, viewed on 19 December 2020, www.eastasiaforum.org/2020/04/24/persistent-danger-plagues-bangladeshs-garment-industry/

Saxena, SB (ed.) 2020b, *Labor, Global Supply Chains, and the Garment Industry in South Asia: Bangladesh After Rana Plaza*, Routledge, Oxon.

Schüßler, E, Frenkel, S, Ashwin, S, Kabeer, N, Egels-Zanden, N, Alexander, R, Huq, L, Oka, C, Lohmeyer, N, Rahman, S, & Rahman KM 2019, 'Garment Supply Chains since Rana Plaza: Governance and Worker Outcomes', *Garment Supply Chain Governance Project*, viewed 29 December 2020, www.researchgate.net/profile/Elke_Schuessler/publication/335609392_Garment_Supply_Chains_since_Rana_Plaza_Governance_and_Worker_Outcomes/links/5d6fe316299bf1cb8087fe7e/Garment-Supply-Chains-since-Rana-Plaza-Governance-and-Worker-Outcomes.pdf

Society for Labour and Development 2020, *Garment Workers in India's Lockdown*, viewed on 22 December 2020, https://media.business-humanrights.org/media/documents/files/documents/Garment-Workers-in-Indias-Lockdown11.pdf

Stanton, A 2020, 'Underpaid in the Pandemic: A Close Look at Garment Maker Wager Gaps During Covid-19', *ReMake*, viewed 18 December 2020, https://remake.world/stories/news/under-paid-in-the-pandemic-a-close-look-at-garment-maker-wage-gaps-during-covid-19/

United Nations Conference on Trade and Development 2020, 'Global Trade Impact of the Coronavirus (COVID-19) Epidemic', *Trade and Development Report Update*, viewed 18 December 2020, https://unctad.org/system/files/official-document/ditcinf2020d1.pdf

United Nations Development Programme 2020, 'Human Rights Due Diligence and COVID-19: Rapid Self-Assessment for Business', United Nations Development Programme, viewed December 14 2020, www.undp.org/content/undp/en/home/librarypage/democratic-governance/human-rights-due-diligence-and-covid-19-rapid-self-assessment-for-business.html

United Nations General Assembly 1948, *Universal Declaration of Human Rights*.

United Nations Office for the High Commissioner for Human Rights (OHCHR), 'OHCHR and the right to social security', viewed 18 December 2020, www.ohchr.org/EN/Issues/RightSocialSecurity/Pages/SocialSecurity.aspx

United Nations Office of the High Commissioner for Human Rights (OHCHR) 2011, 'Guiding Principles on Business and Human Rights', viewed 18 December 2020, www.ohchr.org/documents/publications/guidingprinciplesbusinesshr_en.pdf

Vogel, D 2008, 'Private Global Business Regulation', *Annual Review of Political Science*, vol. 11, pp. 261–282.

Workers' Rights Consortium (WRC) 2020, 'Covid-19 Tracker: Which Brands are Acting Responsibly toward Suppliers and Workers?', viewed 27 October 2020, www.workersrights.org/issues/covid-19/tracker/

16

CAMPAIGNING FOR BOTH INNOVATION AND EQUITABLE ACCESS TO COVID-19 MEDICINES

Brook K. Baker

Ending the COVID-19 pandemic while maximizing human well-being and accelerating economic and social recovery will require rapid development of safe and effective vaccines and medicines and their equitable distribution across the globe. Vaccines, if made widely available, can prevent infection, reduce adverse outcomes, and promote herd immunity. Similarly, medicines can prevent infection, mitigate disease severity, and address long-term sequelae of the disease. Human rights norms can and must be used to advance access to these vital health resources.

This chapter will outline the COVID-19 relevant human rights of access to medicines and to the benefits of scientific progress under the International Covenant on Economic, Social, and Cultural Rights, authoritative General Comments, and reports by Special Rapporteurs for health and for culture. It will explore well-established rights and duties, but also newer human rights claims and more expansive applications that might be pursued in human rights campaigns for (1) better prioritized and more collaborative open-science research and product development, (2) strengthened human rights mandates in clinical trials, (3) continued commitment to safety, efficacy, and quality of medicines even with respect to emergency uses, (4) broad registration and rigorous post-marketing surveillance, (5) expanded supply, and (6) equitable and affordable access to medicines for all.

1 Human right of access to medicines and to the benefits of scientific progress and its medicines-related applications

This section first addresses the basic human right of access to medicines set forth in key human rights instruments and then addresses more specific and actionable duties arising both from the right to health and the right to the benefits of scientific advancement its applications.

1.1 Basic duties

Since the formation of the United Nations more than seventy years ago, and particularly since the adoption of the Universal Declaration of Human Rights, the international community has recognized the fundamental human rights to health and to the health-related benefits of scientific advancement. Article 25.1 expressly recognizes that every person has a right to a standard of living adequate for his or her health and medical care. Article 27.1 guarantees the right to share in the benefits of scientific progress and its applications (United Nations General Assembly 1948). The right to health was further elaborated in Article 12 of the International Covenant on Economic, Social, and Cultural Rights (ICESCR 1976) to recognize 'the right of everyone to the enjoyment of the highest attainable standard of physical and mental health' and the right to 'prevention, treatment and control of epidemic, endemic, occupational and other diseases', and ensured access to medical service and medical attention in the event of sickness.

There is an affirmative duty of progressive realization of the right to health and its subsidiary obligations to the maximum of available resources (ICESCR 1976, art. 2(1)). In 2000, the Committee on Economic, Social, and Cultural Rights (CESCR) issued General Comment 14 formally recognizing the core right of immediate access to essential medicines as defined by the World Health Organization (para. 12(a)). The right of equal and timely access to health goods includes appropriate treatment of prevalent disease and the affordable supply of essential drugs (CESCR 2000, para. 17). States are obligated to take 'steps [which] must be deliberate, concrete and targeted towards full realization', States must 'move as expeditiously and effectively as possible', and States must avoid 'retrogressive measures' (CESCR 2000, paras. 30–32).

Over time, the right of access to medicines has developed further in reports of Special Rapporteurs for health (Hunt 2006, 2008; Grover 2009). Hunt specified that 'access to medicines forms an indispensable part of the right to the highest attainable standard of health' (Hunt 2006, para. 40). The core duty to immediately deliver 'essential medicines' does not mean that there are no human rights obligations with respect to securing access to non-essential medicines (Hunt 2006, para. 58). Recognition of this duty is critically important in the context of COVID-19 because access to medicines and vaccines will be needed well before completion of the arduous process of being added to WHO or national essential medicines lists.

The ICESCR also codified a right to the benefits of scientific progress. The ICESCR holds that '[s]tate parties to the present Covenant recognize the right of everybody … to enjoy the benefits of scientific progress and its applications' (art. 15(1)(b)). In 2020, the CESCR drafted General Comment 25, which clarifies that the right to the benefits of science extends to its material manifestations, including medical applications, as well as to scientific knowledge and information (CESCR 2020, paras 7–8). States have duties to ensure that scientific progress takes place through funding and other means, that science focuses on better and more accessible means for the prevention, control, and treatment of disease, and that its fruits are widely distributed and available to vulnerable and marginalized groups (CESCR 2020, paras. 16, 17, 23, 25, 28–40, 67). Paragraph 37 has particular poignancy:

> As equality is at the core of human rights, States must make every effort to break this vicious circle between substantive inequality and unequal access to the right to participate in and to enjoy the benefits of scientific progress and its applications. … States should prioritize scientific and technological innovations that serve especially the needs of persons living in poverty and ensure that these people have access to the technological innovations.

Likewise, Paragraph 47 clarifies the duty to ensure access to the fruits of science:

> The obligation to fulfil is particularly important in creating and guaranteeing access to the benefits of the applications of scientific progress. States should use the maximum of their available resources to overcome hurdles that any person may face to benefit from new technologies or other forms of applications of scientific advancements. This is particularly relevant for disadvantaged and marginalized groups. Scientific progress and its applications should be, as far as possible, accessible and affordable to persons in need of specific goods or services.

There is also a core obligation 'that in the allocation of public resources, priority is given to research in areas where there is the greatest need for scientific progress in health' (CESCR 2020, para. 52).

While admitting that the right to the benefits of science may depend in part on research carried out by business enterprises and non-state actors, General Comment 25 declares that 'large-scale privatization of scientific research without any other consideration might sometimes have negative effects on the enjoyment of this right' (para. 58). Private scientific research has been associated with the development of international and national intellectual property (IP) regimes, with some positive effects in stimulating innovation. However, General Comment 25 identifies three negative effects of IP: (1) distortions of funding towards commercially profitable investments and away from neglected diseases, (2) limitations on the dissemination of scientific information, and (3) high prices arising from the right to exclude competition (para. 61). Accordingly, States must ensure that the exercise of IP rights are not detrimental to the right to health:

> [I]ntellectual property regime[s] should be interpreted and implemented in a manner supportive of the duty of States 'to protect public health and, in particular, to promote access to medicines for all'. Thus, States parties should use, when necessary, all the flexibilities of the TRIPS Agreement, such as compulsory licences, to ensure access to essential medicines, especially for the most disadvantaged groups.
>
> *(para. 69)*

The Special Rapporteur in the field of cultural rights, Farida Shaheed, issued a key report that addresses the interplay between the right to the benefit of scientific progress and patent rights, affirming the distinction to be made between the two and emphasizing that there is no human right to patent protection. The right to protection of moral and material interests of authors cannot be used to defend patent laws that inadequately respect the right to enjoy the benefits of scientific progress and its applications, to scientific freedoms, and the right to health. Where patent rights and human rights are in conflict, human rights must prevail (Shaheed 2015).

Focusing on the misuse of patents, Shaheed condemned patent trolling and patent thickets that hinder future research, legitimate competition, and access, as well as the use of patents to exclude competitors from producing an improved, dependent technology (Shaheed 2015, paras. 26, 59). She noted with concern that 'intellectual property laws have failed to promote innovation to treat diseases that primarily affect low- and middle-income countries (LMICs)' (paras. 51, 56). She worried that patent-seeking by universities and public research institutions often results in transfers to private entities and that the culture of university research was trending towards commercial interests rather than public good and human advancement (para. 58). The Special Rapporteur recommended instead that universities and public research institutions adopt licensing approaches that serve their social-benefit mission and that they and public and charitable funders of research should ensure that resulting technologies are made widely available (paras. 111, 109). She reasoned that the 'conjoined human right to science and culture should be understood as including a right to have access to, use, and further develop technologies in self-determined and empowering ways' (para. 55), a right that also supports people's right to direct research, drug development, and adapted technologies towards targeted needs. In areas with high social need but low commercial prospects, she recommended the adoption of new incentive models, including 'government grants and procurements, advance purchase commitments, tax incentives for research and development, prizes, and other means' (paras. 91, 108). She urged the adoption, protection, and use of trade related aspects of intellectual property rights (TRIPS) flexibilities (paras. 63–72, 102–107) and reaffirmed the importance of public participation and transparency in intellectual property policymaking and transparency about the costs of drug development (paras. 73–76, 92–94).

2.2 Specific duties

At its most basic level, meaningful access to medicines refers to the ability of all persons to receive the medicines they need and that these medicines are available, accessible, acceptable, and of good quality (CESCR 2000, paras. 12, 16, 17). *Availability* requires sufficient quantities of the medicine (para. 12(a)), meaning that needed medicines must be procured and stock-outs avoided. *Accessibility* entails (1) physical accessibility 'within safe physical reach', (2) economic accessibility – medicines 'affordable for all', and (3) informational accessibility, including 'the right to seek, receive and impart information and ideas concerning health issues'. All such accessibility must be provided without discrimination, especially for the most vulnerable and marginalized sections of the population (para. 12(b)). *Acceptability* refers to the need to 'be respectful of medical ethics' and sensitive to the cultural norms of individuals and communities (CESCR 2000, para. 12(c)). Finally, the medicine 'must also be scientifically and medically appropriate and of good *quality*' (para. 12(d)), an obligation also arising under the right to the benefit of scientific progress where States are enjoined to ensure the quality via science-based regulation and certification of scientific technologies (CESCR 2020, para. 18).

General Comment 14 also clarifies that States have clear obligations to respect, protect, and fulfill the right to health:

> [T]he obligation to fulfil contains obligations to facilitate, provide and promote. The obligation to *respect* requires States to refrain from interfering directly or indirectly with the enjoyment of the right to health. The obligation to *protect* requires States to take measures that prevent third parties from interfering with article 12 guarantees. Finally, the obligation to *fulfil* requires States to adopt appropriate legislative, administrative, budgetary, judicial, promotional and other measures towards the full realization of the right to health.
>
> *(CESCR 2000, para. 33)*

A State's duty to respect the right to health includes duties 'to refrain ... from marketing unsafe drugs' (para. 34), 'to control the marketing of medical equipment and medicines by third parties', and to 'ensure that third parties do not limit people's access to health-related information and services' (para. 35). The duty to protect requires regulating domestic activities of drug companies to prevent them from violating the right to health of others (para. 51). The duty to fulfill the right to health requires States to promote medical research, health education, and information campaigns (para. 36), to support people in making informed health choices (para. 37), and to reduce inequitable distribution of medicines (para. 52). Special Rapporteur Hunt emphasized that the duty to make medicines affordable might require countries to use TRIPS flexibilities, including compulsory licenses (Hunt 2006, para. 47). Pursuant to their duties to ensure the benefits of scientific progress, States should: (1) adequately fund scientific research and provide other incentives such as market entry rewards in neglected fields that 'delink remuneration of successful research from future sales', (2) achieve a better balance in promoting 'open access to and sharing of scientific knowledge and its applications', and (3) prevent 'unreasonably high costs for access to essential medicines' (CESCR 2020, para. 62).

Special Rapporteur for health Grover addressed additional steps that States must take to fulfill access to medicines duties, including establishing essential medicines lists (Grover 2013, paras. 40–46, 73), assuring efficient procurement (paras. 47–53, 74) and distribution systems (paras. 54–56, 74), and promoting rational and appropriate use of medicines (paras. 57–60). First, medicines must be adopted onto WHO and national essential medicines lists based on health needs not patent status or price, and thereafter incorporated into WHO and national treatment guidelines. Second, countries must procure the right quantity of medicines at best sustainable prices and distribute medicines to the right place at the right time in the right quantities. Third, rational use of medicines requires that patients receive medications and doses appropriate to their needs at the lowest cost. It requires proper prescribing and concerted action to minimize patients' out-of-pocket expenses. Fourth, rational use of medicines requires health literacy, informed consent, and appropriate personal, psycho-social, systemic supports for adherence.

Even though primary responsibility for the domestic rights of access to medicines and to the benefits of science falls on the State, States have duties to each other, and private entities also have responsibilities. States must be health-cognizant 'when entering into bilateral or multilateral agreements with other States, international organizations and other entities, such as multilateral corporations' (CESCR 2000, para. 50). Foreign States, especially resource-rich States, have a duty to respect the enjoyment and realization of the right to health in other countries, including access to essential health goods and services (CESCR 2000, para. 39). A State's failure to regulate pharmaceutical corporations to prevent them from violating rights to health abroad is a breach of the obligation to protect the right to health (para. 51). Noting that 'gross inequality' in health status between people in developed and developing countries is 'politically, socially and economically unacceptable', paragraph 38 (CESCR 2000) also emphasizes the obligations of powerful States 'to take steps, individually and through international assistance and cooperation, especially economic and technical, towards the full realization of … the right to health'.

Special Rapporteur Hunt noted that, 'States are required to take effective measures to promote the development and availability of new drugs, vaccines and diagnostic tools for those diseases causing a heavy burden in developing countries' (Hunt 2006, para. 47). Similarly, General Comment 25 imposes obligations on wealthy countries to ensure access to medicines in developing countries (CESCR 2020, para. 79). Furthermore, 'the benefits and applications resulting from scientific progress should be shared, with due incentives and regulations, with the international community, particularly with developing countries' (para. 80). In a prescient statement, General Comment 25 emphasized the need for global cooperation and sharing in the face of pandemics, such as the world is facing with COVID-19 (para. 82).

In many ways, the biopharmaceutical industry wields more power over access to medicines than governments, especially in States captive to corporate interests. In response, General Comment 14 clarifies that the private business sector has 'horizontal' responsibilities regarding the realization of the right to health (CESCR 2000, paras. 42, 48, 64). These responsibilities were explored at length in Special Rapporteur Hunt's 2008 'Human Rights Guidelines for Pharmaceutical Companies in relation to Access to Medicines'. There, he recommended that pharmaceutical companies increase their research commitments on neglected diseases (Hunt 2008, paras. 23–25). He urged pharmaceutical companies to grant non-exclusive voluntary licenses, to waive data exclusivity, and to avoid applying for patents in LMICs for insignificant or trivial modifications of existing medicines (paras. 30–32). With respect to pricing, Hunt recommended that pharmaceutical companies ensure that medicines are affordable to as many people as possible, mentioning differential pricing, voluntary licenses, donation programs, and public-private partnerships that take into account a country's economic development and differential purchasing power (paras. 33–35). Finally, each company should share information bearing upon safety, efficacy, and possible side effects of a medicine so that individuals can make informed decisions and have responsible drug promotion and marketing policies (paras. 39–41).

Efforts to put real teeth into the recognition and enforcement of private enterprises' human rights obligations have been fraught with disappointment (Blitt 2017, pp. 52–54). A 2005 UN mandate on the human rights obligations of businesses resulted in a new Framework for Business and Human Rights in 2008 and Guiding Principles to implement the Framework in 2011 (Ruggie 2008, para. 9; Ruggie 2011). Ruggie's efforts basically maintain the *status quo* by articulating an aspirational 'Protect, Respect, and Remedy' framework but no hard, substantive rules or remedial procedures (Aaronson & Higham 2013). Subsequently, in 2014, following a highly contested vote, the Human Rights Council established an open-ended working group to develop 'an international legally binding instrument to regulate, in international human rights law, the activities of transnational corporations and other business enterprises' (Human Rights Council 2014). In July 2019, a revised draft of such an instrument was published (OEIGWG 2019), though its prospects seem highly uncertain.

2 Human rights-based campaigns for access to medicines in the context of COVID-19

Having addressed basic human rights frameworks on access to medicines, it is now time to apply those frameworks to actionable campaigns responding to the COVID-19 pandemic.

2.1 Promoting open-science research and product development targeting unmet COVID-19 needs and future pandemic risks

The COVID-19 pandemic caught the world flatfooted despite warnings of pandemic risks in general and coronavirus risks in particular. Many commentators sounded the alarm, and some preliminary steps were taken, but for the most part the scientific community was far behind where it should have been in preparing for COVID-19. This has resulted in a massive human rights failure that must be addressed now and for future pandemic risks. Basic science pre-2020 largely ignored research on coronaviruses, though there were two mini-boom and bust cycles following SARS in 2002–2003 and MERS in 2012 (Branswell & Thielking 2020). Had States, public and private universities, public research institutes, and private biopharmaceutical companies prioritized and funded a needs-driven research and development (R&D) agenda, we would not be experiencing our chaotic rush to viral preparedness. Moreover, instead of the current approach that still prioritizes research silos, secrecy, and exclusive ownership rights once commercial applications are identified, the world needs a razor-sharp focus on the COVID-19-related needs of all populations and collaborative, open-science approaches to discovery and innovation. Any resulting medical products should not just be appropriate for use in well-resourced countries – they should be well adapted for use in resource-poor settings.

General Comment 14 pays little attention to the need to prioritize research and development (R&D) to address unmet and emergent needs, but it does enjoin States to promote medical research (CESCR 2000, para. 36). Special Rapporteur Hunt urged greater attention to neglected R&D, arguing that States 'have a responsibility to take reasonable measures to ensure that much-needed new medicines are developed and thereby become available' (Hunt 2006, para. 48). In his 2008 Report, he concluded States are obligated:

> to generate health research and development that addresses … the health needs of disadvantaged individuals, communities and populations. Health research and development includes classical medical research into drugs, vaccines and diagnostics, as well as operational or implementation research into the social, economic, cultural, political and policy issues that determine access to medical care and the effectiveness of public health interventions.
>
> *(Hunt 2008, para. 95)*

Commentary on the right to the benefits of scientific progress specifies 'that in the allocation of public resources, priority is given to research in areas where there is the greatest need for scientific progress in health' (CESCR 2020, paras. 46, 52). Recognizing that private entities ignore R&D on pandemic risks because of uncertain financial returns, States should adequately fund scientific research and provide other incentives such as market entry rewards in neglected fields that 'delink remuneration of successful research from future sales' (paras. 61–62). They should cooperate with other States facing pandemic risks and share scientific knowledge 'to mitigate the impact of the disease and to expedite the discovery of effective treatments and vaccines' (para. 82).

States have further duties to ensure that open science is promoted, including the publication of publicly funded research results (CESCR 2020, para. 16):

> [O]pen science cannot be achieved by the State alone. It is a common endeavour to which all other stakeholders should contribute, nationally and internationally, including scientists, universities, publishers, scientific associations, funding agencies, libraries, the media and non-governmental institutions. All these stakeholders play a decisive role in the dissemination of knowledge, especially when it comes to outcomes of research financed with public funds.
>
> *(para. 49)*

2.2 Addressing human rights and ethical issues in COVID-19 clinical trials

Human rights norms recognize the right of informed consent to medical experimentation (CESCR 2000, paras. 8, 50) and the risk of exploitation of human subjects. An important human rights issue in clinical trials is whether trials inclusively recruit population groups that might need the medicines being studied. History reveals consistent underrepresentation and thus impermissible discrimination against women, children, seniors, people with chronic diseases, and people with disabilities in clinical trials (Frieden 2018; Spong & Bianchi 2018). Women, especially pregnant and lactating women, are disproportionately underrepresented in clinical trials (Feldman et al. 2019). There is systemic discrimination against children both because of misplaced safety concerns (Bavdekar 2013) and lack of commercial prospects. Similarly, clinical trials often exclude or underrepresent older people (Lockett et al. 2019). These historic concerns about underrepresentation of diverse populations in clinical trials have extended to COVID-19 where trials have under-enrolled, for example, participants of color and pregnant women (Chastain et al. 2020; Farrel et al. 2020).

Another clinical trial discrimination issue arises concerning the under-enrollment of populations from low- and middle-income countries (LMICs) in COVID-19 clinical trials where there is a need to study investigational medicines in varied human populations with different patterns of disease and where people's ultimate entitlement to the benefits of scientific progress might be denied in the absence of local trials (COVID-19 Clinical Research Coalition 2020; Brotherton et al. 2020). Under-enrollment must be counterbalanced to avoid using people from poor countries as guinea pigs for research primarily benefiting the Global North (Weigmann 2015; Pasic et al. 2018). An additional human rights concern is whether beneficial health products will be made available in LMICs where clinical trials are performed (Weigmann 2015, p. 569). There is growing appreciation of the right of participation and consultation with people living with the researched disease and people living where clinical trials are conducted.

There are also critiques of longstanding flaws in clinical trial design, including reliance on commercial trials rather than truly independent, government-financed trials (Baker 2008), reluctance to compare investigational medicines against existing medicines for evidence of superiority (Garattini & Bertele 2007), and failure to investigate treatment regimens instead of single medicines (Médicines sans Frontières 2016). The chaos in uncoordinated and underpowered COVID-19 studies reinforces the need for research collaborations, pooling of research findings, and more direct comparisons between competing products so that the best clinical options can be identified (Bach 2020; Nature Editorials 2020; Petkova et al. 2020).

2.3 Establishing a human right to science-based registration and post-marketing surveillance of medicines by national medicines regulatory authorities and a duty for companies to register their medicines broadly

Although the duty to undertake a valid scientific assessment of the safety, efficacy, and quality of a medicines is well established (CESCR 2000, paras. 12(d), 34, 35; CESCR 2020, para. 18; Hunt 2006, paras. 51, 71–73) the duty of biopharmaceutical companies to seek marketing approval of their medicines promptly in all countries is not. Countries must weigh beneficial efficacy against safety risks and render registration decisions in a timely manner so that access to needed medicines is not needlessly delayed. To fulfill this obligation, countries with weak and slow national regulatory authorities might have duties to permit fast-track registration based on WHO prequalification (WHO 2020a) and registration by a stringent regulatory authority, and might also be required to join and use the WHO Collaborative Registration Procedure (WHO 2013). And, to increase efficiency of registration procedures and to incentivize broad registration by manufacturers, countries need to strengthen their medicines regulatory authorities, seek out international collaboration to harmonize regulatory standards, and allow collaborative and expedited registration procedures based on valid regulatory assessments elsewhere.

However, on the opposite side of the equation, pharmaceutical companies are putting increased pressure on regulators to expedite marketing approval and to relax rigorous assessment of safety and efficacy; they are promoting greater reliance on post-marketing studies and clinical experience, thereby putting patients at increased risk for little proven benefit (Puthumana et al. 2018; Kesselheim et al. 2015). With respect to COVID-19, there has been a troubling turn to overly lax and politicized emergency use authorizations for hydroxychloroquine and convalescent plasma in the United States (Zhai et al. 2020; Sharfstein 2020). Even more concerning, Russia and China are rolling out COVID-19 vaccines without large-scale studies proving efficacy and safety (Petersen et al. 2020; Mahase 2020) and President Trump was reported to have been putting pressure on the FDA to expedite emergency use authorization of vaccines before the November election (Dyer 2020). Relaxing standards and an inadequate assessment of longer-term safety and efficacy results violates human rights duties of countries and companies to only market medicines based on reliable scientific evidence.

Authorities must also enforce Phase IV study obligations, establish easy-to-use and reliable pharmacovigilance systems with stringent reporting requirements, and perform regular post-marketing surveillance to ensure the continuing quality and safety of medicines throughout the supply chain (Grover 2013, paras. 61–66). Where countries make registration conditional on the completion and reporting of Phase IV clinical trials in broader patient groups and over a longer period of time, they should ensure that registrants conduct such trials and report results promptly and transparently (Naci et al. 2017). Countries should also utilize robust pharmacovigilance with rigorous reporting requirements to collect information on unexpected adverse side effects (WHO 2014). Given accelerated market entry of COVID-19 related medicines and vaccines, countries must rigorously enforce COVID-19 Phase IV studies, pharmacovigilance, and post-marketing surveillance.

States are obligated to ensure that medicines are accessible and affordable to their populations, but manufacturers of medicines, not governments, initiate applications for marketing approval. Both originators and generic companies consistently neglect registering in poorer and smaller markets, leaving people in those countries without medicines they need. Part of the problem is failure of capacity, inefficiencies, corruption, and other barriers to registration that countries are obligated to address. Regrettably, States have no viable mechanism to force a biopharmaceutical company to enter their market. Moreover, where a comparator originator product has not yet been registered, registration of a generic equivalent is much harder, meaning that the generic licensee might have to conduct costly, time-consuming, and potentially unethical repetitive clinical trials to gain the data needed for registration. The most immediate work-around would be for countries to adopt registration rules allowing them to rely on the fact of registration elsewhere to register a generic product domestically.

The risk of needlessly delayed registration is frankly abhorrent and will be doubly so in the context of the COVID-19 pandemic. Access-to-medicines activists will need to champion a new human rights principle that both originator and generic companies have enforceable duties to register their COVID-19 vaccines and medicines broadly in all countries. This human rights claim can be strengthened by reference to the right to the benefit of scientific progress, a right that remains unrealized if medicines are not registered. Similarly, the right to protection against discrimination should include the right of the population of entire countries to avoid being denied authorized use of new medicines.

2.4 Guaranteeing availability, accessibility, affordability, and equitable distribution of COVID-19 medicines and vaccines

Historically, access-to-medicines campaigns have focused on affordability with efforts to reduce the number of patents on medicines and to promote generic competition. This competition has reduced the price of antiretrovirals in most low- and many middle-income countries by 99+ percent, which has been key to the enormous expansion of treatment from the hundreds of thousands in 2000 to over twenty-five million in 2020 (UNAIDS 2020a). There are some indications of price moderation in the pricing of COVID-19 vaccines, including by Johnson & Johnson, which has promised a non-profit price of $10 for its single dose vaccine, and by Oxford University/AstraZeneca, which have promised a price as low as $6 for a two-dose regimen. However, other vaccine innovators are projecting much higher prices for a two-dose vaccination: Sinopharm $145, Moderna $74, Pfizer $39, and Novovax $32 (Cao 2020). Similarly, Gilead's remdesivir, a repurposed antiviral which has shown only limited benefit shortening hospital stays and easing moderate infection, is priced between $2,340 and $3,120 for a five-day course of treatment (Herper 2020). Given the billions of people needing COVID-19 vaccines and the tens of millions that might require access to therapeutics, the public and private budget implications of over-priced medicines are staggering.

The COVID-19 pandemic, however, is teaching new lessons about the negative impacts of exclusivities on access to medicines. Not only do exclusivities lead to high prices, but they also lead to artificially limited supply. Although vaccine and medicines companies are taking steps to increase their production capacity and are entering into agreements with contract manufacturing organizations to meet rich country demand (O'Sullivan et al. 2020), they are studiously avoiding efforts to more broadly license their medicines with full technology transfer to all qualified generic and biosimilar producers. In the wake of anticipated shortages, the world is experiencing an explosion of vaccine and therapeutic nationalism by the United States, the UK, the European Union, Japan, and other rich countries that have entered into preferential advance purchase agreements locking up the majority of initial vaccine supplies for several years (Launch and Scale Speedometer 2020). This state of affairs results from the perverse synergy of IP and market fundamentalism, whereby governments grant exclusive rights at the same time that they leave commercialization decisions entirely in the hands of IP rightholders, who thereafter give preferential market access to rich countries that race to the front of the line and can afford premium prices. Once again, the risk is that the Global South will be left behind and the human right of every global citizen to equitable access to life-saving and life-enhancing medicines and vaccines will be eviscerated.

In response to the risk of high prices, inadequate supplies, and inequitable access, access-to-medicines campaigners have reacted vigorously to promote open licensing and technology transfer of COVID-related IP, data, and information rights and to ensure that sufficient supplies of affordable medicines and vaccine are equitably distributed. This call has a new urgency given evidence that death rates will be two times higher if vaccines are hoarded rather than shared globally (Arntsen 2020). WHO, Unitaid, over forty countries, and civil society activists rallied early behind a proposal of Costa Rica that the WHO establish a COVID-19 Technology Access Pool (COVID-19 Technology Access Pool 2020). Such a pool would facilitate the development of new medical technologies, ensure open licensing to qualified producers, and guarantee equitable distribution and ethical allocation of supplies (Abbas 2020), but uptake and implementation thus far has been weak. Other academics, scientists, and organizations have promoted an Open COVID Pledge (Open COVID Pledge 2020) and several universities have promised to openly license their COVID-19-related technologies (COVID-19 Technology Access Framework 2020).

In addition to the pursuit of voluntary measures, there has been advocacy: (1) from South Africa and India at the WTO to waive recognition and enforcement of IP rights on COVID-19 health products until herd immunity is achieved (WTO 2020); (2) to use national security measures in international trade law to suspend the recognition and enforcement of COVID-19-related intellectual property protections during the pandemic (Abbott 2020); (3) to establish a new binding agreement under the WHO to redesign global health governance for health R&D (Velásquez 2020); and (4) to adopt and implement compulsory licensing and other measures to overcome IP exclusivities on medicines (Boru 2020; Wong 2020). Several countries have independently adopted laws and policies permitting easier or automatic use of compulsory licensing mechanisms to access COVID-19 medicines and vaccines (Public Citizen 2020). There have also been multiple calls for global solidarity and for equitable access to COVID-19 health products at the UN and WHO (United Nations General Assembly 2020a; United Nations General Assembly 2020b; WHO 2020b). Global partners also established the Access to COVID-19 Tools Accelerator where equitable access is a foundational commitment (WHO 2020c) and other global leaders have championed a People's Vaccine (UNAIDS 2020b). Unfortunately, the rhetoric of sharing COVID-19 resources and technologies is eclipsed by stingy realities on the ground.

3 Conclusion

Human rights provide one of the most compelling moral, ethical, and legal frameworks for campaigns claiming innovation and adaptation of new COVID-19 medicines responsive to the needs of people in LMICs and claiming expanded and equitable access to affordable medicines and vaccines for all people in all countries. Words alone will not deliver the realization of human rights – instead, such goals will be achieved only through vibrant campaigns of people fighting for their lives and for health in their communities.

References

Aaronson, S & Higham, I 2013, '"Re-righting Business": John Ruggie and the Struggle to Develop International Human Rights Standards for Transnational Firms', *Human Rights Quarterly*, vol. 35, no. 2, pp. 264–333.

Abbas, M 2020, 'Treatment of the Novel COVID-19: Why Costa Rica's Proposal for the Creation of a Global Pooling Mechanism Deserves Serious Consideration?', *Journal of Law and the Biosciences*, vol. 7, no. 1, pp. 1–10.

Abbott, F 2020, 'The TRIPS Agreement Article 73 Security Exceptions and the COVID-19 Pandemic', *South Centre*, viewed 20 September 2020, www.southcentre.int/wp-content/uploads/2020/08/RP-116-reduced_1.pdf

Arntsen, E 2020, 'If Rich Countries Monopolize COVID-19 Vaccines, It Could Cause Twice as Many Deaths as Distributing Them Equally', *News@Northeastern*, viewed 28 September 2020, https://news.northeastern.edu/2020/09/14/if-rich-countries-monopolize-covid-19-vaccines-it-could-cause-twice-as-many-deaths-as-distributing-them-equally/

Bach, P 2020, 'We Can't Tackle the Pandemic without Figuring Out Which Covid-19 Vaccines Work the Best', *STAT*, viewed 24 September 2020, www.statnews.com/2020/09/24/big-trial-needed-determine-which-covid-19-vaccines-work-best/

Baker, D 2008, 'The Benefits and Savings from Publicly Funded Clinical Trials of Prescription Drugs', *International Journal of Health Services*, vol. 38, no. 4, pp. 731–750.

Bavdekar, S 2013, 'Pediatric Clinical Trials', *Perspectives in Clinical Research*, vol. 4, no. 1, p. 89.

Blitt, R 2017, 'Beyond Ruggie's Guiding Principles on Business and Human Rights: Charting an Embracive Approach to Corporate Human Rights Compliance', *Texas International Law Journal*, vol. 48, no. 1, pp. 33–62.

Boru, Z 2020, 'Equitable Access to COVID-19 Related Health Technologies: A Global Priority', *South Centre*, viewed 20 September 2020, www.southcentre.int/wp-content/uploads/2020/06/RP-114.pdf

Branswell, H & Thielking, M 2020, 'Fluctuating Funding and Flagging Interest Hurt Coronavirus Research, Leaving Crucial Knowledge Gaps', *STAT*, viewed 20 September 2020, www.statnews.com/2020/02/10/fluctuating-funding-and-flagging-interest-hurt-coronavirus-research/?utm_source=STAT+Newsletters&utm_campaign=dcab17d49e-Pharmalot&utm_medium=email&utm_term=0_8cab1d7961-dcab17d49e-149648021

Brotherton, H, Usuf, E, Nadjm, B, Forrest, K, Bojang, K, Samateh, A, Bittaye, M, Roberts, C, d'Alessandro, U, & Roca, A 2020, 'Dexamethasone for COVID-19: Data Needed from Randomised Clinical Trials in Africa', *The Lancet Global Health*, vol. 8, no. 9, pp. e1125–e1126.

Cao, S 2020, 'Here's How Much COVID-19 Vaccines Will Cost From The 5 Frontrunners', *Observer*, viewed 24 September 2020, https://observer.com/2020/08/covid19-vaccine-price-comparison-moderna-pfizer-novavax-johnson-astrazeneca/

Chastain, D, Osae S, Henao-Martínez A, Franco-Paredes C, Chastain, J, & Young H 2020, 'Racial Disproportionality in Covid Clinical Trials', *New England Journal of Medicine*, vol. 383, no. 9, p. e59.

Committee on Economic, Social and Cultural Rights (CESCR) 2000, *General Comment 14: The Right to the Highest Attainable Standard of Health (Art. 12)*, UN Doc. E/C.12/2000/4.

Committee on Economic, Social and Cultural Rights (CESCR) 2020, *General Comment No. 25 on Science and Economic, Social and Cultural Rights (Article 15 (1) (b), (2), (3) and (4) of the International Covenant on Economic, Social and Cultural Rights)*, UN Doc. E/C.12/GC/25.

COVID-19 Clinical Research Coalition 2020, 'Global Coalition to Accelerate COVID-19 Clinical Research in Resource-limited Settings', *The Lancet*, vol. 395, no. 10233, pp. 1322–1325.

COVID-19 Technology Access Framework 2020, *MIT Technology Licensing Office*, viewed 28 September 2020, https://tlo.mit.edu/engage-tlo/covid-19/covid-19-technology-access-framework

Dyer, O 2020, 'Covid-19: Pharma Companies Promise Not to Bow to Political Pressure to Rush Vaccine Production', *BMJ*, 9 September, p. m3512.

Farrell, R, Michie, M, & Pope, R 2020, 'Pregnant Women in Trials of Covid-19: A Critical Time to Consider Ethical Frameworks of Inclusion in Clinical Trials', *Ethics & Human Research*, vol. 42, no. 4, pp. 17–23.

Feldman, S, Ammar, W, & Lo, K 2019, 'Quantifying Sex Bias in Clinical Studies at Scale with Automated Data Extraction', *JAMA Network Open*, vol. 2, no. 7, p. e196700.

Frieden, J 2018, 'Clinical Trials Needs to be More Inclusive Experts Say', *Medpage Today*, viewed 20 September 2020, www.medpagetoday.com/publichealthpolicy/clinicaltrials/72400

Garattini, S & Bertele, V 2007, 'Non-inferiority Trials Are Unethical because They Disregard Patients' interests', *The Lancet*, vol. 370, no. 9602, pp. 1875–1877.

Grover, A 2009, *Report of the Special Rapporteur on the Right of Everyone to the Enjoyment of the Highest Attainable Standard of Physical and Mental Health*, UN Doc. A/HRC/11/12.

Grover, A 2013, *Report of the Special Rapporteur on the Right of Everyone to the Enjoyment of the Highest Attainable Standard of Physical and Mental Health*, UN Doc. A/HRC/23/42.

Herper, M 2020, 'Gilead announces long-awaited price for Covid-19 drug remdesivir', *STAT*, viewed 24 September 2020, www.statnews.com/2020/06/29/gilead-announces-remdesivir-price-covid-19/

Human Rights Council 2014, *Elaboration of an International Legally Binding Instrument on Transnational Corporations and Other Business Enterprises with Respect to Human Rights*, UN Doc. A/HRC/Res/26/9.

Hunt, P 2006, *Report of the Special Rapporteur on the Right of Everyone to the Enjoyment of the Highest Attainable Standard of Physical and Mental Health*, UN Doc. A/61/338.

Hunt, P 2008, *Human Rights Guidelines for Pharmaceutical Companies in Relation to Access to Medicines*, UN Doc. A/63/263.

International Covenant on Economic, Social, and Cultural Rights (ICESCR) (1976) Opened for Signature 16 December 1966, 993 UNTS 3.

Kesselheim, A, Wang, B, Franklin, J, & Darrow J 2015, 'Trends in Utilization of FDA Expedited Drug Development and Approval Programs, 1987–2014: cohort study', *BMJ*, p. h4633

Launch and Scale Speedometer, *Duke Global Health Innovation Center*, viewed 10 November 2020, https://launchandscalefaster.org/covid-19

Lockett, J, Sauma, S, Radziszewska, B, & Bernard M 2019, 'Adequacy of Inclusion of Older Adults in NIH-Funded Phase III Clinical Trials', *Journal of the American Geriatrics Society*, vol. 67, no. 2, pp. 218–222.

Mahase, E 2020, 'Covid-19: Russia Approves Vaccine without Large Scale Testing or Published Results', *BMJ*, 13 August, p. m3205.

Medicines sans Frontières, 2016, 'Issue Brief: The 3P Project – Accelerating Innovation and Access to Medicines for Tuberculosis', *MSF Access Campaign*, viewed 20 September 2020, https://msfaccess.org/3p-project-accelerating-innovation-and-access-medicines-tuberculosis

Naci, H, Smalley, K, & Kesselheim, A 2017, 'Characteristics of Preapproval and Postapproval Studies for Drugs Granted Accelerated Approval by the US Food and Drug Administration', *JAMA*, vol. 318, no. 7, p. 626.

Nature Editorials, 2020, 'Coronavirus Drugs Trials Must Get Bigger and more Collaborative', *Nature*, vol. 581, no. 7807, p. 120.

OEIGWG Chairmanship Revised Draft (2019), viewed 20 September 2020, www.ohchr.org/Documents/HRBodies/HRCouncil/WGTransCorp/OEIGWG_RevisedDraft_LBI.pdf

Open COVID Pledge 2020, *Frequently Asked Questions*, viewed 28 September 2020, https://opencovidpledge.org/faqs/

O'Sullivan, C, Rutten, P, & Shatz, C 2020, 'Why Tech Transfer May be Critical to Beating COVID-19', *McKinsey & Company*, viewed 27 September 2020, www.mckinsey.com/~/media/McKinsey/Industries/Pharmaceuticals%20and%20Medical%20Products/Our%20Insights/Why%20tech%20transfer%20may%20be%20critical%20to%20beating%20COVID%2019/Why-tech-transfer-may-be-critical-to-beating-COVID-19-vF.pdf

Pasic, M, Vidrih, B, Sarac, H, Pasic, H, Vujević, L, Koruga, A, & Rajič, F 2018, 'Clinical Trials in Developing Countries – Ethical Considerations', *Psychiatria Danubina*, vol. 30, no. 3, pp. 285–291.

Petersen, E, Wejse, C, & Zumla, A 2020, 'Advancing COVID-19 Vaccines – Avoiding Different Regulatory Standards for Different Vaccines and Need for Open and Transparent Data Sharing', *International Journal of Infectious Diseases*, vol. 98, pp. 501–502.

Petkova, E, Antman, EM, & Troxel, AB 2020, 'Pooling Data From Individual Clinical Trials in the COVID-19 Era', *JAMA*, vol. 324 no. 6, pp. 543–545.

Public Citizen 2020, 'People over Patents: How Governments are Preparing to Make COVID-19 Medicines Accessible', *Public Citizen*, viewed 28 September 2020, www.citizen.org/wp-content/uploads/Global-survey-of-IP-and-COVID-final.pdf

Puthumana, J, Wallach, J, & Ross, J. 2018, 'Clinical Trial Evidence Supporting FDA Approval of Drugs Granted Breakthrough Therapy Designation', *JAMA*, vol. 320, no. 3, p. 301.

Ruggie, J 2008, *Special Representative of the Secretary-General, Protect, Respect and Remedy: a Framework for Business and Human Rights*, UN Doc. A/HRC/8/5.

Ruggie, J 2011, *Special Representative of the Secretary-General, Guiding Principles on Business and Human Rights: Implementing the United Nations 'Protect, Respect and Remedy' Framework*, UN Doc. A/HRC/17/31.

Shaheed, F 2015, *Report of the Special Rapporteur in the Field of Cultural Rights: Cultural Rights*, UN Doc. A/70/279.

Sharfstein, J 2020, 'How the FDA Should Protect Its Integrity from Politics', *Nature*, vol. 585, no. 7824, p. 161.

Spong, C & Bianchi, D 2018, 'Improving Public Health Requires Inclusion of Underrepresented Populations in Research', *JAMA*, vol. 319, no. 4, p. 337.

United Nations General Assembly 1948, *Universal Declaration of Human Rights*, UN Doc. A/810.

United Nations General Assembly 2020a, *Resolution Adopted by the General Assembly on 20 April 2020*, UN Doc. A/RES/74/274.

United Nations General Assembly 2020b, *Draft Resolution Submitted by the President of the General Assembly, Comprehensive and Coordinated Response to Coronavirus Disease (COVID-19) Pandemic*, UN Doc. A.74/L.92*.

UNAIDS 2020a, 'Global HIV & AIDS Statistics – 2020 Fact Sheet', *UNAIDS*, viewed 27 September 2020, www.unaids.org/en/resources/fact-sheet

UNAIDS 2020b 'The People's Vaccine', *UNAIDS*, 14 May, viewed 28 September 2020, www.unaids.org/en/resources/presscentre/featurestories/2020/may/20200514_covid19-vaccine-open-letter

Velásquez, G 2020, 'Rethinking R&D for Pharmaceutical Products After the Novel Coronavirus COVID-19 Shock', *South Centre*, viewed 20 September 2020, www.southcentre.int/wp-content/uploads/2020/04/PB-75-Rethinking-RD-after-COVID-19-Shock-REV.pdf

Weigmann, K 2015, 'The Ethics of Global Clinical Trials', *EMBO reports*, vol. 16, no. 5, pp. 566–570.

WHO 2013, 'WHO Launches the PQP Collaborative Registration Procedure', *WHO Drug Information*, vol. 27, no. 4, pp. 325–331.

WHO 2014, 'Reporting and Learning Systems for Medication Errors: The Role for Pharmacovigilance Centres', *WHO*, viewed 28 September 2020, https://apps.who.int/iris/bitstream/handle/10665/137036/9789241507943_eng.pdf?sequence=1

WHO 2020a, 'Prequalification of Medicines by WHO', *WHO*, viewed 28 September 2020, www.who.int/news-room/fact-sheets/detail/prequalification-of-medicines-by-who

WHO 2020b, 'COVID-19 Technology Access Pool', *WHO*, viewed 27 September 2020, www.who.int/emergencies/diseases/novel-coronavirus-2019/global-research-on-novel-coronavirus-2019-ncov/covid-19-technology-access-pool

WHO 2020c, 'Access to COVID-19 Tools (ACT) Accelerator: A Global Collaboration to Accelerate the Development, Production and Equitable Access to New COVID-19 diagnostics, therapeutics and vaccines', *WHO*, viewed 28 September 2020, www.who.int/who-documents-detail/access-to-covid-19-tools-(act)-accelerator

WTO 2020, Waiver from Certain Provisions of the TRIPS Agreement for the Prevention, Treatment and Containment of COVID-19, Communication from India and South Africa, Council for Trade Related Aspects of Intellectual Property Rights, IP/C/W/669.

Wong, H 2020, 'The Case for Compulsory Licensing during COVID-19', *Journal of Global Health*, vol. 10, no. 1, p. 010358.

Zhai, M, Lye, C, & Kesselheim, A 2020, 'Need for Transparency and Reliable Evidence in Emergency Use Authorizations for Coronavirus Disease 2019 (COVID-19) Therapies', *JAMA Internal Medicine*, vol. 180, no. 9, p. 1145.

17

IS COVID-19 FRUSTRATING OR FACILITATING SUSTAINABILITY TRANSFORMATIONS?

An assessment from a human rights law perspective

Claudia Ituarte-Lima

The COVID-19 pandemic has exacerbated the ongoing degradation of a healthy environment, preventing people from the full realization of human rights, such as rights to food, clean water, and sanitation. The enjoyment of many of our human rights depends on a safe, clean, healthy, and sustainable environment. We all rely on the environment and the living world for the air we breathe, the food we eat, the water we drink, and many other contributions that nature provides to people. Nature's contributions to people include regulating environmental processes that filter pollutants to provide clean air and potable water, and sequestering carbon, which is important for a safe climate (IPBES 2019). At the same time, sustainable environmental governance and associated collective action require respect for human rights, such as the right to freedom of peaceful assembly and association.

Hence, human rights and the environment are indivisible and interdependent. The standards and content of this interdependency principle in the environmental context has been clarified by former UN Special Rapporteur on Human Rights and the Environment, John Knox (2018), who presented the Framework principles on Human Rights and the Environment to the UN Human Rights Council. These principles included:

> 1. States should ensure a safe, clean, healthy and sustainable environment in order to respect, protect and fulfil human rights. 2. States should respect, protect and fulfil human rights in order to ensure a safe, clean, healthy and sustainable environment.

However, human rights are increasingly under threat by the compounded challenges of climate change, biodiversity loss, and the rise of pandemics. While the climate change and healthy ecosystems crises consistently show how people, ecosystems, and other living beings around the world are intertwined, COVID-19 has made this connection even more obvious. The COVID-19 pandemic is the tip of the iceberg, signaling much deeper and systemic challenges.

COVID-19 is a symptom of major structural problems, such as climate change, environmental deterioration, social inequalities, displacement and migration, and consumer and production patterns (Castro et al. 2020). Degradation of our planet's health is one of the root causes of zoonotic diseases – diseases originating from pathogens that transfer from animals to humans – such as COVID-19, SARS, yellow fever, and Avian influenza, with more likely to emerge in the future (WHO n.d.; Bonilla-Aldana et al. 2020; IPBES 2020). As many as 2.5 billion cases of human illness and 2.7 million deaths are due to zoonotic diseases each year (Gebreyes et al. 2014).

Research shows that disrupting natural host-pathogen dynamics increases the risk of pandemics (IPBES 2020). This disruption occurs by exponentially increasing anthropogenic change such as shifts in land-use, agricultural expansion and intensification, wildlife trade, and unsustainable consumption. Rather than blaming animals, it is unsustainable human-generated changes that affect the contacts among wildlife, livestock, people, and their pathogens. Moreover, climate change is one of the anthropogenic drivers triggering the movement of people and animals, generating new and increased contact among species of animals, as well as between animals and humans, and causing the spread of pathogens (IPBES 2020).

New solutions are needed to address the combined biodiversity, climate change, and pandemic crises. In response, the concept of transformation towards sustainability has come to the forefront of scientific and policy initiatives. For example, through policy-relevant knowledge generation, the IPBES report on biodiversity and pandemics (2020), the IPBES global assessment (2019), the 2018 Intergovernmental Panel on Climate Change (IPCC) report on the impacts of global warming of 1.5 °C, all seek to understand and support societal transformations towards sustainability. The IPCC Special Report on Extreme Events (2012, p. 5) defines transformation as 'the altering of fundamental attributes of a system (including value systems; regulatory, legislative, or bureaucratic regimes; financial institutions; and technological or biological systems)'. Both the United Nations 2030 Agenda for Sustainable Development and the parties to the Convention on Biological Diversity – in the negotiations of the post-2020 global biodiversity framework – have called for a transformative approach to address current sustainability challenges (Ituarte-Lima 2017; Ituarte-Lima & Schultz 2019; Bennett et al. 2019).

Human rights have a track record of sparking transformative societal change (Boyd 2020). From the end of slavery and apartheid to contributing to building world peace in turbulent times, human rights have played a powerful role in deep systemic and structural shifts challenging assumptions, values, government regimes, development paradigms, and power relations.

In 1948, the United Nations General Assembly adopted the Universal Declaration of Human Rights (UDHR) recognizing the fundamental rights of all peoples, of all nations. In commemorating seventy-two years of the UDHR and reflecting on the critical challenges of COVID-19 and climate change, the Special Rapporteurs,

Independent Experts, and Working Groups that comprise the Special Procedures of the United Nations Human Rights Council underscored the centrality of the UDHR as a guiding framework for humankind in uncertain times. They argued that 'human rights are transformative, provide solutions, and speak directly to each and every individual, as reaffirmed in the Call to Action for Human Rights issued by the Secretary General of the United Nations' (UN HRC 2020).

The research questions framing this chapter are: how has COVID-19 reinforced or changed our understanding of the connections between human rights and a healthy environment? To what extent is COVID-19 frustrating or facilitating sustainability transformations? How might advances and innovations in the right to a healthy environment contribute to societal transformations to address COVID-19 and environmental crises?

To address these questions, I use the concepts of interdependency and indivisibility to frame the analysis of COVID-19, human rights, and the environment. The interdependence of human rights recognizes that the enjoyment of one human right often depends, entirely or in part, upon the realization of other human rights (UN Development Group 2003; Grant 2007). Although in theory this interdependency is widely acknowledged, the levers needed to operationalize it in practice in the environmental context are not well understood.

In this chapter, advances on a stand-alone right to a healthy environment will be used to provide insights in understanding the role of human rights in contributing to transformative approaches to the combined environmental and COVID-19 crises. The right to a safe, clean, healthy, and sustainable environment – recognized in at least 155 UN Member States through their domestic laws, international agreements, or both – has substantive and procedural elements. Boyd describes the substantive elements of this right as: 'a safe climate, clean air, clean water and adequate sanitation, healthy and sustainably produced food, non-toxic environments in which to live, work, study and play, and healthy biodiversity and ecosystems' (2018, p. 13). Procedural elements include access to information, public participation in environmental decision making, and access to justice and effective remedies. Heightened obligations toward people in vulnerable situations are also part of duty-bearers' obligations concerning a healthy environment.

The substantive and procedural human rights obligations concerning a healthy environment and other interconnected rights are indivisible and interdependent as highlighted in various studies (Ituarte-Lima & McDermott et al. 2017; Ituarte-Lima & Schultz 2019; Knox 2017; Ebbesson and Hey 2013). For example, Shelton (1991) argues that procedural access to information interpreted in the context of environmental decision making can effectively protect a healthy environment only if coupled with substantive regulation. Substantive regulations include human rights obligations concerning the right to life, right to health, and right to enjoy the benefits of scientific progress.

Section 1 examines the impact of COVID-19 on the environment-related rights of people in vulnerable situations as well as the levers connected to the right to a healthy environment that might contribute to transformations towards sustainability. The section focuses on three substantive elements of the right to a healthy environment, specifically healthy ecosystems and biodiversity, clean air and clean water, and sanitation. Section 2 addresses the connections between building forward better, the rights of future generations, and the sustainability transformations. A concluding section follows.

A legal interpretation method and systemic interpretation approach are used to address this chapter's research questions (McLachlan 2005). As both Multilateral Environmental Agreements and human rights law include relatively open-ended provisions, resolutions of the Conference of the Parties to the Convention on Biological Diversity and UN Human Rights Council contribute to clarifying the interpretation of the provisions. I also build on the IBPES Conceptual Framework and IBPES and IPCC assessments and reports because they are helpful for understanding the state of biodiversity, ecosystems, and climate.

1 The right to a healthy environment in the midst of COVID-19 and systemic challenges

1.1 Healthy ecosystems and biodiversity

The UN Special Rapporteur on Human Rights and the Environment acknowledges the global agreement that human rights norms apply to a broad range of environmental issues, including biodiversity, i.e., the full variety of life on Earth and healthy ecosystems which are the foundation upon which all life depends (Boyd 2020).

Prior to COVID-19, the international community had recognized the connections between healthy ecosystems, biodiversity, and human rights in international fora in the 2016 Cancún Declaration on Mainstreaming the Conservation and Sustainable Use of Biodiversity adopted at the thirteenth meeting of the Conference of the Parties to the Convention on Biological Diversity. The Human Rights Council also recognized the need for mainstreaming the conservation and sustainable use of biodiversity for wellbeing, explicitly referring to the Cancún Declaration (UN HRC 2020; Ituarte-Lima and Schultz 2019). Yet the urgent need to move from the recognition of rights to ensuring that these rights can be enjoyed in practice has become painfully evident in the midst of tragic events such as the COVID-19 pandemic.

COVID-19 has demonstrated that biodiversity crises can have large-scale multiplying effects across all nations. The Secretary General of the Convention on International Trade in Endangered Species of Wild Fauna and Flora, Ivonne Higuero, highlights that degradation of healthy ecosystems removes vital buffer zones between people and wild fauna, making it more likely that animal pathogens come into contact with humans (Pérez 2020). This degradation also increases the contact between distinct wildlife species that were not previously in contact, thereby increasing the risk of spread of zoonotic diseases. In cases of illegal trade, sanitary standards are less likely to be enforced, increasing the risk of spread of diseases. Addressing these challenges cannot only be reactive, but must be preventive and systemic. We must raise the quality and enforcement of healthy ecosystems and biodiversity standards and regulations which can help reduce the risks that led us to this global pandemic.

Paradoxically, instead of adopting a transformative approach to address COVID-19 and environmental unprecedented challenges, the opposite trend is emerging in various countries. The UN Special Rapporteur on Human Rights and the Environment and the Special Rapporteur for Economic, Social, Cultural and Environmental Rights from the Inter-American Commission on Human Rights note that instead, many countries have loosened environmental standards in the name of making it easier for businesses to operate in the context of COVID-19 (IACHR 2020). Lowering environmental standards due to COVID-19 can increase the risks to the already fragile state of the diversity of life on Earth, including damaging impacts to human wellbeing.

Contrary to the principle of non-retrogression in human rights and environment law, various countries have used COVID-19 as an excuse to reduce environmental enforcement, by placing holds on environmental monitoring and limiting public participation (Boyd 2020; Global Witness 2020). These measures result in significant negative impacts on a wide range of human rights from rights to life and health to rights to water, culture, food, as well as the right to live in a healthy environment.

By lowering environmental standards in response to COVID-19, significant ecosystem services that underpin the economy are affected in ways that are often not appreciated or valued in economic terms (TEEB 2010). Yet, the economic impacts of COVID-19 are revealing the higher costs of a business-as-usual reactive approach, rather than a transformative approach that would benefit the health of people and the planet. Pandemics and zoonotic diseases (both existing and emerging) are likely to cause more than a trillion dollars in economic damage annually (IPBES 2020). Rather than reacting to pandemics, global strategies to prevent pandemics through reducing wildlife trade and land-use change, along with increasing One Health[1] approaches are estimated to cost from US $22 to $31.2 billion (IPBES 2020). This amount is reduced even more (US$17.7 to $26.9 billion) if benefits of reduced deforestation on carbon sequestration are considered (IPBES 2020). Instead of lowering environmental standards, a transformative initiative in line with the human rights-based and One Health approaches that question unsustainable development paradigms and consider the interdependency of the health of people and ecosystems is needed.

Some governments have used COVID-19 to roll-back environmental safeguards and fast track projects that Indigenous peoples and local communities have long opposed (FIAN 2020). Lowering environmental standards in favor of business interests, under the excuse of COVID-19, is already affecting those in the most vulnerable situations. In relatively remote areas such as in the Amazon rainforest, people are especially at risk of COVID-19, not only as individuals, but as people with specific cultural practices and ecological knowledge. In the early seventeenth century, some estimate that as many as 90 percent of the Indigenous population in the Americas died of flu and measles, among other diseases brought by Europeans (Koch et al. 2019). Indigenous people, such as isolated Indigenous groups in Brazil, are highly vulnerable to these non-native diseases. In the Brazilian Amazon, environmental depletion is fast-paced and social inequalities are high; illegal loggers and miners pose threats not only of environmental degradation, but also of spreading COVID-19 among Indigenous peoples and local communities.

While highly vulnerable to the effects of COVID-19, Indigenous peoples and local communities are not passive victims. The Amazon is a biologically rich and culturally diverse region where many Indigenous peoples and local communities hold alternative views of nature and social relations, which can contribute to rethinking our present and reshaping our future (Castro et al. 2020). Strategies used by certain Indigenous peoples involve using the law together with other strategies to enact changes that transform power relations and development paradigms. For example, Nemonte Nequimo, the first female leader of the Waorani Nation, and cofounder of the Ceibo Alliance (a confederation of Amazonian Indigenous nations) led a legal action claiming a violation of Waorani's right to prior consultation. The case resulted in a court ruling protecting 500,000 acres of Amazonian biocultural diverse rainforest and Waorani territory from oil extraction. Nequimo also led an international campaign to petition to the Ecuadorian government in defense of Indigenous rights.

COVID-19 provides fertile ground to question assumptions regarding where sustainable and healthy food can be produced so that urban migrants can enjoy their right to a healthy environment. For countries in eastern Africa, COVID-19 is combined with already existing climate change and threats to healthy ecosystems. In 2019, abnormal rainfall and floods destroying crops were followed by a locust outbreak predicted to come back stronger in future growing seasons. These social-ecological challenges have contributed to people's migration to urban and peri-urban areas. Supporting urban and peri-urban farming would help respond to the devastating effects of COVID-19. With proper implementation, peri-urban and urban farming could be a major strategy to bridge some of the food gaps. Moreover, it may accelerate much-needed employment creation, contributing to the enjoyment of the right to work, particularly for the many women who completely or partially lost their jobs due to COVID-19. Questioning assumptions of food production and consumption patterns can inform transformations towards sustainability.

While home gardening is certainly not a new phenomenon, COVID-19 has made its value more visible, not only in terms of food production, but also in terms of mental health. Home gardening – which has been on the rise since COVID-19 – provides a renewed opportunity for strategies that produce healthy and sustainable food, a substantive element of the right to a healthy environment. Whether it is in an urban or rural setting, gardening can contribute to emotional wellbeing and mental health. For example, one study conducted in the Twin-Cities region of Minnesota, USA, found that for low-income women, practicing gardening is associated with higher emotional wellbeing (Ambrose et al. 2020). Thus, COVID-19 has both reinforced and made us rethink social norms regarding where food is produced and how it is shared and distributed. COVID-19 has also made more visible how the right to food, the right to work, and the right to health, including mental health, are interconnected with the healthy biodiversity and ecosystems dimension of the right to a healthy environment.

From the local to the global, COVID-19 has challenged the way we view geographic scales and jurisdictional borders. Regulation and decisions that affect the health of the environment in one geographical location at one time can have impacts across many regions both now and into the future (IPBES 2019). It is well known that when there are significant impacts on air quality, they can be felt in other regions, depending on air flows. Similarly, impacts on water quantity and quality can be felt downstream. Yet, the way COVID-19 affects these dynamics – and thereby the enjoyment of human rights – is not well understood. The sections below focus on how COVID-19 has either reinforced or modified our understandings of the connections between human rights and healthy ecosystems by examining the clean air and clean water and sanitation elements of the right to a healthy environment.

1.2 Clean air

For COVID-19 responses to be effective in the long term, laws and norms that protect a healthy environment need to be at the heart rather than on the periphery. Whether in an urban or rural setting, vegetation is vital for the air we breathe. Nature contributes to air quality by sequestering air pollutant emissions. Vegetation also has the potential to prevent air emissions by protecting soils and avoiding air dust emissions, as well as by trapping air pollutants in plant parts, and retaining air pollutants on leafy surfaces. In particular, tropical forests are incredibly important for these ecosystems services (IPBES 2019).

Globally, air quality has declined due to the increase in pollutants in the air. It is well established that deforestation, biomass burning, and intensive agriculture release air pollutants (IPBES 2019). The World Health Organization (2018) estimates that around seven million people die each year from outdoor and household air pollution including exposure to PM2.5. The PM2.5 particle, caused largely from fuel combustion from cars, refineries, and power plants pollutes the air causing diseases that span from stroke to lung cancer and respiratory infections (Rodríguez-Urrego & Rodríguez-Urrego 2020). Only about one tenth of the global population is estimated to breathe clean air, which causes an estimated 3.3 million premature deaths annually, particularly in Asia (IPBES 2019).

COVID-19 revived the need to strengthen existing air pollution regulations to protect human health both during and after social-ecological crisis and pandemics (Wu et al. 2020). People who enjoy a healthy environment are in a better position to be resilient to emerging threats such as COVID-19. Legal advances at national and regional levels on the right to a healthy environment can help support people's claims to support duty-bearers' action to safeguard clean air. For example, the Philippines recognizes the right to a healthy environment and its Clean Air Act echoing this right recognizes the right of citizens to breathe clean air (Boyd 2018). The ASEAN Declaration on Human Rights recognizes the right to a safe, clean, and sustainable environment and the ASEAN Socio-Cultural Community Blueprint covers clean air under its ambition to establish environmentally sustainable cities (Ituarte-Lima et al. 2020).

Yet, COVID-19 not only confirmed what we already knew about the impacts of air pollution on the enjoyment of people's right to a healthy environment, but also magnified the negative impacts of breathing polluted air. A study of nine cities in Asia showed that past exposures to high levels of air pollution over a long period correlates significantly with COVID-19 mortality (Gupta et al. 2020). The cities in the study included three cities from China, one from Indonesia, two from Pakistan, and three from India. Furthermore, not everyone is affected in the same way by air pollution, which disproportionately harms people living in conditions of poverty. Temporary settlements, refugee camps, and low-quality housing coincide with areas severely affected by air pollution (Boyd 2020). The developing brains and bodies of children living in urban and rural areas are particularly vulnerable to the adverse impacts of poor air quality. Women in low-income countries and rural areas suffer from long exposure to poor air quality because many have a primary role in cooking and use biomass like fuelwood or animal dung to cook (WHO 2016). Recent research from the World Bank has found that exposure to household air pollution is linked to higher COVID-19 mortality rates (Mani & Yamada 2020).

However, inequality in exposure to poor air quality is not only an issue in middle-income and low-income countries, but also in high-income countries. In the United States, disparities in the distribution of air pollution based on race and poverty became more visible due to COVID-19 (Mikati et al. 2018). While the disproportionate impacts of pollution on minority groups have been discussed for many years in the United States, debates concerning the connection between COVID-19, racism, and air pollution are bringing the issue to the forefront. New scrutiny of suffocating patterns of discrimination and increased traction for the environmental justice demands of a broad range of people can contribute to transformative change and the enjoyment of human rights without discrimination.

Like advancing healthy ecosystems and biodiversity, legal tools relevant to making clean air an element of the right to a healthy environment may help trigger transformative change. In Britain, for the first time, a coroner directly linked a specific person's death to air pollution. The victim was Ella, a nine-year-old British girl who was Black. In his conclusion, the coroner recommended that people living in highly polluted areas receive more information about the risks they face. The death shined a new spotlight on how pollution disproportionately affects minorities and families living in deprived conditions (Peltier 2020). The mayor of London, Sadiq Khan, has made air pollution a major fight of his tenure and has included measures to provide more space to cyclists and pedestrians across London in an effort to encourage 'green and sustainable travel' and prevent a spike in car use and pollution after the lockdown. Mayor Khan is one of the city leaders representing more than 750 million people who have published a 'statement of principles', making a commitment to place equality and climate resilience at the heart of their recovery plans (Taylor 2020).

As new dynamics emerge with COVID-19, the pandemic is challenging established social norms concerning working lifestyles. Long-distance commuting by car, which generates significant air pollution, to work in offices is no longer taken for granted. COVID-19 lockdowns and quarantines contributed to temporary automobile demobilization, which reduced air pollution in various capitals. The fifty most polluted capital cities in the world benefited on average from a decrease of 12 percent of PM2.5 (Rodríguez-Urrego & Rodríguez-Urrego 2020). As a result of the dynamics generated by COVID-19, big businesses such as Facebook, Twitter, and Shopify plan to let a significant number of their staff work from home permanently, even after the pandemic (Dwoskin 2020). City mayors, national level officials, business leaders, and right-holders have an important role in reshaping social norms in a way that contributes to the enjoyment of the clean air element of the right to a healthy environment.

1.3 Clean water and sanitation

Similar to air-related challenges, nature is our silent ally in tackling water-related challenges that prevent the enjoyment of human rights. All the water we drink as well as the water we use to clean our hands to prevent the spread of COVID-19 comes from ecosystems. Nature's contributions to people also include water purification, which is essential for sanitation (Boyd 2020; IPBES 2019). Ecosystems such as wetlands can contribute to addressing the global water crisis because of their role within the hydrological cycle (Shine & Klem 1999). For many, COVID-19 has highlighted the vitality of water in our lives.

According to the OHCHR, around 884 million people do not have access to improved sources of drinking water, while 2.5 billion people lack access to improved sanitation (2010). Among the groups severely affected by lack of access to clean water and sanitation are women and girls in refugee camps. Research and legal advances concerning the right to water and sanitation have focused on access to water and appropriate sanitation facilities without discrimination. COVID-19 has reinforced the importance of access to water and sanitation. Lack of access to clean water and sanitation can multiply the negative effects on people's health by the spread of COVID-19.

Complementary to State obligations to provide sufficient and affordable water leaving no one behind (see more in Chapter 13 in this volume), other important dynamics brought by COVID-19 are not as straightforward, yet are equally important. The clean water and sanitation element of the right to a healthy environment offers an insight to these dynamics focusing on the systemic issues affecting clean water and sanitation: polluted water, water scarcity, and too much water.

To properly understand the effects of COVID-19 on the clean water and sanitation element of the right to a healthy environment, this element needs to be placed in the context of its interdependency with healthy biodiversity and ecosystems. For example, water polluted by plastic waste and microplastics makes it more challenging for the State to provide access to clean water so people can wash their hands frequently to prevent the spread of COVID-19. Furthermore, water polluted by plastics has become a major health risk which criss-crosses national borders posing health risks to humans and non-human beings through food chains.

Various studies revealing the seriousness of plastic pollution and other types of water pollution were conducted prior to COVID-19. While these findings are still valid, policy makers must consider the effects of COVID-19 responses on consumption patterns and associated pollution impacts. COVID-19 has increased the use of single use plastic such as disposable cups. Moreover, COVID-19 has added new polluting plastic products used at a massive scale. Masks, gloves, and bottles of hand sanitizer add to the usual plastic and other litter threatening the health of people and non-human beings. Wild marine animals, such as dolphins, risk confusing 'COVID-19 waste' with food. A French politician characterized 'COVID-19 waste' as an ecological timebomb for the long-term consequences of masks, which have a lifespan of approximately 450 years (Kassam 2020). As water pollution has increased as a result of the COVID-19 response, environmental laws and policies need to adjust to these challenges.

A lever for transformative change relevant for clean water and sanitation builds on legal advances of human rights, not only within one State's national borders, but also beyond. Water is not static; it flows across national borders. Sixty percent of global freshwater flow comes from transboundary basins (UNECE n.d.) Challenges that have emerged concerning clean water and sanitation during the pandemic call for more multilateralism and solidarity. The State is the primary duty-bearer with the obligation to respect, protect, and fulfil the right to safe drinking water and sanitation within its own borders. Yet, international human rights law also generates collective obligations addressed to all States that go beyond their respective borders with two main features. On the one hand, a State that finds itself unable to meet its obligations related to the human right to water and sanitation has a responsibility to seek help from other States. On the other hand, States that are able to support other States in fulfilling their duties have an obligation to do so.

2 Where in 'building forward better' is the right to a healthy environment of future generations?

The UN Special Rapporteur on the right to physical and mental health, the UN Special Rapporteur on the human rights to water and sanitation, the UN Special Rapporteur on human rights and environment, as well as other UN Special Rapporteurs and independent experts view COVID-19 as a serious international crisis and a 'wake-up call for the revitalization of universal human rights principles' (OHCHR 2020). UN Secretary General António Guterres reaffirmed that COVID-19 recovery demands strengthening human rights protection and addressing root causes of inequality, political instability, and displacement (Guterres

2020). He also made a Global Call for Action on Human Rights. Under the 'rights of future generations' theme, the UN Secretary calls for universal recognition of 'the right to a safe, clean, healthy and sustainable environment', and for increasing the focus on protecting the rights and supporting the work of environmental human rights defenders (United Nations Secretary General 2020). This Global Call for Action highlights that '[o]ur enduring challenge is to transform the ambitions of the Universal Declaration into real-world change on the ground' and identifies 'seven areas where concerted effort can achieve a quantum leap in progress or avert the risk of backsliding' (United Nations Secretary General 2020).

For a thriving future, preventive action is needed. Human rights must be understood in the context of systemic social-ecological challenges with sudden shocks that may have long-term effects. Jamison Ervin from UNDP highlights the importance of preventive action and considering tipping points to address the COVID-19 and nature crises: 'early actions have exponential benefits, late actions are exponentially more difficult, and actions beyond the point of no return may have little or no benefit at all' (Ervin 2020). This means that actions by the current generation may have exponential benefits for future generations, while the cost of inaction may be catastrophic – not only for the current generation, but also for future generations and other living beings.

Youth are calling for a new relationship with the Earth for today and in the future, which entails addressing the climate and biodiversity crises. Just as older people are disproportionately vulnerable to COVID-19, young people and future generations are disproportionately vulnerable to the effects of climate change, biodiversity loss, and the degradation of ecosystems. Because the measures to address COVID-19 and safeguard nature are both vital, it is important to generate and share information about the interconnected ways these crises affect people's human rights. Youth are often in the frontlines of environmental mobilizations, and the risks are heightened by COVID-19. For example, in Colombia, death squads taking advantage of COVID-19 lockdown murdered three activists (Parkin 2020). Human Rights Watch documented arrests of seventeen critics for sharing information about COVID-19, including a fourteen-year-old girl who expressed fears on social media about rumors of coronavirus cases at her school and in her province (Human Rights Watch 2020). Environmental rights defenders need to cope with these challenges and the fact that media coverage is focusing on COVID-19 at the expense of other topics.

COVID-19 is combined with other threats, ranging from violent conflict to climate-related migration. Girls and boys displaced from their lands lose vital connections, which affects their enjoyment of the healthy ecosystems and biodiversity element of the right to a healthy environment.

Youth are actively participating in environmental matters during COVID-19 through increased use of social media and online platforms. The concept of 'building back better' and 'building forward better' is being espoused by the United Nations and others for COVID-19 recovery; like UNESCO, I prefer using the latter. The concept of 'building forward better' can be infused with inclusive meaning not least through children and youth exercising the public participation element of the right to a healthy environment. In multilateral environmental fora, young people are raising their voices and highlighting that no one is too young to make a difference. Children and youth are also active in the International Convention on Biological Diversity negotiations, notably through the Global Youth Biodiversity Network (GYBN), an international network of more than 300 youth organizations, from every region of the world, who share the common goal of preventing and halting the loss of biodiversity. In the UN Biodiversity Summit conducted virtually due to COVID-19, the GYBN highlighted the need of transformative action, intergenerational equity, and the protection of environmental defenders.

Children and youth are often perceived as vulnerable groups, but many of them are also environmental human rights defenders and agents of change increasingly making their voices heard. Children and youth have a transformative role to play, not only as the future generation that will inherit an Earth in crisis, but also as today's agents of change that can help to build the future we want.

3 Conclusions

COVID-19 has in some ways reinforced, and in others challenged, our understanding of human rights and the environment. The pandemic has placed the spotlight on the healthy ecosystems and biodiversity element of the right to a healthy environment. The healthy ecosystems and biodiversity element of the right to a healthy environment is possibly the least understood element of the right to a healthy environment. One of the reasons is a narrative that reduces biodiversity to its aesthetic aspects – only one among nature's contributions to people. While ecosystems' degradation can be progressive, the sudden negative effects that a pandemic can have on the enjoyment of the right to a healthy environment is just starting to be understood by human rights scholars and practitioners.

From being on the periphery of legal developments, COVID-19 is prompting us to view healthy ecosystems and biodiversity at the heart of this right. Healthy ecosystems and biodiversity are the foundation of life. Safeguarding nature can have multiplying positive effects in the enjoyment of human rights. Conversely, the ecosystems' degradation and biodiversity loss can have multiplying negative consequences on other elements of this right, as well as in a broad spectrum of other human rights. The interdependency is not only between human rights, but also between human rights and healthy ecosystems. There is also interdependency between the distinct substantive and procedural elements of the right to a healthy environment. International fora such as the CBD and the World Charter for Nature, also recognize the intrinsic values of nature. National legal instruments and jurisprudence in some countries have recognized the rights of nature, in addition to the value of healthy ecosystems and biodiversity in their own rights.

As debates on transformations towards sustainability and on building forward better intensify, including in the post-2020 global biodiversity framework to be adopted in 2021, this chapter has revealed benefits that can derive from weaving together human rights and environmental law. While an increased call to connect human rights and environmental law is beneficial, it is the contention of this chapter that COVID-19 and social-ecological crises require the implementation of human rights principles informed by a deeper understanding of the principle of interdependence and indivisibility of human rights. Recognizing and supporting the transformative agency of groups in vulnerable situations, rather than framing them as passive victims, is also at the core of human rights-nature solutions.

Only concerted multilateral action and solidarity in line with human rights will enable us to address these unprecedented challenges and to become more resilient for the benefit of present and future generations. This chapter has shown that solidarity is not only negotiated in high-level meetings by duty-bearers but is also rooted and reinvigorated by right-holders including women, Indigenous peoples, migrants, youth, and children in vulnerable situations who, even in times of the pandemic crises, stand up for human rights and a healthy environment.

Just as the United Nations General Assembly was able to adopt the UDHR more than seven decades ago, humanity can come together to apply human rights to the biodiversity, climate, and COVID-19 crises now that these threats and the possibilities of world collective action are becoming more tangible. When COVID-19 has passed, instead of continuing to reinforce patterns that destroy nature and a safe climate and frustrate sustainability transformations, let us learn from these turbulent periods and transform our economic and legal systems in a way that ensures that today's and tomorrow's children, youth, and other living beings can thrive.

Note

1 One Health is a conceptual approach to public health that aims to integrate human health, animal health, and environmental health.

References

Ambrose, G, Das, K, Fan, Y, & Ramaswami, A 2020, 'Is Gardening Associated with Greater Happiness of Urban Residents? A Multi-activity, Dynamic Assessment in the Twin-Cities Region, USA', *Landscape and Urban Planning*, vol. 198.

Bennett, NJ, Blythe, J, Cisneros-Montemayor, AM, Singh, GG, & Sumaila, UR 2019, 'Just Transformations to Sustainability', *Sustainability*, vol. 11, no. 14.

Bonilla-Aldana DK, Quintero-Rada K, Montoya-Posada JP, Ramírez-Ocampo S, Paniz-Mondolfi A, Rabaan AA, Sah R, & Rodríguez-Morales AJ 2020, 'SARS-CoV, MERS-CoV and Now the 2019-Novel CoV: Have We Investigated Enough about Coronaviruses? A Bibliometric Analysis', *Travel Medicine and Infectious Disease*, vol. 33.

Boyd, D 2018, *Report of the Special Rapporteur on the Issue of Human Rights Obligations Relating to the Enjoyment of a Safe, Clean, Healthy and Sustainable Environment*, A/73/188.

Boyd, D 2020, *Report of the Special Rapporteur on the Issue of Human Rights Obligations Relating to the Enjoyment of a Safe, Clean, Healthy and Sustainable Environment: Human Rights Depend on a Healthy Biosphere*, A/75/161.

Castro, F, Lopes, GR, & Brondizio, E, 2020, 'The Brazilian Amazon in Times of COVID-19: From Crisis to Transformation?', *Ambiente & Sociedade* [online] vol. 23, e0123.

Ebbesson, J & Hey, E 2013, 'Introduction: Where in Law is Social-ecological Resilience?' *Ecology and Society*, vol. 18 no. 3.

Dwoskin, E 2020, 'Americans Might Never Come Back to the Office, and Twitter is Leading the Charge', *Washington Post*, viewed 29 December 2020, www.washingtonpost.com/technology/2020/10/01/twitter-work-from-home/?arc404=true

Ervin, J 2020, 'Applying the Hard Lessons of Coronavirus to the Biodiversity Crisis', *UNDP*, viewed 29 December 2020, www.undp.org/content/undp/en/home/blog/2020/applying-the-hard-lessons-of-coronavirus-to-the-biodiversity-cri.html

FIAN (2020) Monitoring Report on the Right to Food and Nutrition during covid-19, Monitoring Report June 2020, viewed 16 March 2021, www.righttofoodandnutrition.org/monitoring-report-right-food-and-nutrition-during-covid-19

Gebreyes WA, Dupouy-Camet J, Newport MJ, Oliveira CJ, Schlesinger LS, & Saif YM, 2014, 'The Global One Health Paradigm: Challenges and Opportunities for Tackling Infectious Diseases at the Human, Animal, and Environment Interface in Low-resource Settings' *PLOS Neglected Tropical Diseases*, vol. 8 no. 11.

Global Witness 2020, *US COVID-19 Bailouts Gave Bonuses to Fossil Fuel CEOs While Workers and Planet Suffer*, viewed 29 December 2020, www.globalwitness.org/en/blog/covid-19-bailouts-and-bonuses-for-fossil-fuel-ceos/

Grant, E 2007, 'Accountability for Human Rights Abuses: Taking the Universality, Indivisibility, Interdependence and Interrelatedness of Human Rights Seriously: Conference Papers', *South African Yearbook of International Law*, vol. 32, pp. 158–179.

Gupta, A, Bherwani, H, Gautam, S, Anjum, S, Musugu, K, Kumar, N, Anshul, A, & Kumar, R 2020, 'Air Pollution Aggravating COVID-19 Lethality? Exploration in Asian Cities Using Statistical Models', *Environment, Development and Sustainability*.

Guterres, A 2020, 'Building Back Better Requires Transforming the Development Model of Latin America and the Caribbean', *United Nations*, viewed 29 December 2020, www.un.org/en/coronavirus/building-back-better-requires-transforming-development-model-latin-america-and-caribbean

Human Rights Watch 2020, *List of Arrests and Persons in Detention for COVID-19 Related Offenses*, viewed 29 December 2020, www.hrw.org/video-photos/interactive/2020/03/23/list-arrests-and-persons-detention-covid-19-related-offenses#

Inter-American Commission on Human Rights (IACHR) 2020, 'The Americas: Governments Should Strengthen, not Weaker, Environmental Protection During COVID-19 Pandemic', *Organization of American States*, viewed 29 December 2020, www.oas.org/en/iachr/media_center/PReleases/2020/198.asp

IPBES 2019, *Global Assessment Report on Biodiversity and Ecosystem Services of the Intergovernmental Science-Policy Platform on Biodiversity and Ecosystem Services*, viewed 30 December 2020, www.ipbes.net/global-assessment

IPBES 2020, *Workshop Report on Biodiversity and Pandemics of the Intergovernmental Platform on Biodiversity and Ecosystem Services*, viewed 30 December 2020, www.unenvironment.org/resources/report/ipbes-workshop-report-biodiversity-and-pandemics

IPCC 2012, *Summary for Policymakers. Managing the Risks of Extreme Events and Disasters to Advance Climate Change Adaptation: Special Report of the Intergovernmental Panel on Climate Change*, viewed 30 December 2020, www.ipcc.ch/site/assets/uploads/2018/03/SREX_FD_SPM_final-3.pdf.

Ituarte-Lima, C 2017, 'Transformative Biodiversity Law and 2030 Agenda: Mainstreaming Biodiversity and Justice through Human Rights', in B Hutter (ed.), *Risk, Resilience, Inequality and Environmental Law*, Edward Elgar Publishing, Cheltenham, pp. 84–107.

Ituarte-Lima, C & McDermott, C 2017, 'Are More Prescriptive Laws Better? Transforming REDD+ Safeguards into National Law', *Journal of Environmental Law*, vol. 29 no. 3, pp. 505–536.

Ituarte-Lima, C & Schultz, M (eds.) 2019, *Human Right to a Healthy Environment for a Thriving Earth: Handbook for Weaving Human Rights, SDGs, and the post-2020 Global Biodiversity Framework*, SwedBio/Stockholm Resilience Centre, International Development Law Organization, Office of the High Commission of Human Rights-Special Procedures, UN Environment and Natural Justice.

Ituarte-Lima, C, Bernard, V, Paul, D, San, S, Aung, MM, Dany, C, Chavisschindha, T, Paramita, D, Aung, TM, & Saenphit, N, 2020 'Prosperous and Green in the Anthropocene: The Human Right to a Healthy Environment in Southeast Asia', *The Raoul Wallenberg Institute of Human Rights and Humanitarian Law.*

Kassam, A 2020, 'More Masks than Jellyfish: Coronavirus Waste Ends Up in Ocean' *The Guardian*, viewed 30 December 2020, www.theguardian.com/environment/2020/jun/08/more-masks-than-jellyfish-coronavirus-waste-ends-up-in-ocean

Knox, J 2017, *Report of the Special Rapporteur on the Issue of Human Rights Obligations Relating to the Enjoyment of a Safe, Clean, Healthy and Sustainable Environment*, A/HRC/34/49.

Knox, J 2018, *Framework Principles on Human Rights and the Environment: Report of the Special Rapporteur on the Issue of Human Rights Obligations Relating to the Enjoyment of a Safe, Clean, Healthy and Sustainable Environment*, A/HRC/37/59.

Koch, A, Brierley, C, Maslin, M, & Lewis, L 2019, 'European colonisation of the Americas killed 10 percent of world population and caused global cooling', *The Conversation*, viewed 30 December 2020, https://theconversation.com/european-colonisation-of-the-americas-killed-10-of-world-population-and-caused-global-cooling-110549/

Mani, M & Yamada, T 2020, 'Is Air Pollution Aggravating COVID-19 in South Asia?', *World Bank Blogs*, viewed 30 December 2020, https://blogs.worldbank.org/endpovertyinsouthasia/air-pollution-aggravating-covid-19-south-asia

McLachlan, A 2005, 'The Principle of Systemic Integration and Article (31)(3)(C) of the Vienna Convention', *The International and Comparative Law Quarterly*, vol. 54, no. 2, pp. 279–319.

Mikati, I, Benson, AF, Luben, TJ, Sacks, JD, & Richmond-Bryant, J 2018, 'Disparities in Distribution of Particulate Matter Emission Sources by Race and Poverty Status', *American Journal of Public Health*, vol. 108, no. 4, pp. 480–485.

Parkin, D 2020, Colombian death squads exploiting coronavirus lockdown to kill activists, The Guardian, 23 March 2020, viewed 16 March 2021, www.theguardian.com/world/2020/mar/23/colombian-groups-exploiting-coronavirus-lockdown-to-kill-activists

Pérez, F 2020, 'There Are No winners in the Illegal Trade in Wildlife', *UN Environment Programme*, viewed 29 December 2020, www.unenvironment.org/news-and-stories/story/there-are-no-winners-illegal-trade-wildlife?fbclid=IwAR1tYpJSa7kVYrgY-UQX-GH9-3EpMF_Q5GART7yOwbKyJgLgqqKn9wi6gjs.

Peltier, E 2020, 'In Landmark Ruling, Air Pollution Recorded as a Cause of Death for British Girl', *The New York Times*, viewed 30 December 2020, www.nytimes.com/2020/12/16/world/europe/britain-air-pollution-death.html#:~:text=the%20main%20story-,In%20Landmark%20Ruling%2C%20Air%20Pollution%20Recorded%20as%20a%20Cause%20of,person's%20death%20to%20air%20pollution.

Rodríguez-Urrego, D & Rodríguez-Urrego, L 2020, 'Air Quality During the COVID-19: PM2.5 Analysis in the 50 Most Polluted Capital Cities in the World', *Environmental Pollution*, November.

Shelton, D 1991, 'Human Rights, Environmental Rights and the Right to Environment', *Stanford Journal of International Law*, vol. 28, no. 103.

Shine, C & Klemm, C 1999, 'Wetlands, Water and the Law: Using Law to Advance Wetland Conservation and Wise Use', *IUCN Enivornmental Law Centre*, viewed 30 December 2020, https://portals.iucn.org/library/sites/library/files/documents/eplp-038.pdf.

Taylor, M 2020, 'World Cannot Return to "Business as Usual" after Covid-19, Say Mayors', *The Guardian*, viewed 30 December 2020, www.theguardian.com/environment/2020/may/07/world-cannot-return-to-business-as-usual-after-covid-19-say-mayors

TEEB 2010, 'The Economics of Ecosystems and Biodiversity: Mainstreaming the Economics of Nature: A Synthesis of the Approach, Conclusions and Recommendations of TEEB', viewed 30 December 2020, http://teebweb.org/publications/teeb-for/synthesis/.

United Nations Development Group 2003, *The Human Rights Based Approach to Development Cooperation: Towards a Common Understanding Among UN Agencies*, viewed 16 March 2021, https://undg.org/wp-content/uploads/2016/09/6959-The_Human_Rights_Based_Approach_to_Development_Cooperation_Towards_a_Common_Understanding_among_UN.pdf

United Nation Economic Commission for Europe (UNECE), *COVID-19: The Role of the Water Convention Protocol on Water and Health*, viewed 30 December 2020, https://unece.org/environment-policy/water/covid-19-role-water-convention-and-protocol-water-and-health

United Nations Human Rights Council (UN HRC) 2020, 'The Universal Declaration of Human Rights: A Guiding Framework for Humankind in Uncertain Times', viewed 17 December 2020, www.ohchr.org/EN/HRBodies/HRC/Pages/NewsDetail.aspx?NewsID=26586&LangID=E

United Nations Office of the High Commission of Human Rights (OHCHR) 2010, *The Right to Water: Fact Sheet 35*, viewed 29 December 2020, www.ohchr.org/documents/publications/factsheet35en.pdf

United Nations OHCHR 2020, *No Exceptions with COVID-19: "Everyone Has the Right to Life-saving Interventions"* viewed 29 December 2020, www.ohchr.org/EN/NewsEvents/Pages/DisplayNews.aspx?NewsID=25746&LangID=E

United Nations Secretary General 2020, *Secretary General's Remarks to the UN Human Rights Council: "The Highest Aspiration: A Call to Action for Human Rights,"* viewed 29 December 2020, www.un.org/sg/en/content/sg/statement/2020-02-24/secretary-generals-remarks-the-un-human-rights-council-%E2%80%9Cthe-highest-aspiration-call-action-for-human-rights-delivered-scroll-down-for-all-english.

World Health Organization (WHO) (n.d.) 'Zoonotic Disease: Emerging Public Health Threats in the Region', viewed 30 December 2020, www.emro.who.int/about-who/rc61/zoonotic-diseases.html

WHO, 2016 'Burning Opportunity: Clean Household Energy for Health, Sustainable Development, and Wellbeing of Women and Children', viewed 30 December 2020, www.who.int/airpollution/publications/burning-opportunities/en/

WHO 2018, '9 out of 10 people worldwide breathe polluted air, but more countries are taking action' News release, 2 May 2018, Geneva.

Wu, X, Nethery, RC, Sabath, MB, Braun, D, & Dominici, F 2020, 'Air Pollution and COVID-19 Mortality in the United States: Strengths and limitations of an Ecological Regression Analysis', *Science Advances*, 6.

Conclusion

18

THE POST-CRISIS HUMAN RIGHTS AGENDA

Morten Kjaerum

In 2005, UN Secretary General Kofi Annan observed that '[t]he human family will not enjoy development without security, will not enjoy security without development, and will not enjoy either without respect for human rights' (UN 2005). This lesson has been borne out through history, as human rights have time and again grown out of responses to wars and disaster or been gained through long and fierce struggles. Each crisis has been a mirror for society, reflecting back its weaknesses and inequalities, the powers that deny freedom and the aspects of society which seriously erode human dignity (Snowden 2019). As the previous chapters have made clear, the COVID-19 crisis has highlighted the existing societal injustices that challenge the dignity of millions of people in the twenty-first century. The crisis being global and existential has in itself become a defining moment for human rights.

The historical expression of human rights culminated in the Universal Declaration of Human Rights (UDHR) following the atrocities of World War II. 'Never again' was the resounding call from the thirty articles of the Declaration. Never again should the world accept the violations that were addressed in each of the articles, referring not only to the atrocities that had taken place in Europe, but also to other harrowing experiences of humankind throughout history and on all continents. Accordingly, the document is not only a reminder of the atrocities of the war, but of the collective experience of humankind of inequality, violence, and oppression.

Throughout history, the drivers for change have been diverse but two overriding phenomena stand out. The first is the wish not to repeat actions that severely undermine the stability of society or that even have the potential of leading to armed conflict and war. Such acts are detrimental to the individual, society, and the economy, which provides a strong incentive for prevention. A second driver, is the moral drive or moral imagination, which can conceive of a better world – a world free of slavery and discrimination, where gender equality prevails and which in other ways is a better place for all (Lauren 2011).

The current COVID-19 crisis is global, profound, and existential, having a severe impact on hundreds of millions of people. It has brought about numerous human rights challenges and has made very visible – and deepened – already existing human rights violations. This situation may constitute a window of opportunity allowing for a serious confrontation of some of the key human rights concerns. Following the massive exposure of injustice, the realities of inequality and human rights deprivation, including the risk of destabilization of societies on a large scale, people may be able to imagine a more equal world and to conceive of the wider societal benefits of creating such a world. In this chapter I will (1) in the light of the current challenges (2) and the critique of human rights (3) explore the key elements of the human rights agenda in the post COVID-19 era and (4) draw some conclusions charting the way forward.

1 Old problems as recurrent challenges

According to the Freedom in the World Index, 2019 was the fourteenth consecutive year that experienced a global decline in freedom (Freedom House 2020, p. 2). This trend has continued and even accelerated in some countries during the COVID-19 crisis. Governments across continents have to varying degrees sidestepped democratic procedures and ruled by decree, through speeches and administrative circulars, or by merely tweeting new orders for how citizens should act. Some countries have applied or adopted emergency legislation, which lacks basic rule of law and human rights safeguards and taken measures going beyond what domestic legislation and international human rights law permit. In addition, the stringent limits on temporary derogations, including strict proportionality and necessity requirements and formal notification procedures in relevant human rights conventions have been disregarded.[1]

These illiberal and authoritarian trends coincide with what seems to become the deepest recession since World War II, more than twice as deep as the recession following the financial crisis (World Bank Blog 2020). Estimates include a potential 4 to 5 percent decline in the global GDP in 2020 with some countries reaching a 10 to 15 percent decline in GDP. Consequently, between seventy and a hundred million people will be pushed into extreme poverty erasing most of the progress that has been made the past five years in reducing extreme poverty, and 177 million people will fall below the international poverty lines (World Bank 2020). More than 250 million people are at risk of acute hunger (World Food Programme 2020). In this scenario, global and local inequality stand out with immense clarity. In some countries, social security schemes provided a safety net for those at risk of unemployment or who lost their jobs long into the crisis, but in the least developed countries hundreds of millions of people have been thrown into situations of extreme precariousness (ILO 2020). Social protection is a human right according to ICESCR; nonetheless, 55 percent of the global population is completely unprotected (ILO 2017, p. xxix). Thus, the global inequality that was already serious prior to the COVID-19 crisis has now been severely deepened.

The crisis has further exposed pre-existing intra-societal inequalities to the extent that they should be difficult to ignore. Local outbreaks of COVID-19 in specific industries such as in the meat industry in Germany and the agriculture sector in Spain have revealed the extremely harsh and exploitative living conditions of migrant workers in these sectors in Europe (Lee 2020) and similar examples can be seen elsewhere (Koh 2020). Poor living conditions pose not only a serious threat to the life and health of workers but also entail a health threat for the entire surrounding community. The disproportional number of migrants and ethnic and racial minorities among those who have been exposed to COVID-19 (Moore et al. 2020) illustrates not only the exploitative working conditions, but also how members of such groups often occupy the most exposed frontline work, working in care homes and hospitals, retail, and other places where contact with other people is high (Drefahl et al. 2020). It also bears witness to the poor housing conditions of many migrants and racial minorities, who may share minimal living space with more people. Recognizing the considerable burden these groups have carried in order to assist others throughout the crisis has made structural racism visible to more people and raised its profile on the global agenda.

Inequality does not exclusively manifest along the lines of ethnicity, race, or migration status, but it also has a clear gender dimension. Women are overrepresented in frontline positions and their vulnerability is accentuated when having an ethnic or racial minority background. During the crisis women often had to support families through increased unpaid labor. At the same time, women faced a higher risk of violence during lockdown. Men, on the other hand, are disproportionally represented in COVID-19 related deaths when they are single, under-educated, and make minimum or no income (Drefahl 2020 et al.). Finally, persons who have been detained, imprisoned, or live in care homes for older people or persons with disabilities have faced extremely precarious situations. Indeed, many thousands have died due to lack of professional care, resources, or simply due to neglect of their situation.

The combined challenges caused by the COVID-19 crisis – of declining respect for basic rule of law principles, deepening economic inequality, and intense exposure to structural discrimination in relation to gender, ethnicity, race, age, and disability – calls for a serious global conversation about the strengthening of all human rights in the years to come and to what extent new rights should be developed.

2 Is there a future for human rights?

An obvious first question is: to what extent will human rights play a role in the building back of societies after the COVID-19 crisis? This leads to the larger existential question: is there a future for human rights at all? This has been debated in academic circles at length with book titles such the *End Times for Human Rights* (Hopgood 2013) and *Evidence for Hope* (Sikkink 2017). A central point of critique is the relatively weak standing of human rights in relation to economic and social inequalities, despite the centrality of socio-economic issues to people's everyday existence. Samuel Moyn (2018) argues that human rights may have addressed the 'status inequality', i.e., non-discrimination and gender equality, but fundamentally failed to address the 'distributive inequality', meaning economic inequality. Moyn's critique cannot be ignored; little attention has been paid to economic, social, and cultural rights, and the needs of socially marginalized groups have not attracted much interest apart from the perspective of status inequality. However, as Kathryn Sikkink argues, the entire human rights system should not be dismissed simply because it does not live up 'to the ideal of full compliance with the letter of the law', ignoring the many gains human rights have brought about for people on all continents (Sikkink 2017, p. 35).

Samuel Moyn, however, perceives human rights as part of the problem, stating that human rights were '[b]orn in the assertion of the "power of the powerless,"' but eventually 'became bound up with the power of the powerful' (Moyn 2010, p. 227) meaning the neoliberal agenda. Manfred Nowak takes the opposite view in outlining the human rights consequences of neoliberal policies. He argues that human rights are rooted in a social welfare model rather than in neoliberal thinking and are thus part of the solution rather than the problem for those living on the fringes of society (Nowak 2016). Kathryn Sikkink argues that conceptually 'the ways in which human rights and neoliberalism focus on the individual are quite different' (Sikkink 2017, p. 39). Whereas, human rights focus on the wellbeing of the individual in the broadest sense, neoliberal individualism is about self-maximization and self-interest as motivation for economic production. Human rights place individual human beings at the center, meaning that legislation, policies, and strategies need to take into consideration a specific policy's impacts on individuals, as opposed to focusing primarily or exclusively on the economy. This contrasts with the new public management models that have been developed with only a remote perspective on ordinary citizens.

Further, human rights adopt an inclusive approach bringing those left behind to the forefront and adding gender and equality perspectives, whereas the neoliberal agenda will either ignore or disregard the groups falling outside the traditional economic space.

Finally, while the neoliberal economy considers the market to be the optimal regulator and therefore endorses deregulation in the economic field and the minimization of taxation, human rights underscores the important role of democratic structures in ensuring an equal level of education, health, social security, and justice for all. Thus, regulation and taxation are pre-conditions for human rights to be fully protected, respected, and fulfilled, and thereby realized. A future human rights agenda addressing inequality and challenging key parameters of the neoliberal economic agenda will not be incongruous with the historic raison d'être of human rights, but will further its consistent development.

3 Elements for the post COVID-19 agenda

3.1 *Address inequality or vanish*

For the past thirty years the link between human rights and inequality has surfaced in the human rights agenda, but with only limited traction. Following the financial crisis and the adoption of the SDGs in 2015, the momentum is stronger. With SDG 10, states commit to 'reduce inequality within and among countries'. With the backdrop of SDG 10, the COVID-19 crisis may constitute a powerful mirror exposing the hyper-inequality and creating such a strong disruption of societies and the economy that the need for changes no longer can be brushed aside. Underpinning the importance of this momentum are the ground breaking studies of Thomas Piketty (2014, 2019) analyzing how unequal societies have higher rates of homicide and are more prone to social unrest and conflict with immense negative impact on human rights and social cohesion. His conclusions are well illustrated by the massive demonstrations in many cities on all continents in the aftermath of the financial crisis and most clearly revealed by the social unrest in Chile in 2019 with protesters explicitly targeting the neoliberal constitution adopted under the Pinochet regime.

The UN Trade and Development report of 2020 expresses the same concerns and, in light of the COVID-19 crisis, fears a 'spiral of growing in-equality' (UNCTAD 2020, p. 75) or what could be labeled hyper-inequality. UNCTAD underscores the challenges for the traditional economist rethinking of what creates value in society including such elements as social welfare systems:

> These systems are treated more as consumption goods than investments in the future. Moreover, they are systematically undervalued (and underpaid) largely because they are considered to be women's work.
>
> *(UNCTAD 2020, p. 76)*

The overwhelming negative impact on the realization of human rights for the individual and the destabilizing effect on society of hyper-inequality accentuated by the COVID-19 crisis should commit the human rights system to the project of growing and maturing the attempts that have been made the past thirty years to moving inequality high on the world's agenda. In 2015 Philip Alston, as Special Rapporteur on human rights and extreme poverty, made the statement that 'a human rights framework that does not address extreme inequality as one of the drivers of extreme poverty and as one of the reasons why over one quarter of humanity cannot properly enjoy human rights is doomed to fail' (UN Human Rights Council 2015).

The poverty and inequality agenda following in the slipstream of the COVID-19 crisis will encompass many dimensions depending on the communities that are the target of the discussion. However, with the adoption of the SDGs, states not only committed to address inequality but also to '[e]nd poverty in all its forms everywhere'. Contrary to the Millennium Development Goals, the SDGs contribute to establishing a common global agenda rather than dividing the world into developing and developed countries. This has offered a unique opportunity to challenge inequality and poverty on all continents, not limiting the efforts to the developing countries with traditional development approaches but rather open for a global dialogue on how to jointly tackle poverty and inequality where it prevails.

One key element to address is how to create resilience by supporting and strengthening the capabilities of people falling into poverty as a long-term complementary factor to the short-term relief (Sen 1999). The COVID-19 crisis had led to more than 500 million people losing their jobs and thereby hundreds of millions of people falling from positions in society where their capabilities were recognized into poverty and idleness. This offers an opportunity for a breakthrough in basing future poverty strategies on people's personal strengths and capabilities rather than having the main focus be on their vulnerability. The polarization that the job losses will create in most societies will demand new human rights-based approaches where all parties to the challenges jointly look for ways forward including the relevant social partners (employers and employees), local authorities, states, and civil society.

In order to ensure that the necessary changes can be realized the funding base for communities must be strengthened. The two ways of achieving this are (1) through taxation and (2) by optimizing the use of available funds (fighting tax evasion, corruption, and economic crimes). Tax issues will therefore be further integrated in the human rights agenda in years to come since there will be a high demand on states to be able to deliver health and other services with fewer casualties than has been the case during the COVID-19 crisis. The European Union and some of its member states have consistently linked financial support to companies facing challenges due to the COVID-19 crisis to whether companies paid taxes to the local community as opposed to locating parts of their business in tax-havens (Meredith 2020). The EU's blacklist of uncooperative tax jurisdictions has however been criticized for being too weak to stop millions in COVID-19 bailouts from ending up channeled to corporate tax dodgers (Oxfam International 2020). Until this is rectified, half-measures to prevent tax evasion are only paying lip-service to the issue.

Another key element to address is corruption. In the health sector, corruption alone costs an estimated $500 billion per year and dramatically impacts the quality of care (Transparency International 2019). The COVID-19 crisis has exposed corruption in a new way since, in some countries, frontline personnel caring for the sick could not get the required number of facemasks, other basic equipment, or life-saving medicine due to severe overpricing or diversion of funds or goods. This presumably cost the lives of many frontline personnel and patients. In a crisis situation, funding is often made available at short notice and the control systems that are normally in place are bypassed or relaxed. When the result is fraudulent and corrupt practices, entire communities become victims.

Corruption often thrives in societies where there is a concentration of power in the executive branch and weak or non-existent checks and balances. It thrives where there is poor transparency regarding executive decisions, restricted access to information, weak systems of oversight and enforcement, and an absence of free media and civil society. Corrupt practices are often perceived to be 'business-as-usual' and are still not sufficiently stigmatized, one reason being that corruption is perceived as a crime without victims, an 'invisible crime'. In the SDGs' target 16.5

states have committed themselves to 'substantially reduce corruption and bribery in all its forms' since corruption is not only an obstacle to realizing the SDGs, but also seen in many societies as the single most important impediment to realizing human rights (Raoul Wallenberg Institute 2018). Corruption is generally not perceived as a human rights violation. However, a growing number of scholars such as Moyo (2021) argue that corruption is not only an impediment to the realization of human rights but a human rights violation in its own right. The Inter-American Commission on Human Rights has framed its work on anti-corruption around the assertion that 'acts of corruption can constitute a human rights violation' (CIDH 2019). UN human rights mechanisms increasingly raise issues related to corruption (Raoul Wallenberg Institute of Human Rights and Humanitarian Law 2018) and the OHCHR has added the issue to its list of frontline issues, meaning issues that have the potential to move into the core business of the office.

In recognizing the severe impact of corruption and with an increased focus on inequality and economic and social rights, the act of corruption should be construed more explicitly as a human rights violation on the future human rights agenda. Further, it should be built into anti-corruption initiatives since human rights illuminate corruption in a manner that has the potential to mobilize people and to complement the traditional anti-corruption agenda. A human rights-based perspective brings visibility to the victims of corruption, such as persons who cannot realize their rights to health or life since funding made available for purchase of personal protective equipment, medical devices, or relevant medicine either vanished through corruption or was not available in the first place due to tax evasion.

3.2 New social contract

An increased focus on fulfillment of economic and social rights in the post COVID-19 crisis period harmonizes well with the inclusion of human rights in the sustainability agenda. The UN Secretary General (2020) has addressed it in his call for a New Social Contract and New Global Deal. The COVID-19 crisis has highlighted where the current social contract has failed and where it is being eroded. Being mindful of the vast differences between countries and regions it can be said that the current social contract builds to a large extent on the traditional structures of the labor market as it was developed since the second half of the nineteenth century. The globalized economy, including global supply chains, automation, artificial intelligence, the gig economy, and the demise of labor organizations, have eroded traditional structures and contractual relations which historically contributed to a sense of security and trust among workers. The COVID-19 crisis has made this clear with millions of people losing their income now working in the precariat; losing their jobs in the garment sector or other industries in the Global South due to supply chain disruption; and experiencing deep inequalities along ethnic and gender lines. Where is the global or local responsibility for these people? States have failed; social partners have not delivered or do not care sufficiently about equality issues; and market forces have shown their incapacity to be entrusted with creating a system based on solidarity and equality. The crisis has illustrated how vast numbers of people have been at the fringes of the existing social contract. As underscored by the UNSG, the new social contract has to build on lessons learned and address status and economic inequality simultaneously.

The new social contract must however go beyond that, since it should also include elements to address what has been labeled the inequality of attention or poverty of satisfaction (Kennedy 1968). This encompasses the feeling of not belonging or being listened to, either because the person was not given the skills needed to succeed in the modern world or the person's skills were not utilized. Feeling unheard and invisible is an important driver for the success of the populist movements in the Global North (Müller 2016). People at the extreme right as well as other extremist groups build their understanding of their place in society around the feeling of being excluded or a feeling of poverty of satisfaction (German 2007). In the Global South the same sense of not belonging has in some studies been seen as a driver behind migration flows (UNDP 2019) because people leave, not exclusively due to lack of work, but rather because they lack agency to impact society and their own lives due to discrimination, gender inequality, or corruption. These weaknesses in governance systems limit people's potential and make decisions of authorities non-transparent with little or no accountability. The feeling of no future and no way to impact the situation is an important driver for anger and the desire to leave.

Inclusion, higher levels of economic equality as well as equality of attention are alongside civil and political rights as key components of the new social contract. Philip Alston wrote in his final report as Special Rapporteur on extreme poverty:

> Social justice commitments are nowhere better reflected than in the fiscal system, and coordinated global tax reform that reduces mass avoidance and evasion will be crucial. Fair and equitable taxation can lay the foundations for a society that respects and promotes well-being for all.
>
> *(UN Human Rights Council 2020b, para. 68)*

This is echoed in the analysis of UNCTAD: 'the role of the State, including enhanced public spending, in saving lives and livelihoods has returned to the center stage in response to the COVID-19 shock' (UNCTAD 2020).

3.3 Accountable governance structures

SDG 16 calls for 'peace, justice and strong institutions'. In target 16.6, States commit to 'develop effective, accountable and transparent institutions at all levels'. To realize a well-functioning fiscal system and build trust with the aim to fulfill human rights for all after the COVID-19 crisis, accountable governance structures need to be in place. During the COVID-19 crisis two trends have emerged that address this issue. While in some countries power has been centralized, in others local authorities closest to the citizens have taken the lead. In the post COVID-19 period, both trends should be part of the future although they seem contradictory. Building back, it is important to strengthen relevant State structures, in particular in the health and social welfare area to allow them to better deliver the protection of the right to health, life, and not least social security. At the same time, it is important to ensure that strengthened governance structures are operating within the established human rights framework, building upon democratic principles and the rule of law, while avoiding carrying forward the authoritarian elements developed during the crisis.

The need for the dual approach of well-functioning institutions and a value-based legal framework is a historical lesson well depicted by Timothy Snyder (Snyder 2015) in his book *Black Earth* where he analyzes why Jewish communities were better protected during the Holocaust in some states than in other. The book was written in light of undemocratic and authoritarian developments, eroding institutions and neglect for the rule of law which were prevalent before the COVID-19 crisis and have in many countries been consolidated during the crisis. Based on his studies, Snyder underscores that it is a misunderstanding to believe 'that freedom is the absence of state authority' (Snyder 2015, p. 337) while stressing that institutions and the legal framework is what protect vulnerable groups and minorities in any society. He concludes that 'effective prevention of mass killings is incremental and its heroes are invisible' (Snyder 2015, p. 342). Laws, institutions, officials, and judges provide the strongest bulwark against any form of human rights violations and they are often indispensable in fulfilling human rights. An important element going forward is to ensure properly funded institutions established according to law, with clear mandates and working with a human rights-based approach.

In many countries local authorities at different levels have during the COVID-19 crisis stepped up their engagement with, and protection of, the citizens in the local community through the local health and care systems. Local authorities have also struggled to fulfill, for instance, the right to education for children sent home from schools, and the rights to food and housing for the most marginalized and disempowered persons in the local community. The fact that many education and care facilities were unable to meet COVID-19 challenges should make local authorities explore the human rights-based approach when delivering services. This includes accountability structures such as simple complaint procedures when a person is not receiving the assistance to which he or she feels entitled. From media reports and discussions in the human rights city movement in particular during the World Human Rights City Forum 2020 (Gwangju 2020), there are good reasons to believe that some of the deaths in care homes for older persons and among ethnic and linguistic minorities during the COVID-19 crisis could have been avoided if human rights had been part of the standard toolbox for municipalities and care homes. The human rights-based approach, including non-discrimination and gender equality, provide strong tools for analyzing who would be at the highest risk in concrete situations and establishing accountability procedures that could have brought some of the inadequacies to the forefront. The human rights-based approach identifies those who are at risk of being left behind. In the end, the COVID-19 crisis may well demonstrate the unsustainability of institutions as we know them today. In his article in this volume the Special Rapporteur on the rights of persons with disabilities calls for closure of care institutions to be replaced by community living. It will be a key discussion for the coming years in relation to the social protection of older people and persons with disabilities.

As part of the new social contract, the right to participate should be an integral element. Local communities have the power to make this right genuine by realizing a duty to engage citizens including those most at risk of marginalization and discrimination in the decisions about their lives individually and in the community. In a time of crisis where fear and insecurity prevail it is important that trust has been built in order for citizens to follow the instructions given, such as social distancing and other precautionary measures that have been communicated throughout the pandemic. Fulfilling the right to participate is an obvious instrument to reconnect citizens and authorities and offer the local community a sense of control and influence. New models for participation and engagement should be explored further, particularly at the local level and 'measures should be taken to build mutual respect, understanding and trust between public authorities and civil society actors' (UN Office of the High Commissioner for Human Rights 2018).

That local authorities engage more on human rights does not mean that states can or should abandon their responsibilities, but rather that the implementation of human rights is more deeply embedded in the society (UN Human Rights Council 2020a). The more human rights are implemented in practice at the very local level where people live, the more they will also take color and shape from that locality and become more appealing in the particular cultural contexts (Merry & Lewitt 2017). If not, they may easily be perceived as irrelevant and be disregarded. So, on the one hand, bringing human rights closer to the local realities may lead to a loss of some universal uniformity, while on the other hand, human rights may regain credibility that may have been lost due to being perceived as remote from the realities and problems of disempowered people. Research will have to look into this in the coming years, however the role of local authorities and institutions should remain high on the future human rights agenda (Oomen et al. 2016).

A particular effect of the COVID-19 crisis key to the right to participation is the rapid uptake of the digitalization of people's everyday private and work life. The crisis has in record time made the world more digitally connected. Local communities and individuals in remote places were suddenly given the opportunity to take part in exchanges and webinars with high-level people in capitals. This has greatly contributed to pulling the world closer together, facilitating national and global dialogue on some of the key issues attached to agendas such as the UN call to Build Back Better. Webinars on issues of concern to the most vulnerable groups, such as trafficked women and indigenous peoples, have made their concerns more visible and lifted them to the global level. However, there is still a long way to go until the world is anywhere close to providing equal access to such opportunities. There are still major obstacles for persons with disabilities, the elderly, linguistic minorities, and others who must be part of the global or local digital dialogue. There is a linguistic dominance and a clear preference for the technologies that appeal to dominant groups. Only 47 percent of people in developing countries and 19 percent in least developed countries, have access to the internet. Even so, the access may not be with a bandwidth that permits any real participation in a digital workshop. In the Global North the corresponding number of people with internet access is 86 percent (Statista 2020). Those not on the internet are left behind in global and national developments. Bringing the remaining 14 percent in the Global North and 81 percent in the least developed countries online and making online content accessible for all must be prioritized. In the future, substantive access to the internet will make up an increasingly important part of the right to participation.

4 Conclusion

The magnitude, severity, and global impact of the COVID-19 crisis entails a profound impact on the future of local, regional, and global interactions including how human rights unfold. It is a defining moment in history with more than 1.6 million deaths attributable to COVID-19 by the end of 2020. Global leaders had to address the urgencies of the crisis while at the same time planning for a different future to avoid a collapse in social cohesion and a deepening of authoritarianism. The COVID-19 response resembles what leaders in the past were called to do during and after profound crises such as World War II.

Throughout the pandemic, human rights have in some countries guided decisions, including determining how far decision makers would go in introducing new restrictions while fulfilling their duty to protect the rights to life and health. However, more often new policies, legislation, and actions have been devoid of rights language, or considerations on the impact of measures taken on minority groups or gender aspects. Processes have lacked transparency, democratic inclusion, or accountability mechanisms. Inequality in relation to status, economy, and attention has been exposed in novel ways and has been aggravated by the crisis.

The post COVID-19 era offers an opportunity to use these insights to build stronger communities based on human rights and democratic principles. In order for this to happen in a coherent manner the human rights mechanisms at all levels, from the UN to regional bodies, national structures, and local communities, need to be better joined up around the core themes outlined above. The erosion of the UN and regional human rights bodies that has been prevalent in recent years, should not be used to marginalize them even further in frustration over their incapacity to perform optimally. Instead, their very raison d'être should be recalled and the institutions reinforced in terms of funding and personnel.

In the UN, human rights, development, and peacebuilding are seen as the three equal cornerstones necessary to creating a peaceful world. Nonetheless human rights receives only 3 percent of the overall UN budget and severely lags behind in terms of capacity. The lack of funding has to be corrected since the human rights bodies must play a crucial role in the rebuilding of societies after the COVID-19 crisis by providing a platform for states to meet and discuss pertinent issues including with civil society and other actors; to develop a globally inclusive narrative for the new social contract; to monitor states parties' implementation of international conventions while they are rolling back crisis measures; to assist states in fulfilling their human rights obligations; and finally to provide a remedy for victims of human rights violations. As a novel feature, local level authorities have to become part of the human rights ecosystem in order to recreate this wide legitimacy and relevance (UN 2020). In this way the human rights mechanisms can provide guidance and inspiration to all actors – duty bearers as well as rights holders.

In parallel to this, monetary and financial institutions such as the World Bank, the IMF, as well as the European Central bank and other financial institutions need to integrate human rights into their policies and strategies. Hitherto they have at best only paid lip-service to human rights. Going forward, new human rights-based approaches must be developed. Hyper-inequality is an integral part of the problem facing the post COVID-19 world and hyper-inequality is why the financial sector must in broad terms pronounce itself to be part of the solution. If the financial world does not embark upon the post COVID-19 agenda of building back better, including a new social contract, it will be very difficult to establish any real changes.

Human rights and the structures created in the aftermath of World War II still have validity and legitimacy to guide global developments in the post COVID-19 era. Their very purpose is to avoid the repetition of actions that severely undermine the stability of any society and they can build on the strong global imagination that a more equal and democratic world is achievable; however, commitment and devotion is required at all levels of government and civil society to fully explore the openings that the current crisis offers.

Note

1 The data has been derived from the pilot project *Evaluating Legal and Policy Responses to Covid-19 from a Human Rights Perspective in Developing Countries* implemented by the Raoul Wallenberg Institute of Human Rights and Humanitarian Law in cooperation with the UN Office of the High Commissioner for Human Rights. The results of the study are forthcoming in 2021.

References

Comisión Interamericano de Derechos Humans (CIDH) 2019, 'Corrupción y derechos humanos', 6 December, viewed 27 December 2020, www.oas.org/es/cidh/informes/pdfs/CorrupcionDDHHES.pdf

Drefahl, S, Wallace, M, Mussino, E, Aradhya, S, Kolk, M, Brandén, M, Malmberg, B, & Andersson, G 2020, 'Socio-demographic Risk Factors of COVID-19 Deaths in Sweden: A Nationwide Register Study', *Stockholm Research Reports in Demography*.

Freedom House 2020, 'Freedom in the World 2020: A Leaderless Struggle for Democracy', viewed 27 December 2020.

German, M 2007, *Thinking Like a Terrorist: Insights of a Former FBI Undercover Agent*, Potomac Books, Washington DC.

Gwangju 2020, World Human Rights City Forum, viewed 29 December 2020, www.whrcf.org/bbs/board.php?bo_table=eng_p4_06_2020&sca=2020&page=1
Hopgood, S 2013, *The Endtimes of Human Rights*, Cornell University Press, Ithaca.
Hopgood, S, Snyder, J, & Vinjamuri, L 2017, *Human Rights Futures*, Cambridge University Press, Cambridge.
International Labor Organization (ILO) 2017, 'World Social Protection Report 2017-19: Universal Social Protection to Achieve the Sustainable Development Goals', viewed 27 December 2020, www.ilo.org/wcmsp5/groups/public/---dgreports/---dcomm/---publ/documents/publication/wcms_604882.pdf
ILO 2020, 'ILO Monitor: COVID-19 and the World of Work. Sixth Edition, Updated Estimates and Analysis', *International Labour Organization*, 23 September, viewed 27 December 2020, www.ilo.org/wcmsp5/groups/public/@dgreports/@dcomm/documents/briefingnote/wcms_755910.pdf
Kennedy, R 1968, 'Remarks at the University of Kansas, 18 March 1968', *JFK Library*, viewed 27 December 2020, www.jfklibrary.org/learn/about-jfk/the-kennedy-family/robert-f-kennedy/robert-f-kennedy-speeches/remarks-at-the-university-of-kansas-march-18-1968.
Koh, D 2020, 'Migrant Workers and COVID-19', *Occupational & Environmental Medicine*, vol. 77, no. 9, pp. 634–636.
Kose, A & Sugawara, N 2020, 'Understanding the Depth of the 2020 Global Recession in Five Charts', 15 June, viewed 27 December 2020, https://blogs.worldbank.org/opendata/understanding-depth-2020-global-recession-5-charts
Lauren, PG 2011, *The Evolution of International Human Rights: Visions Seen*, University of Pennsylvania Press, Philadelphia.
Lee, G 2020, 'Coronavirus: What Went Wrong at Germany's Gütersloh Meat Factory?', *BBC News*, 25 June, viewed 27 December 2020, www.bbc.com/news/world-europe-53177628
Meredith, S 2020, 'These European Countries Are Refusing to Offer Bailouts to Companies Linked to Offshore Tax Havens', *CNBC*, 19 May, viewed 27 December 2020, www.cnbc.com/2020/05/19/coronavirus-eu-countries-deny-bailouts-to-firms-linked-to-tax-havens.html
Merry, S & Levitt, P 2017, 'The Vernacularization of Women's Human Rights', in S Hopgood, J Snyder & L Vinjamuri (eds.), *Human Rights Futures*, Cambridge University Press, Cambridge, pp. 213–236.
Moore, JT, Ricaldi, JN, Rose CE, et al. 2020, 'Disparities in Incidence of COVID-19 Among Underrepresented Racial/Ethnic Groups in Counties Identified as Hotspots During June 5–18, 2020 — 22 States, February–June 2020', *Centers for Disease Control and Prevention: Morbidity and Mortality Weekly Report*, vol. 69, no. 33, pp. 1122–1126.
Moyn, S 2010, *The Last Utopia: Human Rights in History*, The Belknap Press of Harvard University Press, Cambridge.
Moyn, S 2018, *Not Enough: Human Rights in an Unequal World*, Harvard University Press, Cambridge.
Moyo, K 2021, 'As a Human Rights Violation', in M Davis, M Kjaerum, & A Lyons (eds.), *Human Rights and Poverty*, Edward Elgar Publishing.
Müller, J 2016, *What is Populism?*, University of Pennsylvania Press, Philadelphia.
Nowak, M 2016, *Human Rights or Global Capitalism: The Limits of Privatization*, University of Pennsylvania Press, Philadelphia.
Oomen, B, Davis, M, & Grigolo, M 2016, *Global Urban Justice: The Rise of Human Rights Cities*, Cambridge University Press, Cambridge.
Oxfam International 2020, 'Weak EU Tax Haven Blacklist Allows Corporate Tax Dodgers to Pocket Millions of Euros in Bailouts', 5 October, viewed 27 December 2020,

www.oxfam.org/en/press-releases/weak-eu-tax-haven-blacklist-allows-corporate-tax-dodgers-pocket-millions-euros

Piketty, T 2014, *Capital in the Twenty-First Century*, 2014, The Belknap Press of Harvard University Press, Cambridge.

Piketty, T 2019, *Capitale et idéologie*, Éditions du Seuil, Paris.

Raoul Wallenberg Institute of Human Rights and Humanitarian Law 2018, 'The Nexus Between Anti-Corruption and Human Rights', *Raoul Wallenberg Institute*, viewed 27 December 2020, https://rwi.lu.se/app/uploads/2018/10/Nexus-report-online.pdf

Roosevelt, FD 1941, 'Transcript of President Franklin Roosevelt's Annual Message (Four Freedoms) to Congress (1941)', viewed 27 December 2020, www.ourdocuments.gov/doc.php?flash=false&doc=70&page=transcript

Sen, A 1999, *Development as Freedom*, Oxford University Press, Oxford.

Sikkink, K 2017, *Evidence for Hope: Making Human Rights Work in the 21st Century*, Princeton University Press, Princeton.

Snowden, F 2019, *Epidemics and Society: From the Black Death to the Present*, Yale University Press, New Haven.

Snyder, T 2015, *Black Earth: The Holocaust as History and Warning*, 2015, Tim Duggan Books, New York.

Statista 2020, *Percentage of Global Population Accessing the Internet from 2005 to 2019, by Market Maturity*, viewed 29 December 2020, www.statista.com/statistics/209096/share-of-internet-users-in-the-total-world-population-since-2006/

Transparency International 2019, *The Ignored Pandemic: How Corruption in Health Care Delivery Threatens Universal Health Coverage*, viewed 27 December 2020, http://ti-health.org/wp-content/uploads/2019/03/IgnoredPandemic-WEB-v3.pdf

UNCTAD 2020, 'Trade and Development Report 2020: From Global Pandemic to Prosperity For All: Avoiding Another Lost Decade', viewed 27 December 2020, https://unctad.org/system/files/official-document/tdr2020_en.pdf

UNDP 2019, *Scaling Fences: Voices of Irregular African Migrants to Europe*, viewed 27 December 2020, www.undp.org/content/undp/en/home/librarypage/democratic-governance/ScalingFences.html

UN General Assembly 1993, *Vienna Declaration and Programme of Action*, A/CONF.157/23.

UN General Assembly 2005, *In Larger Freedom: Towards Development, Security and Human Rights for All*, A/59/2005.

UN General Assembly 2015, *Transforming Our World: The 2030 Agenda for Sustainable Development*, A/RES/70/1.

UN Human Rights Council 2013, *The Negative Impact of Corruption on the Enjoyment of Human Rights*, A/HRC/RES/23/9.

UN Human Rights Council 2015, *Report of the Special Rapporteur on Extreme Poverty and Human Rights*, A/HRC/29/31.

UN Human Rights Council 2020a, *Local Government and Human Rights*, A/HRC/45/L.27.

UN Human Rights Council 2020b, *The Parlous State of Poverty Eradication*, A/HRC/44/40.

UN Office of the High Commissioner for Human Rights 2018, 'Guidelines for States on the Effective Implementation of the Right to Participate in Public Affairs', viewed 27 December 2020, www.ohchr.org/EN/Issues/Pages/DraftGuidelinesRighttoParticipationPublicAffairs.aspx.

UN Secretary General António Guterres 2020, 'Opening Remarks at Nelson Mandela Lecture: Tackling the Inequality Pandemic: A New Social Contract for a New Era', 18 July, viewed 27 December 2020, www.un.org/sg/en/content/sg/speeches/2020-07-18/remarks-nelson-mandela-lecture-tackling-the-inequality-pandemic-new-social-contract-for-new-era

World Food Programme 2020, 'COVID-19 Will Double Number of People Facing Food Crises Unless Swift Action is Taken', 21 April, viewed 27 December 2020, www.wfp.org/news/covid-19-will-double-number-people-facing-food-crises-unless-swift-action-taken

World Bank 2020, viewed 4 March 2021, www.worldbank.org/en/topic/poverty/brief/projected-poverty-impacts-of-COVID-19

World Bank Blog 2020, Understanding the Depth of the 2020 Global Recession in Five Charts, June 2020 (Online), viewed 18 October 2020, https://blogs.worldbank.org/opendata/understanding-depth-2020-global-recession-5-charts

INDEX

Note: Page numbers in *italics* indicate figures.

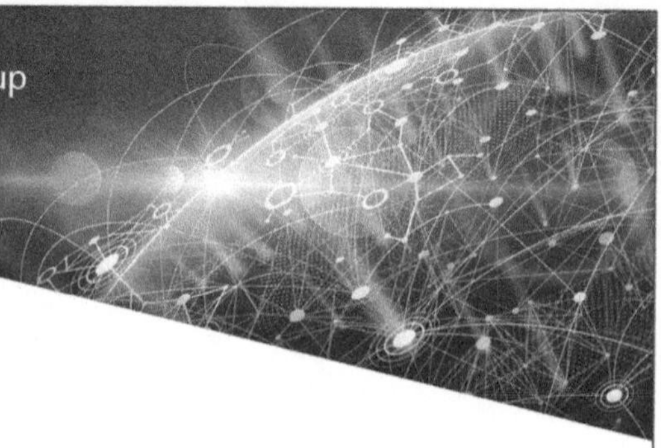